Cynthia W. Cooke, MD is Assistant Clinical Professor of Obstetrics and Gynaecology at the University of Pennsylvania. She is a consultant on contraceptives to the US Government and has a private practice in Philadelphia.

Susan Dworkin is a contributing editor to *Ms.* Magazine as well as a political speechwriter and playwright in New York.

Jill Turner is an award-winning medical journalist and freelance contributor to *The Times, The Guardian* and the BBC. She has been the health and social services correspondent of *New Society* and is currently Editor of a new *Times* weekly health supplement.

Wendy Savage is Senior Lecturer in Obstetrics and Gynaecology at London Hospital Medical College and has also practised in Kenya, Nigeria, New Zealand and the United States. She is a member of Doctors for a Woman's Choice on Abortion.

"Well written and well organized . . . a level-headed guide to women's health" NEW YORK DAILY NEWS

"Valuable for its scope and painstaking detail'
PUBL

D1382050

CONTENTS

Preface to the British Edition

This guide and reference book is concerned primarily with the good health of women, for most of us are healthy most of the time, and secondarily with our ill health. We want women to enjoy a positive sense of well-being. We would like them to feel in control of their bodies and treatment. We hope this book will calm the initial fears ignorance breeds and tell you when you need to see a doctor. Next, it should help you to understand what the doctor says and suggest what to ask. Finally, it should explain what the doctor didn't and answer the questions you forgot to ask. *The Good Health Guide for Women* was originally published in the United States of America, compiled by an eminent gynaecologist and equally eminent journalist. But while women's bodies round the world function in much the same way, our terminology, our medical systems and sometimes our treatment is different. It has been our privilege to anglicize and, where necessary, update and rewrite the American edition to make this valuable friend available to women in Britain, Australia, New Zealand and other countries. We are a medical journalist and a consultant gynaecologist, and we hope that we have done the book justice.

We offer heartfelt thanks to Patricia Tudor, who made the initial British alterations, to Toni Belfield of the Family Planning Association who answered endless questions and checked the proofs for any idiocies that had slipped through, to Anne Woodham who provided the information on the Australian and New Zealand health systems, to Nancy Duin who painstakingly, patiently and knowledgeably read the proofs, raised further queries, researched the abortion laws in Australia and New Zealand and collated corrections and references, to Nina Shandloff who had the thankless task of bullying us, and to Gail Rebuck who commissioned us. Our gratitude also goes to Jean Ellison, Susan Curzon-Hope, the Department of Health, the British Medical Association and the Pharmaceutical Society, who answered our queries, and to the Family Planning Association for allowing us to reproduce the charts in Chapter 3. It is only now, looking back, that we notice that from beginning to end this has been a book by women.

Jill Turner and Wendy Savage

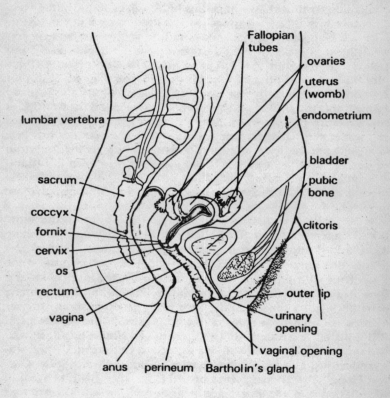

Fallopian tubes

ovaries

uterus (womb)

endometrium

lumbar vertebra

bladder

pubic bone

sacrum

clitoris

coccyx

fornix

cervix

os

rectum

outer lip

vagina

urinary opening

vaginal opening

anus   perineum   Bartholin's gland

FEMALE REPRODUCTIVE SYSTEM

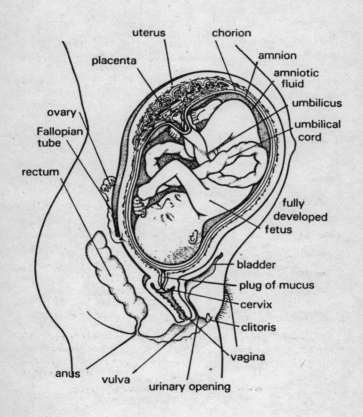

uterus | chorion | placenta | amnion | amniotic fluid | umbilicus | umbilical cord | ovary | Fallopian tube | rectum | fully developed fetus | bladder | plug of mucus | cervix | clitoris | vagina | anus | vulva | urinary opening

PREGNANCY AT AN ADVANCED STAGE

1

WELL-WOMAN CARE

Relationships between doctors and patients are changing fast. Patients know more than they have ever known before about the functioning of their bodies. The first cracks have appeared in the mystification of medicine, yet we still don't know enough to treat ourselves. It is important to recognize the limits of one's own knowledge: to know when to consult a doctor. But a little learning – recognized as such – can help you ask the right questions.

We have tried to guide our readers; to bring them safely through the complexity and confusion. We believe women must take advantage of the information explosion and hold themselves as responsible as their doctors for knowledge of their bodies and maintenance of their own good health. No longer can the patient cower behind her own ignorance, praising her doctor for what goes right and blaming her doctor for what goes wrong. Doctors too must abandon any remaining preference of omniscience in order to avoid disillusion and distrust among the public.

A more egalitarian division of power between patient and doctor requires that the language barrier between them be broken. On the one hand, the woman has to learn the medical terms; on the other hand, her doctor has to learn to speak in plain English as much as possible.

Throughout this book we have written out the medical terms phonetically, and we ask our readers to say them out loud a couple of times whenever they appear. Only in this way can medical language be desanctified, so that words like osteoporosis and prostaglandin become merely words, instead of insurmountable barriers between people who should be talking to each other more, not less.

The old-style paternalistic family doctor may once have been a comforting figure, and even the strongest of us may harbour a nostalgia unworthy of us for that comfortable old dependency on doctors – a concomitant of all the other outworn and outdated dependencies of women. But what happens when the doctor is a woman, as we hope half of our medical graduates soon will be? Doesn't that focus the mind on what we really need from our doctors?

The need for each one of us to understand and take responsibility for our own health care becomes clearer all the time. In the following chapters we have tried to explain the workings of the body, the physiology, to women in the sort of detail which has until now been reserved for doctors. A full understanding of how our bodies work is a stage in a progress that has already taken us a long way. After all, there was a time when women didn't even look at their bodies, let alone talk about or understand them.

This progress has been made in part through the efforts of the women's movement, but is also linked to a greater openness in Western society. The women's movement has been influential in making it clear to the medical profession that women are just as concerned about their bodies as men are – that breast cancer or abortion are just as important as coronary heart disease or ulcers. All the professions in this country, including the medical profession, are conservative by nature and, being dominated by men, have tended to ignore the needs of women. There *are* signs that medical schools and the students emerging from them now are less conservative than their predecessors, although it is still true that 95 per cent of medical students come from the top two socio-economic classes and have to make an enormous effort to understand the real social problems faced by the majority of their patients.

The power of the medical profession, reinforced by the bureaucracy of the National Health Service, makes change exceedingly slow. It is therefore important for women (in particular) to make their needs known to their doctors in an attempt to improve the service at a grass roots level. It *can* be done. For example, induction of labour had become so common that 40 per cent of women in England and Wales were having their labour induced until their outcry brought about a change in obstetric practice.

CHOOSING A DOCTOR

It is up to you to choose your National Health Service general practitioner. You can get the full list of doctors in your area from your local family practitioner committee. The list – or at least the address of your FPC – should be available at your main post office, library or Citizens' Advice Bureau. The list will also show which doctors provide contraceptive and maternity care.

The FPC list includes a doctor's qualifications. The basic medical qualification is MBBS (Bachelor of Medicine, Bachelor of Surgery). If somebody has not got their medical degree from a university, they might in the past have qualified by taking conjoint. This examination bestows more letters – MRCS, LRCP (which mean Member of the Royal College of Surgeons and Licentiate of the Royal College of Physicians). Another qualification is called LMSSA (Licentiate in Medicine and Surgery, Society of Apothecaries, London). Some doctors may have collected all these letters after their names. This does not mean that they are any better qualified than those who have the MB.

After doctors have qualified, they have to spend a year in hospital before being registered. During that time they are called house officers. After registration they may take further exams, which are compulsory for those who wish to specialize, for example in surgery. Nowadays a doctor who is intending to do obstetrics as a GP may have the DRCOG (Diploma of the Royal College of Obstetricians and Gynaecologists). Some doctors may have done more training and obtained their MRCOG (Membership of the Royal College) but decided not to become hospital gynaecologists and to go into general practice instead. These doctors should have a special interest in obstetrics and gynaecology.

Doctors interested in paediatrics may take the DCH (Diploma in Child Health). Sometimes doctors who have done work with children take a special paediatric course as part of their MRCP (Member of the Royal College of Physicians). Surgeons will become Fellows of the Royal College of Surgeons (FRCS) and anaesthetists must have a FFARCS (Fellow of the Faculty of Anaesthetists, Royal College of Surgeons).

Doctors with the letter C after their name in the FPC list are willing to provide contraceptive services, for which they receive extra payments. *It does not mean that they necessarily have any training in contraception.* Look for a doctor who holds the certificate in contraception, which used to be issued by the Family Planning Association and is now issued by the Joint Committee on Contraception. Campaign to make this training compulsory for doctors who want to provide contraceptive services.

MRCGP (Membership of the Royal College of General Practitioners) is a voluntary examination which GPs are likely to take if they are interested in providing a high standard of care. Those who do a lot of research may become fellows (FRCGP).

Your local community health council, whose task it is to represent your interests as a consumer of the National Health Service, is in a good position to know which doctors in your area are good and which not so good. Choose a doctor with qualifications which will be useful to you and your family. Choose one who is near your home. Ask your neighbours for their experience of local doctors. Ask them how easy the doctor is to contact and how pleasant the receptionist is: these are useful pointers to what the doctor is like. Another way of finding a doctor who is considered competent is to ask your local health visitor orr district nurse who *her* doctor is.

You have a right to meet your doctor before you decide to register. They have the right to refuse to admit you, though this is rarely done. But it is quite likely that an established good doctor will have a full list and will be unable to accept any more patients.

If you have difficulty finding a doctor, ask the FPC to help. They will make sure you are registered with an NHS doctor near you.

You can change your doctor if you are dissatisfied, even if you have not moved house. Your medical card has details about how to change your doctor printed on it. The quickest way is to get your doctor to give consent in writing – usually on your medical card – to your leaving his or her list. If you don't want to confront your doctor (or don't see why you should have to get permission), you should send your card to the FPC and tell them you want to change your doctor. You do not have to give a reason.

If you are away from home, you can get NHS treatment from another doctor either as an emergency patient (for not longer than twenty-four hours) or as a temporary patient for three months.

Most doctors now work in group practices and health centres. Although you have some say about which doctor you see, there will be times when "your own doctor" is simply not available. Doctors, like the rest of us, need some time off. They also, incidentally, need their sleep. Don't call your doctor out if you can wait till morning. On the other hand, if it is a genuine emergency or you are feeling rapidly worse, make it clear to your doctor that you really need attention. Because they get unnecessary night calls, some doctors use an emergency (deputizing) general practitioner service all the time. This is a service where telephone calls are accepted on a central switchboard and are referred to doctors working on a sessional basis. In some towns this works well, but in others the deputizing service takes on too many doctors' lists and too much night work compared with the number of doctors available to see patients. In these cases patients suffer long delays. If necessary, dial 999 and ask an ambulance to take you to the nearest hospital accident and emergency department.

If you need a doctor to visit you during the day because you cannot get to the surgery, let the receptionist know early in the day so that the doctor can plan to include you in the round before starting out.

Visits to the surgery are often rushed. The average time taken is, astonishingly, only six minutes. More and more doctors are using appointment systems, while others simply take patients from the waiting room in turn. Decide which system suits you best, and try to choose a doctor who works in that way. Doctors with appointment systems usually reserve some time for patients who need longer visits.

Appointment systems are run by receptionists caught between anxious patients and doctors wishing to control their workload. Not surprisingly, they often adopt a dragon-like tone. If you really feel you need to see a doctor that day, do not be put off with an appointment two or three days later. If you still fail to get an appointment, go to your nearest accident or emergency department. Let your doctor know of your concern and, if necessary, change your doctor.

Don't let the doctor's hurry stop you raising all the questions worrying you. But do think what you want to say and what you want to ask before you go in. List your symptoms, in your own mind if not on paper, work out how long you have had them for, when they occur and what they seem to be connected with. If you think it might be relevant, work out the date of your last period. If your ill health might be to do with your diet, make a list of what you have eaten recently.

Make sure the doctor explains clearly and fully what he or she thinks is wrong with you and why, and what the other possibilities might be. Get the doctor to tell you the range of treatment possibilities, and why one is being recommended over the others. You should understand how the treatment works and be absolutely clear what you have to do. By the time you leave the surgery, you should feel confident about any treatment you are starting.

WORKING WITHIN THE NHS

Under the NHS, women are likely to have their consultant chosen for them by their general practitioner, who writes a letter of referral to one of the local consultants. In many specialties, hospitals operate catchment areas. They will not accept a psychiatric patient who lives on the wrong side of the road, and women seeking abortions may be turned down even by a sympathetic doctor frightened of being overloaded with work at a time of limited resources. Consultants must accept patients from within the area if they are referred by GPs, but they will often give a date some time ahead. If you want to see a particular consultant outside your area and he or she will accept you, you can see that person under the National Health Service. It is not necessary for you to go as a private patient.

You are entitled to a second opinion, which will be arranged by your general practitioner, if you are unhappy about the treatment or advice you have received from the first hospital. It is not fair to use this privilege repeatedly or for minor ailments, but do ask for a second opinion if you are worried about a major problem.

Community health councils, as mentioned earlier, represent the consumers of the National Health Service . If you are dissatisfied with any aspect of your medical care and do not feel that the doctors and nurses have really listened to you, you can complain to the family practitioner committee or hospital administrator. If this still brings no satisfactory action, you can complain to the community health council who may take up your complaint for you. Community health councils have also been active in looking at aspects of health care provision such as maternity, geriatric or psychiatric care. Although they lack the power to force change, community health councils are slowly getting the consumer point of view through to the medical profession. You should write to your Member of Parliament, sending a copy to the Minister of Health, about major problems, such as long waiting lists for operations.

We have not discussed private medicine because we believe in the National Health Service. It is an extremely low-cost and efficient health system in comparison with those of other countries. We spend a smaller proportion of our Gross National Product on health care than almost any other Western country, yet most of the population receives a reasonable standard of care and there are some centres of real excellence. Such centres provide care as good or better than any that can be bought privately.

There is no doubt that the American system, based on health insurance, is cumbersome, bureaucratic and expensive. It also leads to a lack of trust between doctors and patients and rich pickings for lawyers and insurance companies. It does not provide adequate care for the poorest people, the unemployed and the old.

We must fight to protect our National Health Service and not allow it to be run down by cuts in resources. It is currently facing yet another crisis and it is up to us, the public, to make sure we don't lose it.

HEALTH CARE IN AUSTRALIA

Australia has no National Health Service and, according to a national survey by the Australian *Women's Weekly*, nearly nine out of ten Australian women believe health care costs are ridiculously high. They complain that doctors' fees are exorbitant ($A12 to visit the GP) and the health funds are making excessive profits.

Health insurance is currently under re-examination by the Federal Government, but, unlike the practice of some North American insurance companies, Australian women are not asked to pay higher rates because they make more visits for routine gynaecological check-ups. Childbirth and abortion (where medically recommended) are covered for both married and unmarried women, whereas private health funds in Britain and some in the US refuse to insure these peculiarly female conditions, unless there are complications.

At present the Australian Government meets any medical costs in excess of $20, and provides free public hospital treatment (with the doctor of the hospital's choice), so long as the patient is registered, though not necessarily insured, with Medibank or a private health fund.

Nearly three quarters of young—and healthy—women between twenty and twenty-four resent paying the $3.75 to $5 a week for basic health insurance, which covers 85 per cent of all medical bills and intermediate hospital ward treatment; it is a growing trend for them to attend public hospital clinics rather than a private gynaecologist or other specialist. Many prefer to use the family planning clinics run by the Family Planning Association and the Catholic Social Welfare Commission, which are free and government-subsidized.

As a result, people have been withdrawing from the health funds in such droves that many of the funds are finding themselves in financial straits, and hence are lobbying the Government for a change. The Jamison Report of 1981 recommended that Government benefits be limited to those who had *taken out* health insurance—but then what safety net will there be for the old and the poor, those who can least afford and most need health care?

But Australian patients, like patients in Britain, are becoming better-read, less intimidated, and consequently more militant. They ask questions. Doctors are losing their mystique, and the scandals surrounding Medibank frauds and doctors' tax avoidance in the 1970s helped tarnish their image. The NSW Legal Aid Commission reports that applications for legal aid in medical malpractice suits have risen markedly, and it is said that this number has increased from three or four a year in 1977 to over a hundred.

When doctors treat their profession as a business, making fewer home calls and refusing to be available twenty-four hours a day, they must expect their customer-patients to respond in kind. Most malpractice cases are for negligence, but in 1980 a patient succeeded, for the first time in Australian legal history, in a claim against his doctor of assault and battery for medical treatment. Not only that, but three highly qualified doctors testified as witnesses on the patient's behalf—a sign that the "conspiracy of silence" could be breaking down.

But as patients we should be wary of growing so litigious that we risk a situation like that now existing in the United States, where doctors' omnipresent malpractice insurance rebounds on every patient's pocket. This insurance, invented to protect doctors and hospitals against the wrath of injured patients, enriches no one except the insurance companies and the legal profession.

Those who have fought for non-discriminatory practices in Australian medical schools have won a little. Women doctors now make up 18 per cent of the medical workforce. But women should keep in mind that more than 50 per cent of physicians belong to the traditionally conservative Australian Medical Association, although organizations with a new social conscience such as the Doctors' Reform Society have recently become more vocal.

One noticeable and remarkable phenonemon is that Australian women seem to need more hysterectomies than women in any other country except the United States. Why on earth should four times as many Australian wombs need removing as British or Swedish ones? Doctors frequently recommend the operation when a woman complains of heavy menstrual bleeding, often as a result of sterilization, but many women—and progressive doctors—suspect sheer avarice. The Doctors' Reform Society advises any woman who feels her doctor is hustling her off to hospital to rebel, and seek a second opinion.

A women should never decide on a doctor or a mode of treatment of a serious illness without at least one or two other opinions. The opinion of another doctor is fine. When choosing a physician, the opinions of other women who have sought health care or experience the ailment are excellent. Patient self-help groups are invaluable selection aids. Keep in mind that doctors are often reluctant to criticize each other. Don't wait for doctors to become the willing judges of their peers; you could wait a lifetime. Use the best tool available now—the experience of other women who have gone through the same thing.

Already Australian women have proved they can change the system. Expectant mothers at some major city hospitals can hardly believe the revolution in childbirth in as short a time as three years. Bean bags, mirrors, music and birth companions are not merely tolerated but offered to women in labour. Birth centres, where women can have their babies "naturally" in a home-like environment with fathers and other members of the family freer to come and go, have been established at the Women's Hospital, Crown Street, Sydney, at the Royal Women's Hospital and the Queen Victoria Medical Centre in Melbourne, and at the King Edward Memorial Hospital, Western Australia. This development is an undisguised attempt by the hospitals to counter the growing demand for home births and to react to the complaint that hospital maternity wards are clinical and forbidding. Perhaps pioneer days are too fresh a memory for Australian doctors, when a difficult labour on an isolated homestead could be a dangerous nightmare. As it is, candidates for the birth centres are carefully vetted medically, and even then, among apparently healthy mothers, one third are transferred to the hospital's ordinary labour ward.

A few hospitals, like Sydney's Westmead, are experimenting with short-stay maternity patients, who go in for only twenty-four or forty-eight hours and then go home, but one problem has been a lack of nursing sisters to visit the mothers at home.

There is, however, another side of the coin. Many expectant mothers, especially those with two or three children already, look forward to a week in hospital as a rest from family demands. Some at the new self-care unit at the Royal Hospital for Women, Paddington, Sydney, have argued that they *want* the nurse to bath the baby, that they *like* their meals on a tray in bed instead of eating at a table with other new mothers.

Nevertheless, the transformation in childbirth is largely due to women's new awareness and concern for their own health. They are insisting that the facilities they read about in the media—such as ultrasound, now routine equipment at most city hospitals—be made available. Country hospitals (long the poor relations) are increasingly feeling the pressure to provide more sophisticated services.

ADDITIONAL NOTES ON NEW ZEALAND

Like Australia's, the New Zealand health care system is increasingly geared to the private patient, with no-frill public health care offered at hospitals to those who cannot afford doctors' bills or health insurance fund premiums.

The Government makes a contribution towards GP and specialist fees, hospital and maternity care and subsidizes family planning clinics. It will pay $1.25 towards the cost of a visit to the doctor, as much as $4 towards out-of-hours service, and raises this to $8 for children and pensioners. For a trip to a specialist, a Government benefit of $20 is available. Most doctors claim benefits directly from the Department of Health and ask patients for the balance.

New Zealanders have a long tradition of sensible and enlightened baby and child care, and Karitane nurses have acquired an international reputation. This national interest is reflected in the strength of the natural birth and home birth campaigns, which have grown up in opposition to official policies encouraging hospital delivery. The laws covering contraception and abortion are relatively unenlightened. (See p. 205)

In New Zealand, as in Australia and Britain, women are demanding greater participation in decisions relating to their own and their families' health. A growing number of doctors are joining them in this long-term struggle. Although in some ways our campaigns and problems are specific to where we live, basically we all want the same things, and our collective efforts—and increasing confidence in the knowledge of our own bodies—may eventually pay off.

2

PUBERTY,
MENSTRUATION and
ADOLESCENCE

Puberty is the process of maturing physically. In girls, this takes place over a three-to-five-year period, usually between the ages of eight and 17, and establishes the regular cycle of menstruation.

If a girl is completely unprepared for puberty, it may frighten her; when she gets her first period, she may think some terrible internal disorder is causing her to bleed. Even the best-prepared girl may be alarmed and overawed by the enormous changes in her body, so certain basic, positive ideas should be communicated to her from the beginning.

Every healthy young woman in the world menstruates. Nothing is more usual, more routine, more normal. Menstruation is not a curse; it should never be labelled as such, or by any other euphemistic name; it is not to be hidden shamefully from the other members of the family.

The menstrual cycle is a vital indicator of a woman's good health. It tells her as much about her physical well-being as the level of her appetite or the level of her blood pressure. It should never be treated as a disease, or its routine discomforts dealt with as though they were disease symptoms.

With puberty comes *adolescence,* when the girl matures psychologically and socially. It is an emotional time. Its strains on both parents and daughter will be much lessened if everybody deals with its physical aspects forthrightly.

Sex can be discussed separately or together with menstruation. A girl needs to know everything she can about puberty and the menstrual cycle, regardless of whether she has started consciously thinking about sexuality. However, with the great peer pressure toward early sexual relationships, puberty is a logical time to begin discussions of sexuality and contraception, although it is preferable

11

to start earlier. In addition, the years of puberty and adolescence are years of intense sexual drive, so discussions of sexuality are not only appropriate—they are vital. No mother can hope to keep her girl isolated from the explosion of explicit sex at the corner newsagents, in everyday bookshops, in all the media. There is pressure on young people—real social pressure—to be grown-up sexually when they are still kids at heart.

If a parent can take the pressure off a little—by giving her child a sense of self-respect, a sense of the responsibility of sex—that may help to give a girl some extra time to grow up and, at the risk of sounding old-fashioned, to postpone sex until she's ready to enjoy it.

If you can convince your girl to set her *own* sexual agenda—and not allow it to be set for her by some sweet but clearly rapacious teenage boy—then she is well on her way to being a free woman all her life, a woman who will always be in control of her own sexuality.

PUBERTY

1. External signs of puberty

Several key outward changes signify that a girl is maturing sexually:

   a. Breasts begin to develop
   b. Pubic and underarm hair begins to grow
   c. There is a spurt in height and weight
   d. The pelvic bones widen

At the end of this process, menstruation begins.

This is the usual order of the outward changes during puberty. However, *there is nothing at all abnormal if changes occur simultaneously or in a different order, as long as they all occur.* The exception to this is that the menstrual period does not usually start until most of the other development is complete.

2. Breast development in puberty

A girl may normally start developing breasts as early as seven to eight years of age. Initially, only the nipple protrudes from the chest wall. Then glandular tissue begins to grow under the nipple. This is a *breast bud.* Sometimes one breast bud develops before the other. It should not be mistaken for a tumour.

3. Breast soreness during puberty

Breast buds may feel sore because they are composed of gland tissue responsive to the concentrations of oestrogen in the blood,

12

which begin to rise during puberty, prior to menarche—
(me-NAR-ke), the onset of menstruation.

The discomfort is mild, and girls can be assured that it will pass.
Sometimes young girls, curious about their new breasts, will touch
or rub them repeatedly, making the breast bud sore. This too is
nothing to worry about. Only if there is redness or discharge from
the nipple need medical advice be sought.

4. When to start wearing a brassiere

Brassieres are of dubious value except for heavy-breasted
women. So there's no good reason at all for young girls to wear
them. Young girls sometimes like to emphasize the fact that their
breasts are growing by wearing a bra—in fact, fancy bra and panty
sets, imitating the underwear of mature women, are a fad among
many youngsters who are still completely flat-chested.

Try to encourage your girl not to wear a bra before it makes
sense but don't put her down by saying there's no reason to do so.
If you honestly feel that she faces some psychological disadvantage
by going braless, by all means let her have her desire. Peer pressure
is a powerful force when you're growing up. And bras are not a
powerful force for good or ill, at any stage.

5. Pubic hair growth

The first pubic hair usually appears at about the same time the
nipples begin to protrude. First, a few strands of hair appear on the
outer lips of the vagina. These gradually grow more numerous until
they cover the pubic area. Later, the hair grows sideways towards
the upper thighs. At the time of menarche, hair growth is not
complete and usually needs another year for full development. The
woman's pubic hair thus grows in a typical triangle pattern, with a
sharp upper border. Occasionally a light growth of hair will extend
up to the navel.

6. Underarm hair growth

The hair in the underarm regions appears about the same time as
that in the pubic area. This is in response to the same hormonal
process, increased production of androgen by the adrenal glands.
Small amounts of hair around the breasts are also normal.

7. Growth spurt in puberty

By the time menarche occurs, 90 per cent of a girl's pubescent
growth spurt has usually taken place. The average height gain after
the first period is an additional 2¼ inches. Because growth is

steady and continues until menstruation, well-nourished girls who menstruate later are usually taller.

OPINION: The use of high doses of oestrogen to stop the growth of tall girls is a practice to be condemned! Only in extraordinary circumstances should a young girl be exposed to the risks of oestrogen (See p. 334) and certainly not when the goal is only to make her a few inches shorter.

Simultaneously with the spurt in height, girls experiencing puberty usually gain weight as well. By age seven or eight, girls are generally more plump—and taller—than boys. However, parents should carefully distinguish pubescent weight gain from general obesity. An overweight child has developed a greater *total* number of fat storage cells. A child growing plump at the onset of puberty is only experiencing an increase in the fat content of the cells she already has and a change in the *distribution* of fat on her body.

As a rule, children who are fat before puberty experience earlier menarche. This lends support to the idea that sexual development depends partly upon the achievement of a 'critical mass'—a certain weight per unit of height. (Ref. 1) This and many other theories about what causes the onset of puberty are all unproven.

8. Changing body shape

Total body fat increases during puberty, and the bones of the pelvis grow and widen. Together, these developments create a redistribution of body fat on to the thighs and hips. The resulting figure change is more or less pronounced, depending on the individual. If it isn't very pronounced at all, there's nothing to worry about; a quick look back at the female figures on the family tree will usually provide ample explanation.

9. When the first menstrual period occurs

The average age for menarche in the United Kingdom is 13—but the *normal* age range is 10 to 17 years. Over the past century, the average age for menarche has decreased three to four months each decade, probably the result of improved nutrition.

10. Factors influencing the age of first menstruation

    a. *Nutrition:* a poorly fed girl will usually menstruate later.

    b. *Light:* blind girls menstruate earlier.

    c. *Climate:* not a factor.

    d. *Race:* not a factor.

    e. *Altitude:* girls living at high altitudes will usually menstruate later.

f. *Heredity:* this is probably the most important factor of all—if other conditions are equal. Even though the average age of menarche is decreasing, mothers who experienced menarche late in their generation will usually have daughters who experience menarche late within the range for *their* generation.

g. *General physical health:* severe illness during puberty—such as diabetes or rheumatic fever—tends to delay menarche.

h. *General mental health:* when a girl is under great strain during puberty—due to mental illness or a severe shock such as the death of somebody close to her—menarche may be delayed. (Ref. 2)

11. Irregular periods are normal during puberty

Young girls tend to menstruate irregularly at first, and it sometimes takes two or three years for the monthly cycle to establish its lifelong pattern. But a girl should assume she is ovulating and use contraception if she is having sex.

The irregularity is due to the fact that, although the young girl's ovaries are not yet releasing eggs, they are producing high levels of *oestrogen,* the hormone that controls a woman's physical development and secondary sexual characteristics. The oestrogen is building the endometrium (en-do-ME-tree-um)—the lining of the uterus that is eliminated during menstruation. However, no ovulation—egg release—is occurring to govern *the time span* at which this elimination occurs. *Oestrogen production without ovulation leads to irregular menstrual bleeding.*

The same situation often occurs in older women, who have ceased ovulating but whose bodies are still producing oestrogen or who are receiving oestrogen by medication. (See Nos. 43 – 46 below for abnormalities of bleeding)

12. Other changes at puberty

The onset of puberty creates changes in the internal organs of a woman's body.

The uterus gets bigger and changes shape.

The vagina begins to elongate, and a watery secretion appears.

The small inner lips of the vagina—*labia minora* (LA-bia)—begin to grow.

The pelvic bones grow and change shape.

Body cells increase their fat content.

The body's metabolism changes, requiring additional calories and protein. (These nutritional needs are greatest just before menarche and coincide with the body's growth spurt.)

Sweat glands in the underarm area enlarge.

13. Growth of the uterus

Under the influence of oestrogen during early puberty, the uterus enlarges and changes shape. The fundus, or upper part of the organ, grows larger and continues to change shape until young adulthood, when it has become round (or pear-shaped).

14. Growth of the vagina

The vagina begins to grow longer during puberty and its lining thickens. The labia minora—the inner lips of the vagina which are very small before puberty—begin to grow and protrude between the labia majora, the large outer lips of the vagina.

15. Vaginal secretion before menarche

A discharge of vaginal cells may occur as menarche approaches —it is usually thin and watery, whitish or pale yellow. The secretion is a sign of normal growth and good health; only if it is accompanied by severe itching or irritation should medical advice be sought. A slight, yellowish stain on underwear is normal. Cotton pants are advisable.

16. Pelvic bone growth

The bones of the pelvis change their shape early in puberty, laying the skeletal foundation for a new distribution of fat and muscle over the hips and thighs.

17. Growth of sweat glands

Sweat glands in the underarm area enlarge during puberty, leading to an increase in perspiration and odour. Now is the time for a girl to start washing under her arms at least once daily and familiarizing herself with powders, deodorants and antiperspirants. (See p. 225)

MENSTRUATION AND THE HORMONES THAT GOVERN IT

18. What is happening when you menstruate?

Every month, the lining of the uterus (the endometrium) grows thicker, enriched by blood and other nutrients brought to it by chemical and hormonal reactions in your body. Unless and until you decide to become pregnant, your body simply does not need all the cells that have built up inside your uterus, and therefore your body eliminates them—at regular monthly intervals—in the bleeding that appears as menstruation. *This process is a sign of general good health in all women.*

19. How to calculate your menstrual cycle

Count the days of your menstrual cycle from the first day of bleeding, ending it on the day before resumption of bleeding. If you started menstrual bleeding on September 1 and started again on September 30, then your cycle was 29 days long—September 1 to 29.

20. When is a menstrual cycle 'regular'?

A *normal* menstrual cycle is 21 to 35 days long (28 days is the average). A *normal* menstrual flow is one to seven days long. A certain pattern in the length of period and cycle usually establishes itself for each individual woman in the first few years of menstruation. However, a variation of several days either way is common from time to time and does not mean that the period is 'irregular'; nor does it imply ill health.

21. How much bleeding is normal?

The amount of blood loss during a menstrual period varies greatly from woman to woman, *but is usually about the same with each period for an individual woman.* The normal range can require, on the light side, one or two tampons or pads per day, to (on the heavy side) eight to ten tampons or pads per day. The flow should not be so heavy as to gush down a woman's legs. Any marked increase or decrease in flow should be medically evaluated. The amount of blood loss during menstruation is *not* an indicator of fertility.

22. What is a hormone?

A hormone is a chemical substance produced by one part of your body, which enters the blood stream and causes changes in other parts of your body. It is a product of the endocrine or glandular system. The word comes from the Greek—to rouse or set in motion—and that's exactly what a hormone does. Hormones set in motion the whole process of sexual maturation and govern the menstrual cycle.

23. Hormones that make the menstrual cycle work

Six hormones work together in a chain reaction that governs the menstrual cycle.

a. *Oestrogen* (EES-tro-jen), produced primarily by the ovaries, controls much of a woman's growth and physical sexual development.

b. *Progesterone* (pro-GESS-ter-own), produced by the ovaries,

17

alternates with oestrogen for dominant effect during the menstrual cycle.

c. *FSH-RF* are the initials for *Follicle Stimulating Hormone-Releasing Factor.* It is produced by the hypothalamus (hipe-oh-THAL-amus) in the brain (See No. 28).

d. *FSH* is the *Follicle Stimulating Hormone* which FSH-RF activates. It is produced for the pituitary (pit-YOU-it-ary) gland and triggers the growth of follicles—groups of cells surrounding eggs in the ovaries—which then produce oestrogen and progesterone.

e. *LH-RF* are the initials for *Luteinizing Hormone-Releasing Factor,* produced by the hypothalamus. (LH-RF and FSH-RF are actually one substance, called gonadotropin-releasing hormone—GNRH. For clarity they are discussed separately.)

f. *LH, Luteinizing Hormone,* produced by the pituitary gland, is released by LH-RF and triggers ovulation—the release of the egg from the ovarian follicle and the ovary—then changing the broken follicle to a *corpus luteum* (LOOT-ee-um) or yellow body. (Luteinizing means yellowing; lutein is a yellow pigment, another form of which gives an egg yolk its colour.)

24. The ovaries

The word 'ovary' comes from the Latin word *ova*, meaning egg. It is your two ovaries that contain the eggs or germ cells. When a girl is born, each ovary contains 100,000-400,000 eggs. This number progressively decreases throughout a woman's life until menopause, when very few remain. The ovaries also produce oestrogen and progesterone.

25. The ovarian follicles and corpus luteum

Ovarian follicles are clusters of cells surrounding the eggs in each ovary. The cells of the follicles are the major producers of oestrogen and progesterone. After ovulation, the follicle becomes the corpus luteum and produces higher levels of oestrogen and progesterone.

26. What is ovulation?

Ovulation is the process, usually at mid-cycle, by which an ovarian follicle breaks and releases an egg from the ovary into one of the Fallopian tubes.

27. The Fallopian tubes

The Fallopian tubes receive the eggs that are released during ovulation. They are connected to the uterus, and when and if an egg is fertilized by a sperm, it is carried along one of these tubes to the uterus itself.

(The reason Fallopian is written with a capital letter is that the tubes are named after Gabriello Fallopio, a sixteenth-century Italian anatomist who discovered them. He also did some basic work on bone typing and analyzed how our sense of taste works, and is credited with inventing the first sheath.)

28. The hypothalamus

The hypothalamus is a glandular and nerve centre located in the centre of the brain, directly above the pituitary gland. Besides producing FSH-RF and LH-RF, the hypothalamus is thought to be the major control centre for hunger, thirst, sleepiness, sexual appetite, and all the other endocrine systems besides the reproductive system.

Because of its location, the hypothalamus is greatly affected by signals from other parts of the brain. For example, it is very sensitive to general illness and mental stress and often passes these negative signals on through the hormone chain to affect the menstrual cycle itself. *It is for this reason that irregularities in the menstrual cycle may accompany a disorder that has nothing to do with a woman's reproductive system.*

29. The pituitary gland

The pituitary gland is located at the end of a stalk, just below the hypothalamus, at the base of the brain. It is very important in its role of producing all the 'stimulating' hormones for all the glands of the body—in addition to FSH and LH, thyroid-stimulating hormone (TSH) and adrenocorticotropic hormone (ACTH). The pituitary also produces prolactin, important in milk production, and oxytocin, important in milk let-down and uterine contractions after delivery. (See p. 141)

30. How the hormone chain reaction works in the menstrual cycle (This example assumes a 28-day cycle and no fertilization.)

DAY 1   On the first day of menstrual bleeding, oestrogen and progesterone are at their lowest levels in the blood stream. The hypothalamus reacts to these low levels by producing FSH-RF, which triggers production of FSH. FSH stimulates development of *several* ovarian follicles, which then begin producing oestrogen at increased rates.

TO DAY 14	Ovarian follicles continue producing oestrogen for about 14 days until the hormone reaches a high level in the blood stream. This high level causes the hypothalamus to produce a spurt of LH-RF, the hormone that triggers production of LH. LH stimulates ovulation, causing *one* egg (occasionally more) to be released by the ovary. (No one really knows why only one egg is released and the other follicles just degenerate and disappear.)
DAYS 15 AND 16	The egg pops out of the ovary and is picked up by the fimbria, the fringe at the end of the Fallopian tube. For 12 to 36 hours, while the egg is in the Fallopian tube, it is available for fertilization. When it is not fertilized, it disintegrates with *no symptoms or ill-effects*.
TO DAY 28	Meanwhile, the action of LH is changing the ruptured ovarian follicle into the corpus luteum or 'yellow body'. This yellow body produces increasing levels of oestrogen and progesterone for the next 8 to 10 days, with progesterone usually becoming dominant. The yellow body degenerates after this time and the blood levels of oestrogen and progesterone decline unless pregnancy occurs.
DAY 1	When oestrogen and progesterone reach low enough levels in the blood stream, the lining of the uterus (endometrium)—which has thickened in response to the hormonal chain reaction—is shed. Menstruation begins again. The cycle repeats itself.

31. How oestrogen and progesterone affect the endometrium

Oestrogen stimulates the growth of the endometrium, the lining of the uterus.

After ovulation, in the second half of the menstrual cycle, progesterone dominates and thickens the endometrium even more.

Near the end of the cycle, oestrogen and progesterone levels decrease. The endometrial cells stop multiplying and degenerate. The uterus sheds the unneeded cells along with some blood, resulting in menstruation.

32. How oestrogen and progesterone affect the glands of the endometrium

Before ovulation, the glands of the endometrium—viewed through the microscope—are straight. After ovulation, progesterone makes the glands develop and produce mucus. They look long and twisting. The change makes a more hospitable place for the fertilized egg to implant.

The change in the shape of glands is useful in the evaluation of an endometrial biopsy, taken in the investigation of an infertile couple (see Infertility, Chapter Four). The pathologist will be able to detect whether the woman has ovulated if the biopsy is taken in the second half of the cycle.

33. How oestrogen and progesterone affect the Fallopian tubes

Inside the Fallopian tubes are cilia (SIL-ee-a)—wavy, hairlike projections—which, if they have the opportunity, help to push the sperm and egg together and then move the fertilized egg on into the uterus. (The word derives from a Latin word meaning eyelashes.)

Around the time of ovulation, oestrogen and progesterone work to increase the number of cilia and their movement in the tubes.

Oestrogen and progesterone also cause increased mucus production and stronger muscle contractions in the tubes—both aids to the sperm in reaching the egg.

In addition, the muscular contractions of the Fallopian tubes and the ligaments that support the ovaries bring the tubes closer to the ovaries. This means that when ovulation occurs, the Fallopian tube is in a better position to catch the egg.

34. How oestrogen and progesterone affect the cervix

The cervix is the lower part of the uterus that extends into the vagina. Glands in the cervix normally secrete mucus to lubricate the vagina, to protect the endometrium from infection and to facilitate passage of sperm into the uterus at the right time for fertilization.

The amount of mucus is smallest right after menstruation ends.

But as oestrogen levels rise, the cervical glands secrete more and more mucus.

At mid-cycle, the time of ovulation, mucus becomes sticky and so abundant that you may notice it as a vaginal discharge. This sort of mucus has a texture and chemical make-up (alkaline Ph) most welcoming to sperm. (See Chapter Three, No. 131, the cervical mucus method in rhythm birth control.)

Later on in the cycle, progesterone makes the cervical mucus thicker and more impenetrable to sperm, changing it chemically to an acid Ph.

35. The ferning test, a simple lab procedure, can indicate much about a woman's hormonal status

Oestrogen causes an increase in the salt content of the cervical mucus during the first half of the cycle. If a smear of this mucus is taken and analysed, before ovulation when oestrogen levels are high, a *ferning* pattern will appear as the smear dries. The ferning is caused by crystallization of the salt. This is a very simple test.

After ovulation, the rising influence of progesterone causes a decrease in salt content. The dried smear shows a cellular pattern.

By checking how the salt pattern develops, a gynaecologist can tell you if ovulation has occurred. But an endometrial biopsy is a better way of informing a woman whether the corpus luteum is functioning properly. (See p. 93) The ferning test is also used to reassure and monitor progress in a woman who has had several miscarriages.

36. How oestrogen and progesterone affect the vagina

Oestrogen helps the cells lining the vagina to multiply and the cell layers to become thicker. This causes an increase in watery discharge (which includes cervical and vaginal secretions and cells) in the early part of the cycle and before menarche.

Progesterone slows the increase in these cell layers and, as a result, fewer are shed. The amount of discharge towards the end of the menstrual cycle is less than in the earlier weeks.

37. A vaginal smear can indicate a great deal about a woman's hormonal status

There are three kinds of cells in the vaginal lining: basal cells (the deepest layer), intermediate cells (the middle layer), and superficial cells (the outermost layer).

Since oestrogen causes an increase in the number of superficial cells, these should predominate in a smear taken during the first half of the cycle.

Since progesterone reduces the number of superficial cells, intermediate cells should predominate in a smear taken during the second half of the cycle.

If there is anything awry in the normal ebb and flow of these hormones during the menstrual cycle, the cell balance in the smear will show it.

This test may be done during an infertility investigation or around the time of menopause to evaluate the amount of oestrogen still present in the body. It is also done to evaluate children with premature sexual development. (See p. 265)

38. How oestrogen and progesterone affect the breasts

In the early part of the cycle, oestrogen causes an increase in the number of glands and ducts in the breasts. These are mostly milk carriers—although they don't normally function as such until after a delivery.

Progesterone, in the second half of the cycle, has a much more marked effect, causing the swelling of breast glandular tissue and congestion of blood vessels in the breast.

39. Mild breast tenderness is normal before menstruation

Sometimes progesterone and oestrogen cause breast tenderness and swelling toward the end of the cycle. The veins in your breast may appear more prominent at this time, because progesterone is triggering congestion of blood vessels.

The discomfort is usually mild, *a normal sign* of the forthcoming period. Nothing is wrong if it *doesn't* occur.

Severe tenderness may happen as part of premenstrual syndrome. (See p. 311)

40. Menstrual protection: pads or tampons?

There is no intrinsic advantage to one type of protection over another; individual comfort should be the deciding factor. Most girls who are still virginal prefer pads. A young girl should start with the smallest kinds of tampons. Some superabsorbent tampons have recently been withdrawn from the market because of their possible association with Toxic Shock Syndrome. (See p. 237)

41. Regular bathing should continue during menstruation

A girl should be encouraged to continue bathing, showering and washing her hair during her menstrual period just as she would usually. The same goes for swimming and other athletic activities.

42. Dysmenorrhoea (dis-men-or-REE-ah)

Menstrual pain does not usually begin until the second or third year of menstruation, when the young woman begins to ovulate. In many cases, mild to moderate pain-killers bring complete relief. In more severe cases, medical help may be needed. (See p. 312)

43. Irregular periods after menarche are normal

As mentioned before, the first year or two of menses may not be accompanied by ovulation. This means that the levels of oestrogen are high in the body, and changes in this one hormone cause the bleeding which occurs. However, the absence of the high levels of progesterone, which are normally present before menstruation, tends to make the periods irregular. The most usual pattern is to skip several months in between periods. If the length of flow is normal (one to seven days), this irregularity is of no concern during the first few years of menstruation. There are some patterns of menstruation which are not normal during puberty, and these are discussed below.

44. Excessively lengthy menstrual periods after menarche

Once in a while, a girl who has just begun menstruating will experience periods which come infrequently, but last two to three weeks at a time. This usually signifies that she is not ovulating. In some girls this amount of bleeding can cause anaemia (see pp. 356-360), but for most this pattern is just a severe nuisance. A frequent treatment is progestogen tablets, taken for five to seven days each month for several months. The girl will get her period in the few days after stopping the tablets each month. This progestogen therapy will not affect the hypothalamus significantly, nor will it cause ovulation. This pattern of bleeding is called metropathia haemorrhagia.

45. Frequent periods after menarche

In some girls who are not yet ovulating, periods come too frequently—say, every two or three weeks—in addition to lasting too long. (See above) This is not only a nuisance; it can also lead to anaemia.

Tablets of a progestogen, a synthetic form of progesterone, can be taken for two or three weeks to stop the bleeding. Thereafter they can be given for several days every month to regulate menstrual flow. Again, this treatment will not significantly affect the hypothalamus but it will control the bleeding from the endometrium. Some doctors prescribe low-dose combination birth-control pills, if progestogen alone does not work. This is not recommended because it *does* affect the hypothalamus. (See p. 38) Adjusting the progestogen dose usually controls bleeding.

46. Amenorrhoea—prolonged absence of periods

Occasionally, girls who are not yet ovulating miss their periods for very long spans of time—say, six to twelve months. This is called amenorrhoea (ah-men-o-REE-a) or oligomenorrhoea.

If a girl was menstruating irregularly, the amenorrhoea has less significance. It is probably related to the menstrual cycle itself and not to another more serious disease process. If a girl was previously *regular* but misses her period for four to six months, she should receive a physical (*not just a gynaecological!*) examination.

If a girl had *regular* periods previous to the amenorrhoea, an examination is a must. Certain causes must be checked for:

a. Pregnancy

b. Serious illness such as diabetes or thyroid disease

c. Extreme weight loss. If a girl has been on a crash diet and lost a lot of weight quickly, she may also lose her periods. (The most extreme example of this is *anorexia nervosa*—see Nos. 63 – 65 below. But it can happen just from crazy dieting, when the girl is not anorexic at all but simply ill-advised about nutrition.)

d. Extreme weight gain. If the cause is just overeating, then the amenorrhoea should not last long. If another disease process has caused her to gain weight this must be treated with concern.

e. Severe emotional stress. (Life can sometimes be awful or exciting enough to make you miss a period.)

47. Premature or precocious puberty

When a girl experiences the changes of puberty before age seven, she must be examined for other problems such as possible tumours on the ovaries, on the pituitary gland, or hypothyroidism— underactive thyroid gland. In many cases, nothing is wrong. The girl is just ahead for her generation.

48. Premature breast growth

If a little girl is developing breasts at a very early age, with no other signs of puberty, she should be examined for other problems. Usually there are none, and the rest of puberty will proceed normally at a later time.

49. Premature pubic-hair growth

Pubic-hair growth, before other signs of puberty, occurs most often in children with known neurological problems—for example, nervous disorders such as cerebral palsy or seizures. If neurological damage was not previously apparent, then premature pubic-hair growth is *not* a sign of it. As with premature breast growth, puberty usually occurs normally at a later date.

50. Delayed puberty

If the various other stages of puberty are progressing, there is no need to worry if menarche has not occurred before the sixteenth birthday. But if menarche does not occur within the next year, or if the other changes of puberty do not occur, then disease must be suspected.

a. When *no* changes of puberty occur, there may be some congenital abnormality present such as *Turner's Syndrome*. A girl born with Turner's Syndrome has very tiny ovaries or none at all: therefore oestrogen and progesterone are not being produced in sufficient quantities. The disorder is named after Henry H. Turner, an American endocrinologist, who discovered it in the 1930s.

In such cases, oestrogen and progesterone therapy can be used to develop breasts, pubic hair, and other female sexual characteristics, including menstrual periods, so that a woman with Turner's Syndrome can lead a normal life. However, since there is no ovulation, she will not be fertile.

b. When puberty seems to be occurring normally, but there is no menarche, an examination can usually determine the cause. There may be a condition present such as *imperforate hymen* in which the hymen —the membrane that covers the vaginal opening in little girls—must be broken surgically to allow menstrual blood to flow out.

As with all deviations in the menstrual cycle other rare causes of delayed menarche require a general physical as well as a gynaecological examination.

ADOLESCENCE

Strictly speaking adolescence is that period of time when young people (usually in their teens) establish an identity separate and distinct from their parents. It is a tumultuous time, made more so by the soaring sexual and emotional demands of puberty. Parents usually have problems during the adolescence of their children; they have to put up with a lot of rejection (as their ideas are challenged) and fear (as their children go off on their own). It is often very difficult for a parent to distinguish between normal adolescent behaviour and real abnormality. Keep in mind that this time of exploration and experimentation is necessary; that it will probably pass. When you are being driven to despair by your teenagers, remember your own youth and think with sympathy of your own mother. If you are an adolescent, think of your mother now!

51. Temporary homosexual attachments are normal during adolescence

Boys and girls often form passionate attachments to older role models of the same sex in early adolescence, a normal manifestation of the break with parental identification. Girls often have very close friends from whom they are inseparable at this time, with whom they share all their intimacies, sometimes including bodily touching and mutual exploration. This is normal too. Don't make a girl feel guilty about it.

52. Don't wait for your girl to become sexually active to tell her about reproduction, sex and venereal disease

Children should be told the facts of life as soon as they start asking about them. As your child approaches puberty, discuss all aspects of sex with her; open communication between parent and child is vital at this time. Studies have shown that teenagers engaging in sex have less accurate knowledge about vital sexual topics than those who are not. So in this case, knowledge may actually serve as a healthy, intelligent deterrent. *Support sex education in schools.*

53. Sexual arousal and vaginal discharge are normal in adolescence

A watery secretion from the vagina is a normal result of oestrogen influence on the vaginal mucosa at puberty. But it also may be due to fantasies and sexual arousal. (Boys have wet dreams; girls do as well.) If the vagina is not irritated, don't be alarmed. Suggest cotton pants to your daughter; they are more absorbent than nylon and reduce the incidence of conditions like thrush.

54. Masturbation and self-exploration are normal in adolescence

Unless masturbation is obsessive, it is a completely healthy way for a girl to learn about and feel at ease with her body.

55. Sports activities

An adolescent girl should take part in sports whether she is good at them or not, because they build her general health and accustom her to competition. The emotional lessons learned on the field or court spill over to relationships later in life, so that as an adult the girl is less inclined to accept passive, non-competitive roles. Likewise, boys who see girls participating actively in athletics are more likely to grow into men who are unafraid of strong, equal female partners.

56. Early gynaecological examinations

It is unusual in Britain for young women to have a gynaecological examination unless they attend a clinic for contraceptive advice. Routine examinations in a girl who is not sexually active might pick up a symptomless ovarian cyst, but these are uncommon at this age.

It would be a good idea if GPs were to have a talk with young teenagers covering menstruation, contraception and the pros and cons of early sexual activity. If you and your daughter agreed, your own GP or a young people's family planning clinic could give advice, and if necessary carry out an examination.

57. Patient confidentiality and the adolescent

Medico-legally speaking, children become adults at 16 in Britain. They can then give their own consent for contraception, abortion or any other treatment. However, GPs and clinics do respect the confidence of a girl under that age if they are convinced that they are acting in her best interests. This position is supported by the British Medical Association. It is wrong for parents to put pressure on doctors to betray such confidences. In an emergency situation, it is possible for a senior doctor to act *in loco parentis* and sign the consent form for operative procedures.

58. Adolescent pregnancy

Pregnancy among teenagers is on the rise as social attitudes change to allow greater sexual contact among young people. In addition, the age of puberty is decreasing—so the age of fertility starts earlier.

Don't try to cope alone. Talk with the people at the family planning clinic or your GP, who are neither as hurt nor as angry nor as frightened as you are, who know all the options, and who can recommend good counsellors, an invaluable assistance at this time.

59. The options in adolescent pregnancy

a. If the father is known, and the youngsters are over 16 and want to get married, they can do so with your permission. *But if they are very young, this is probably a bad idea.*

b. The girl can have the baby and bring it up with her parents' help. This may be hard on the family financially. *Keep up school attendance.* The social stigma of being an unwed teenage mother is fast declining; even though you may find it horrifying that your daughter is going to school with a big belly, the kids and the teachers have probably witnessed this before and may notice it less than you would have thought. If the head teacher will not allow your daughter to stay at school, ask for home tutoring.

c. Very often, girls who drop out of school because they become pregnant never finish their education. This is a tragedy; it penalizes the girl for ever for something she did when she was very young.

d. The baby may be given up for adoption immediately after birth. Don't choose this option without the wholehearted agreement of all concerned. *Do not choose it without counselling.*

e. While the mother finishes school, the child may be placed in foster care. If the mother keeps in contact and retrieves the baby permanently by the time she is a toddler, the break with the foster parents may be uneventful.

f. If the pregnancy is discovered early enough, the option of abortion should be discussed. *Do not make the decision for abortion without advice.* A young girl may have fears about her future fertility, and qualms about the operation once it is over. Full discussion without pressure is the only way of minimizing these problems.

g. There is no reason why the father and his parents should not share in the decision as to how the pregnancy is handled, and its attendant costs.

h. Teenage pregnancy is often a self-repeating phenomenon, especially if a girl is made to feel guilty and dirty by her parents and friends, and even more so if she drops out of school. So try to see adolescent pregnancy for what it is: something that can happen to anyone, and which has happened to a young woman whose whole life is still before her.

60. Medical aspects of adolescent pregnancy

Teenagers who decide to have their babies experience a higher incidence of
   a. Anaemia
   b. High blood pressure
   c. Prematurity
   d. Caesarean-section delivery

61. Adolescent mothers often do not get good antenatal care

Very often, a teenager who thinks she is pregnant will not know where to turn. She may tell her boy friend before she tells her mother; he may not know where to turn either. If a girl hides her pregnancy until it is well advanced, passing the critical first three months without antenatal care or advice, she creates unnecessary hazards to her baby. In addition, clinics and doctors are often completely unprepared to cope with the emotional complexities of the adolescent personality; they may look down on the girl, condemn her; she may feel uncomfortable with them and neglect to show up for her appointments. If she goes into labour without having had the advantages of routine antenatal attention, the risk of complication grows. Pregnant teenagers need very good antenatal care.

62. Opinion: Venereal disease is a major hazard of teenage sexual activity. Insist that sexual partners use condoms

Other forms of birth control may protect a girl against pregnancy, but they will not protect her against venereal disease. A girl should insist that any man she sleeps with uses a sheath. Teenage boys should be educated to wear them too.

63. Neurotic dieting: anorexia nervosa (an-oh-RECK-see-a nair-VOH-sa)

Teenage girls often diet because they want to be attractive; so do teenage boys. However, there is one condition—anorexia nervosa—when the dieting is obsessive, when a girl feels that she must lose more and more weight, stops eating almost entirely, and *still* thinks she is fat. She keeps on this pattern until she is concentration-camp thin and her body begins to break down and die. Literally, she is starving herself to death for deep-rooted psychological reasons that are still incompletely understood. They are often connected with fear of growing up, stress and pressure at home or work, a difficult relationship with one or both parents, high intelligence and a high level of interest in food within the family. In some cases, especially where the parents are strict or have high expectations of their children, it is a search for approval. Fortunately, anorexia nervosa is rare, although its incidence is increasing; it primarily affects girls aged 16 – 19 but boys can get it too. In older women, it is often connected with a lack of self-confidence and sexual problems.

64. Symptoms of anorexia nervosa

a. A teenager who is on a crash diet will complain of feeling hungry all the time; the anorexic will maintain, no matter that she has virtually stopped eating anything at all, that she feels full and fine. Sometimes she will eat a lot and then vomit. Or she will take laxatives to force elimination of the food.

b. Crash dieters start to eat again eventually, when they've lost enough weight to be satisfied with themselves. The anorexic is never satisfied; she always maintains that she must get thinner, even when she is down to skin and bones.

c. A crash dieter may lose her period, because the hypothalamus is affected by weight loss. (See No. 46 above). This usually worries a girl enough to get her eating properly again. But the anorexic is not scared by the loss of her period; she may even welcome this sign that she has withdrawn from maturity.

ANY ONE OF THESE SYMPTOMS SHOULD TAKE THE GIRL AND HER PARENTS TO A DOCTOR IMMEDIATELY.

65. Treatment of anorexia nervosa

Treatment is frequently extended hospitalization and psychotherapy. The first step is to prevent death from starvation. If the condition is caught early, it is easier to cure. But girls will often go to great lengths to hide their condition and there is a low success rate with chronic anorexics. Families of anorexics may expect to be involved in the therapy, because the roots of this problem are often found in family relationships. Look also for the local branch of Anorexic Aid, a self-help body of mainly former anorexics.

66. Acne: a very common problem of adolescents

Adolescence is accompanied by an increase in hormones—which cause the growth of pubic and underarm hair and increase the oil secretions in the skin pores. Spots, blackheads and whiteheads break out on the face, the chest and the back. No one really knows why one teenager has only a few spots while another may be covered all over. There are two principles in acne treatment:

a. To render it as mild as possible during the adolescent years;

b. To make sure it will leave no scars in the future.

67. Blackheads: the least serious acne lesion

Sometimes a skin pore is blocked by a collection of oils. The tip of the oil collection, exposed to the air, turns black; the rest of the oil in the pore remains whitish. This is called a blackhead. It will not usually leave a scar unless picked or squeezed with dirty fingers and thus become infected. Gentle squeezing *with very clean hands* to release the oil from the pore is probably no danger; or the teenager can use an extractor.

68. Whiteheads: more serious acne lesions

A whitehead forms just like a blackhead except that the pore has no opening to the outside. The oil cannot drain; cysts form underneath the skin; a dot of white pus will indicate infection. The area around a whitehead may be painful, for it is the tip of a small infection, not as with a blackhead, the tip of a blocked pore. Whiteheads should not be squeezed or picked, for this can lead to scarring.

69. Recommended treatment for mild acne

a. Don't pick at the spots. This may lead to infection and scarring.

b. Wash hair two or three times a week, to keep it from becoming oily. Oily hair can aggravate acne, especially on the forehead. Avoid hair creams, sprays, grease.

c. Wash the face two or three times a day. Don't scrub hard. Press a hot flannel over the affected area, then lather gently with an acne soap containing resorcinol, salicylic acid, or benzoyl peroxide.

d. Try going over your face with an ice cube after washing; the cold will help to keep the pores tight and closed.

e. Avoid greasy skin lotions or cosmetics.

f. To cover up the acne, use the special cosmetics that have been developed for this purpose.

g. Astringents like witch hazel or alcohol may be useful in cleaning excess oil from the face.

h. Don't rub the acne lesions or put excess pressure on them. For example, don't lean your chin or your face continually on your hand.

i. Stay away from foods thought to aggravate acne—chocolate, nuts, iodized salt and fizzy drinks. Some dermatologists feel acne sufferers should avoid milk as well. If, after three to four weeks of avoiding these foods, the acne is not improved, then you can conclude that diet is simply not a principal cause of the lesions.

70. For treatment of severe acne, consult your doctor

Don't try to treat severe acne alone. Your GP may refer you to a dermatologist, who is specially trained in skin care.

71. Antibiotics as a treatment for severe acne

If skin infection is present, the doctor may prescribe a broad-spectrum antibiotic such as tetracycline. Usually the dosage is one 250 – 500 mg tablet daily for several months. This treatment appears to affect the skin bacteria and releases enzymes which break down the fats on the skin. Antibiotic creams which are applied directly to the skin are also being tested.

Remember! Antibiotics can cause candidal vaginitis. (See Chapter Eleven) So if vaginal itching occurs while you are on the treatment, tell your doctor.

72. Vitamin A acid as a treatment for severe acne

Vitamin A acid, currently being tested in Britain but already available and popular in the United States, is applied as a solution or in pre-soaked swabs. It works by breaking down the sebum, the fatty substance produced in the pores, thereby drying the skin.

Vitamin A acid is applied when the face is dry, lightly and once a day at first, to see how much can be tolerated. During the first three weeks of treatment, the acne may appear to worsen. Skin may redden, cystic areas enlarge. Thereafter improvement can be expected. The daily treatment is continued for six to eight weeks, then decreased to two or three times per week. Taking vitamin A orally does not have the same effect as applying a solution to the skin, and may be dangerous since this vitamin is stored by the body.

73. Side effects of vitamin A acid
   a. There may be no side effects at all.
   b. People using vitamin A (Retin-A) may become highly sensitive to the sun and sun lamps; some skin tumours have even been reported.
   c. Some people become highly sensitive to soap. As a general rule, avoid sunbathing and excess face washing while under treatment.
   d. Loss of skin pigment may occur, but this reverses itself when treatment stops.

74. Surgery as a treatment for severe acne
A dermatologist may lance very large cysts or whiteheads in the surgery, making a tiny cut right over the lesion so the pus can escape. This only helps for a short time and obviously does not cure the condition.

75. Cryotherapy and dermabrasion as treatment for severe acne
Cryotherapy or cryoslush therapy is the application of a mixture of dry ice (cryo- is from the Greek *kryos* meaning ice-cold) and acetone or liquid nitrogen to affected skin areas with gauze once a week. It makes the outer scarred layers of skin peel off and may help severe acne. (It also removes tattoos.)

Dermabrasion involves 'sandpapering off' the rough top layer with a rotary abrasive.

76. Warning: Do not accept X-ray or ultra-violet light therapy for acne. Both may increase your risk of skin cancer.

77. Opinion: Oestrogen should not be used routinely for acne treatment in adolescents.
When women began taking birth control pills, it was noted that

as a result many no longer suffered from acne. This is because the oestrogen in the pills counteracts the hormones which build up oily skin secretions. Using this knowledge, dermatologists sometimes recommend the pill for young women suffering from bad acne. *All of these hormones are very strong agents, with potential for adverse effects on other parts of the body, so they should not be used routinely or for long periods of time.*

78. Some unavoidable elements which aggravate acne
Acne can be aggravated by:

a. Hot humid weather

b. Strenuous sports, which cause an increase in adrenal hormone production

c. Emotional stress.

There is sometimes no way to avoid emotional stress or hot humid weather, and sports are too important for general health to give up. There is also no way to avoid adolescence, and the parent and teenager trying to cope with these years should remember that they will fade away, like acne, with remarkable haste.

3

BIRTH CONTROL

No single scientific breakthrough has altered our lives so momentously as the discovery and mass use of safe, effective contraceptive methods. These discoveries ended an epidemic of death and chronic illness from unpreventable pregnancy that had always ravaged the women of the world. In days still not completely gone, a woman literally had babies until she died.

Make yourself familiar with as many birth control methods as possible; one type may be good now, but tomorrow, a back-up or alternative method may be required.

Never let anyone else decide what kind of birth control is best for you—not your lover, not your neighbour, not your doctor, not even this book. Many doctors have a particular method they think is best for most of their patients most of the time; magazines and media resound with the opinions of the individuals who think the pill is terrible for everyone, or foams are terrible for everyone. Listen to all this advice the way you would listen to a political candidate. But when you cast your vote, cast it according to what *you* think is best for *you*.

ORAL CONTRACEPTIVES

1. History of oral contraceptives

Since the beginning of recorded history, men and women have been taking potions to render themselves temporarily sterile. Most of these—until the pill—were ineffective. A few, like arsenic, mercury and strychnine, could render the taker sterile by rendering the taker dead.

In 1927 two physiologists in Germany, Bernhard Zondek and Selmar Aschheim, discovered that when the urine of pregnant women was injected into lab animals, the animals went into heat. The Zondek-Aschheim test became an early test for pregnancy; it was also a breakthrough necessary for the discovery of the oestrogens, female hormones, by Adolf Butenandt in Germany and Edward Doisy in America. In the early 1930s the Schering-Kahlbaum Co. in Germany and Parke-Davis in the United States began manufacturing hormones from animal sources, an expensive process. Further research showed that administration of hormones could prevent conception in laboratory animals. Soon it was discovered that cholesterol was the basic substance on which all hormones were built, and this led to the discovery of the androgens, male hormones. In 1937 diosgenin, a chemical used to synthesize androgen, oestrogen, and progesterone, was discovered in large quantities in a Mexican yam. This made it much more feasible and inexpensive to produce hormones for clinical use.

The discovery of the hormones opened up new possibilities for controlling many sexual and reproductive functions. In the 1940s it was learned that oestrogen and progesterone could inhibit ovulation in women, a breakthrough which led eventually to development of the pill.

2. The original 'pill' experiments

In the 1950s G. D. Searle and Co., began work on the synthesis (production in a laboratory) of steroids, a large group of chemical substances that includes hormones, vitamins and other bodily substances. (Cholesterol, cortisone and the sex hormones are all steroids.) In 1952 Norethynodrel, the progestogen in the Enovid pill, was synthesized, along with another progestogen, Norethindrone.

The first large-scale clinic trials in Britain took place in Birmingham in 1960. The medical advisory council of the Family Planning Association approved the use of oral contraceptives in 1966. In 1963 a new progestogen, Norgestrel, was produced. Now steroids can be produced synthetically by constructing three-dimensional molecular models.

Two different types of pill are currently on the market—combined pills (with oestrogen and progestogen) and minipills (with progestogen alone). Current research centres on reducing side effects and dosage levels.

3. Statistical context of the pill

Today, over 3 million British women take the pill. There are about 50 million women using it throughout the world; approximately 20 to 25 per cent of British women between 15 and 40 now use the pill.

4. Warning: if you are taking the pill, tell anyone you see for any health reasons

Like pregnancy, the pill has some effect on virtually all the body systems. (Ref. 1) For example, since the pill can affect your eyes, the optician should be told if you are taking the pill—even if your visit is just to check your glasses.

5. Recommendation: Do not take the pill for longer than five years without a break

Even though it is the most effective form of birth control, the pill—whether the combined pill or the minipill—carries with it a very wide range of known and potential side effects (see below). In addition, there *may* be cumulative effects for women who take the pill over many years, that are now only suspected.

6. Limitations on the pill

a. The pill may be obtained only by prescription from a doctor or family planning clinic.

b. The quantities of oestrogen and progestogen in the pill have been constantly lowered over the years. Doctors should prescribe the *lowest effective* dose of oestrogen and a number of very low-dose pills are now available.

c. There is now no limit on the number of years the pill may be taken (but recent studies suggest that there should be a break at regular intervals—at least every five years). Women who have taken the pill for more than five years have a higher death rate even after stopping than those who never took the pill. (Ref. 2)

7. The combined pill

The combined pill is most widely used in this country. Each pill contains an oestrogen and a progestogen. All pills in the package are identical. The exception to that is the 28-day package, which contains seven inert pills (without active hormonal ingredients).

8. Oestrogenic compounds used in the combined pills

There are two of these—*mestranol* and *ethinyl oestradiol*.

For most practical purposes—including evaluation of side effects—there is little difference between these two oestrogens. Some tests show ethinyl oestradiol to be more potent than mestranol; others find it about equivalent in strength.

9. Progestogenic compounds used in various combined pills

There are five of these (listed in order of potency, the strongest first): *norgestrel, ethynodiol diacetate, norethisterone acetate, norethisterone, norethynodrel.* The reason there are so many progestogens is basically that each company developed its own. All except norgestrel come from the Mexican yam (barbasco root). Norgestrel is synthesized completely in the laboratory.

10. How the combined pills prevent pregnancy

a. They block ovulation.

The hormones block the release of FSH-RF (Follicle Stimulating Hormone-Releasing Factor) from the hypothalamus, and therefore the follicles in the ovary do not mature completely. In addition, hormones in the pill stop the release of LH-RF (Luteinizing Hormone-Releasing Factor) so that there is no spurt of luteinizing hormone at mid-cycle and therefore no ovulation. (See Chapter Two, Menstruation)

b. They change the cervical mucus so that it is thick and relatively impenetrable by sperm—replacing the stringy, watery mucus that is normal at mid-cycle and easily penetrated by sperm.

c. They keep the endometrium (the lining of the uterus) thin, so that implantation of a fertilized egg is much less likely. Because the combined pill keeps the endometrium thin, women who are taking it tend to have lighter menstrual flows.

d. They may slow down the rate at which the egg passes along the Fallopian tube, preventing implantation.

11. If taken correctly, the combined pills are almost 100 per cent effective in preventing pregnancy

Even if some pills are missed and ovulation occurs, the other three factors are at work. The pills with less than 50 mcg oestrogen are a fraction less certain to prevent pregnancy—but still more than 99 per cent effective. (Below 30 mcg the risk is higher—effectiveness drops to 97 – 98 per cent.) The benefits of reducing the oestrogen in the pills and avoiding the side effects may justify running the highly remote risk that the pill will not work (see below).

STOP PRESS: New triphasic pills which mimic the natural rise and fall in the ratio of oestrogen to progesterone are now available. In trials, these were as effective as the fixed-dose combined oral contraceptive, although the sequential (variable dose) pills previously available were not as effective.

While these new pills may be an improvement, the total amount of oestrogen in a monthly cycle is higher than when the 30-mcg pills are taken, even though the amount of progesterone per month has been reduced. Although we don't know what is important about progesterone or what the safe level of oestrogen is per day, there is some evidence from blood-clotting studies that certain combinations of oestrogen and progesterone are safer than others. We will have to wait and see whether these pills are an improvement, as the manufacturers claim.

12. The minipill

The minipill was first marketed in 1973. It contains no oestrogen, only progestogen. There are three kinds of minipills, containing different progestogens. (See table below and, for further information, John Guillebaud's excellent book *The Pill* (Oxford Paperbacks, £1.95). They do not block ovulation, but work by affecting the cervical mucus. The endometrium is also less receptive to any sperm that does penetrate this barrier. It is important to take these pills at the same time each day.

Table 1

Brands of progestogen-only pills available in Britain

Name of pill	Number in packet	Progestogen content (microgrammes)
Neogest	35	DL-norgestrel 75 mcg
Microval Norgeston	35 } 35	levonorgestrel 30 mcg No extra, inactive, hormone and therefore preferable
Micronor Noriday	42 } 28	norethisterone 35 mcg
Femulen	28	ethynodiol diacetate 50 mcg

13. Advantages of the minipill

Because the minipill contains no oestrogen, it is felt to be free from the major side effects that sometimes result from oestrogen action in the pill (see below) and which have caused the major controversies over the other pills.

14. Disadvantages of the minipill

a. The minipills are estimated to be only 97 per cent effective (about the same as the IUD). This is because they do not block ovulation as combined pills do.

b. There is a high incidence of breakthrough bleeding with the minipill, the factor which most women who discontinue it cite for doing so.

c. They offer less protection against ectopic pregnancy. (See p. 164) If the minipill fails, one pregnancy in ten is ectopic.

15. A back-up method should be used during the first 14 days on the minipill

The Family Planning Association recommends that a back-up method—ideally a spermicide or sheath—should be used during the first two weeks of the first pack.

16. When to start taking birth control pills

The pill (all kinds) can be started on day 5 of the cycle. It can be started the day of an abortion, or three to four days after childbirth if the mother is not breast-feeding, though recently there have been warnings to wait two weeks after childbirth. When started at these times, the pill is effective immediately and requires no back-up birth control. The minipill (see No. 15 above) is an exception.

17. 21-day and 22-day pills

When using the 21-day and 22-day pills, take one a day until the pack is finished, wait seven or six days respectively without taking pills, then start a new pack. Since all pills are now recommended to be taken on 28-day cycles, you would always be starting a new pack every twenty-ninth day, on the same weekday each month.

18. 28-day pills

It's somewhat easier to take the 28-day pills because you don't have to remember *not* to take them. Just take them every day, with no breaks between packs.

CAUTION: Remember that you start with the active pills and finish with the 'sugar' pills. If you take sugar pills for two weeks at a time, you can get pregnant.

19. Minipills

The minipills come in packages of 28, 35 or 42 pills. They are taken continuously with no break between packs, starting at the times discussed above. Most women become regulated and bleed only once a month or less often, although they take the pills continuously.

20. Pills should be taken at the same time each day

The best time is after eating. for this prevents nausea, one of the most frequent complaints of women on the pill. Minipills should be taken in the early evening, rather than just before going to bed.

21. What to do if pills are missed

If you forget one combined pill, take it as soon as you remember and carry on normally by taking the next pill due on time. *If your combined pill is more than 12 hours overdue you must not rely on its contraceptive protection.* Complete the course as usual, but *use other contraceptive precautions as well* for 14 days, or until your next period, *whichever is the longer. Women on a progestogen-only pill should take additional precautions for 14 days if their pill is more than three hours overdue.*

WARNING: Severe diarrhoea or vomiting (as in a viral illness) may cause the body to absorb the pill poorly. Use a back-up method for the remainder of the pack if this occurs.

22. When to use a back-up method with the pill

    a. When one or more low-dose pills have been missed
    b. When a combined pill is more than 12 hours overdue
    c. During the first two weeks on the minipill
    d. After a gastro-intestinal illness (vomiting, diarrhoea)
    e. When you are taking any medications listed in No. 50 below.

23. Menstruation while taking the pill

Menstruation is reorganized by the pill. The hormone effects of the pill allow bleeding to occur only at regulated times which can always be anticipated. A woman bleeds as a reaction to her withdrawal from the pill (during the 6 or 7 days she does not take them, with the 21- to 22-day types or during the inert pills in the 28-day type). This kind of controlled menstruation is called 'withdrawal bleeding'.

The absence of oestrogen in the minipill means that you cannot anticipate when bleeding will occur, an inconvenience which may be aggravating but is *not a danger or an indicator of ill health.*

24. Decreased menstrual flow while taking the pill is normal

Many women think that decreased menstrual flow while taking the pill indicates that something is wrong. *This is not true.* The menstrual flow should be only the amount of blood and endometrium that builds up each month. (See Chapter Two) When a woman takes the combined pills, there is less endometrial build-up and consequently less menstrual flow. *Even if bleeding lasts only a day, a few hours, or is limited to spotting, that is sufficient.* Scanty periods occur most frequently when progestogen-dominant pills are used. If for any reason, even a psychological one, additional menstrual flow is desired, then oestrogen-dominant pills can be taken instead. However, high-dose oestrogen pills have other problems. (See below)

25. Breakthrough bleeding

Breakthrough bleeding is usually a light blood flow that surprises the pill-taker by occurring while she is on the active pills and not at the time allotted for menstrual flow during the cycle. *It is a harmless side effect. It does not indicate ill health or that the pill is failing.*

With low-dose pills, breakthrough bleeding is very common in the first one or two cycles. If it amounts only to spotting, then no particular action is indicated. If the bleeding is heavy and troublesome into the second or third cycle, then a woman may conclude that she needs a slightly higher-dose pill and should try a different type.

Occasionally, a woman will experience breakthrough bleeding once or twice a year; this is nothing to worry about.

When changing to another pill because of breakthrough bleeding, a pill with more or a different progestogen should be used.

26. Heavy breakthrough bleeding

If breakthrough bleeding involves a heavy flow, then pills should be stopped and a new pack started on the fifth day of bleeding. Use a back-up method. (See No. 21 above) If the bleeding is very heavy or persistent, or associated with severe pain or fever, consult your doctor.

27. Dysmenorrhoea (pain) during breakthrough bleeding

Breakthrough bleeding sometimes involves dysmenorrhoea. The pain should not be severe, and should not last very long; if it is severe or continuous, consult your doctor.

28. Conditions which the pill can help

a. *Heavy menstrual flow that causes anaemia:* Menstrual flow is usually lighter among women on the pill.

b. *Dysmenorrhoea* is less frequent and less severe among women on the pill. (See p. 311)

c. *Premenstrual syndrome* is rare among women on the pill. (See p. 311)

d. *Acne* is known to improve in women using oestrogen-dominant pills, so much so that some doctors will sometimes prescribe the pills for short periods of time as treatment for acne even when no birth control is desired. (See p. 31)

e. *Ovarian cysts:* Women on the pill experience a definite decrease in functional ovarian cysts. (See p. 328)

All of the above benefits occur because women who are taking the pill do not experience the hormonal changes inherent in an unregulated menstrual cycle, thereby avoiding the discomforts associated with menstruation.

Consider the risks carefully (See Nos. 33 – 51) before accepting the pill as treatment for these conditions.

29. Minor side effects indicating a pill change or discontinuation is in order

Some minor side effects of the pill indicate that the woman is taking the wrong dose pill for her body, and should change to another type.

a. *Breast tenderness:* This is a normal sign of adjustment to a new hormonal cycle in the first two to three months of pills. If it continues or is severe, consult a doctor and change to another type of pill. *Breast tenderness while taking the pill is not a sign of cancer.* If the pain is mild, a bra with better support and some over-the-counter analgesics should relieve it.

b. *Change in breast size:* Some women on the pill report a decrease, some an increase in breast size. Neither is cause for worry. If the change involves a bra size or more, consult a doctor.

c. *Weight gain* is a common complaint among women on the pill; it is thought to be related to the progestogen component. Tests on large numbers of women show little or no weight gain on the average is associated with pill usage, but many women *know* better. So if a woman feels she has gained, or that the fat distribution on her body has changed for the worse, she should switch to a different form of birth control.

d. *Candidal infection of the vagina (thrush)* (See p. 288) is sometimes aggravated by the progestogens in the pill, which increase the glycogen or cell sugar in the cells of the vagina. If these infections recur frequently, try a new pill with lowered progestogen. Many women experience changes in the *amount* of vaginal discharge (either more or less than usual) because of the pill. Unless this really bothers you, it is nothing to worry about.

e. If *headaches* occur repeatedly while taking the pill, try another pill with lower oestrogen. If headaches occur while taking the inert pills, or while off the pills, try a compound with lower progestogen. WARNING: If migraine headaches appear or are aggravated by the pill, it should be discontinued. If there is any doubt as to whether the headache is migraine, make sure; check with a doctor; frequent migraine is an absolute contra-indication for the pills. (See No. 33 below) If any weakness, dizziness, or blurring of vision occur with the headaches, see a doctor immediately. (See No. 39 below) If that is impossible, stop the pills.

f. *Loss of menstrual period:* If no pills have been missed and the period does not occur, the pills should be continued for one more month. If no menstrual period occurs during the second month, this probably indicates that the endometrium-suppressing component in the pill is too strong and the woman should switch to another type of pill. (If no pills have been missed, loss of the period is not necessarily a sign of pregnancy. However, if you've missed two periods, *or* if you have any other signs of pregnancy, have a pregnancy test—just in case.)

g. *Mood changes:* As with the menstrual cycle generally, hormonal changes may cause changes in mood which appear as psychological but are essentially endocrine. Studies on psychological changes among women on the pill show a variety of differing results: no changes; deep depression; improvement in depression; loss of libido or sexual drive. (Ref. 3, 4) Vitamin B6 may offset some of these changes.

Be your own judge. If you are experiencing some change in temperament, if you're feeling *very* bad, the pill may be aggravating a pre-existing condition. Stop the pill and seek further professional advice if the problem persists.

h. Some women on the pill need to take vitamin supplements. (See p. 248)

30. Hair loss

If a woman taking the pill experiences hair loss, she should discontinue using it and see if hair growth begins again. If it does not, investigate other causes and treatments.

31. Skin changes

Aside from the beneficial effect on acne, several unpleasant skin changes are often associated with pill-taking.

a. Some women experience a greater sensitivity to sun and more frequent burning. It is always wise to limit exposure to the sun (See p. 33) and even more so if taking the pill.

b. Moles frequently become darker when the pill is taken. This may be a harmless pill effect. To make sure, check with a doctor.

c. Pre-existing skin conditions, such as rosacea or (a red rash on the chest and face) and eczema (a rash on the neck or in the creases of the elbows and knees) can be aggravated by the pill.

d. Chloasma (mask of pregnancy) is a brownish discoloration on the cheeks, forehead and nose which is deepened by exposure to the sun. (This is very strange since the word chloasma comes from the Greek word meaning to become green.) Very rarely, the pill can cause chloasma; if it does, use another form of birth control.

e. Acne may appear for the first time or become severe during the first few months *after stopping* the pill. Treat it as you would treat other acne. (See p. 32) This problem usually does not more than six months.

32. Delay in return of periods after stopping the pill

After discontinuation of the pill, the first period is usually delayed a few weeks as the body readjusts to a new cycle. This is usually not a cause for concern unless this time is very prolonged. (See No. 45)

33. Who should not take the pill?

Generally accepted, absolute contra-indications to the pill include women who:

a. have a history of blood-clotting disorders (phlebitis, embolus, heart attack, stroke);

b. have severe or frequent migraine headaches;

c. have hypertension (high blood pressure);

d. have hyperlipidaemia (increased fat in the blood);

e. are heavy smokers (especially over age 35);

f. are over age 40;

g. have sickle-cell anaemia or related diseases which predispose to blood-clotting problems;

h. have liver abnormalities or dysfunction as shown by blood tests (recent history of jaundice, hepatitis, glandular fever or idiopathic jaundice of pregnancy);

i. have had cancer of the breast or uterus;

j. are breast-feeding;

k. have grossly irregular menstrual periods until the reason for this is discovered.

OPINION: *The following should also serve as contra-indications to the use of the pill.* They include women who:

a. have *severe* chronic diseases such as heart disease, kidney disease, or asthma;

b. have diabetes;

c. were exposed to DES and/or related compounds before birth (See p. 355)

d. have large fibroid tumours of the uterus or breast;

e. have severe varicose veins;

f. have eye problems such as optic neuritis, glaucoma;

g. suffer from severe depression;

h. are severely overweight;

i. have a history of Sydenham's chorea (sometimes associated with rheumatic fever, see p. 367);

j. have epilepsy;

k. have cystic disease of the breast or a family history of breast cancer (See p. 333).

Of course, any woman who experiences disquieting bodily changes after going on the pill should immediately consider another method of birth control.

34. Thromboembolic diseases (blood clots); the major negative side effects of the pill

The clotting factors in blood give blood its ability to thicken, to clot. They are essential to the healing process. If we did not have them, we might bleed to death from scratches.

However, an *increase* in clotting factors may cause *thrombosis* (thromm-BO-siss)—a thickening or coagulation of the blood inside the veins or arteries. Thrombosis is a very serious health matter, for when it occurs, the flow of blood through the body is obstructed and the system of circulation which nourishes each part of the body is threatened.

Tests in Britain and the United States (Ref. 3, 5) have shown that in a few women, the oestrogen content of the pill somehow increases the number of clotting factors in the blood, increasing the danger of thromboembolic disease. *Therefore, any history of thromboembolic disease is an absolute contra-indication for the pill.* There are several types of thromboembolic disease of major concern:

a. Superficial thromboses
b. Deep-vein thrombophlebitis
c. Stroke
d. Heart attack

35. Symptoms of thromboembolic disorders: See a doctor immediately
a. Severe headaches
b. Blurring or loss of vision (especially if it is in one eye only)
c. Sensation of lights flashing
d. Swelling and pain in the legs
e. Severe chest pain; coughing blood
f. Acute shortness of breath
g. Numbness of the side of the face or in one arm

36. Superficial thromboses
These are clots in the outermost veins of the legs. The symptom is a hot red painful area over a vein. The treatment is bed rest and support. The affected leg should be elevated. Generally, superficial clots are not serious—*but a doctor should always be consulted*. If there is any possibility of deeper clots, heparin, a blood-thinning medication, may be prescribed. The pill must be stopped immediately on recognizing the symptom, but *that will not in itself cure the condition. Further treatment is needed*. This and the following disorders occur in women not on the pill as well, so all women should be aware of the symptoms.

37. Deep-vein thrombophlebitis
This is less common than superficial thrombosis but more serious. Here, the clot forms in the veins deep inside the muscles of the legs and the pelvic area. When it occurs, it carries a risk that the clot will break out of the area and travel through the circulatory system to the lung, causing a pulmonary embolus (a blood clot in the lung) which is very dangerous, sometimes fatal.

The symptoms of deep-vein thrombophlebitis are severe pain, redness and a hot feeling in the leg—usually in the calf muscle. Any woman with any of these symptoms should seek emergency medical care. If the diagnosis is confirmed, the treatment is bed rest in the hospital along with blood-thinning medicine.

38. Varicose veins
This common disorder of women (see p. 370) may be aggravated by the pill. If the varicose veins are mild, then the woman can take

47

the pill. If she notices any increase in the severity of her condition, she should stop taking the pill.

If her varicose veins are severe, the woman should not take the pill. The condition is related to *stasis* of the blood inside the vein—a tendency of the blood to idle, to flow sluggishly. The more pronounced the stasis, the more severe the varicosity, and vice versa—and the more likely it is that the condition could be a prelude to a clotting disorder. So, if you have severe varicose veins, don't use the pill.

39. Stroke

A stroke is caused by a blood clot or haemorrhage in the brain, and occurs more frequently in pill-takers than in other women. The incidence is also much higher in women who take the pill and are over 35, who have taken it for five years or more, have hypertension or are smokers. A stroke is potentially fatal or paralyzing. The symptoms are weakness on one side of the body, numbness, blurry vision, a sensation of seeing bright lights, headache or seizures. *If you have any of these symptoms, stop the pill and see a doctor fast.* In women under age 35 who don't smoke, the risk is only slightly greater than for non-pill takers. (Ref. 2)

40. Heart attack

A heart attack is caused by a clot in the arteries leading to the heart. Conditions which predispose to heart attack are heavy smoking, hyperlipidaemia (high blood fats), hypertension and use of oral contraceptives. When these factors are sorted out, it seems that *smoking* has a dominant role, and compounds the risk of the pill. (Ref. 5, 6) The symptoms of heart attack are severe chest pain, pain in the left arm and shortness of breath. Any of these should take you to a doctor immediately. *The Family Planning Association has strongly urged smokers not to take the pill.*

41. How to minimize the risk of thromboembolic disease as a result of pill-taking

In some cases, there is no obvious predisposing factor towards thromboembolic disease other than taking the birth control pill. However, other pre-existing conditions can cause a greater chance of these disorders. Follow these suggestions:

a. Stop smoking. Smoking is much worse for your health than pill taking.

b. Do not take the pill if you are over 40 years old.

c. Do not take the pill if you have hypertension.

d. Do not take the pill if you have migraine headaches. (These are associated with disturbance of the blood flow to the brain.)

e. Do not take the pill if you have hyperlipidaemia (high-per-lip-ih-DEEM-ia: increased blood cholesterol and other fats). Many fat people and some thin ones have this trouble; *only a blood test can detect it.* Women over 30 who are on the pill should get blood tests for blood cholesterol and fats. (See p. 251)

f. Use a pill containing 50 mcg or less of oestrogen.

g. Do not take the pill if you have severe varicose veins, any previous history of blood clots, heart attacks, or coronary artery disease.

h. Stop the pill if you are about to have major surgery (any operation which will require recuperation in bed for a long period of time). Don't start the pill again until you are completely recovered. Surgery carries an accompanying risk of clotting trouble, which the pill might aggravate.

42. Liver tumours and related problems

There have been reports of a number of liver tumours, called adenomas, occurring, more often in women on the pill than in other women. (Ref. 5, 7) Although these tumours are usually benign, they have caused serious problems with bleeding into the abdomen. These are fortunately very rare, but are very difficult to diagnose. They seem to occur mainly in women who have been on the pill for longer than five years. All the more reason to take periodic breaks from oral contraception.

In other women, the progestogen in the pill may aggravate pre-existing liver dysfunction. In some women, it may slow the elimination of waste products by the liver, allowing bilirubin (a red bile pigment) to build up, causing jaundice. (When deposited in the skin, in jaundice, bilirubin shows up yellow.) *This change is reversible upon stopping the pill.*

Anyone who has had hepatitis or a recent history of glandular fever should have a test to see that liver function is normal before starting the pill. Alcoholic women or drug-dependent women should not take the pill without liver tests. Idiopathic jaundice of pregnancy is an absolute contra-indication to the pill, for the pill generally causes it to recur.

A related disease is the increase in gallstones among women on the pill (about twice normal). (Ref. 3) The progestogen in the pill may cause decreased excretion of cholesterol from the gall bladder, resulting in stones.

43. Other side effects of the pill: hypertension (high blood pressure), eye problems

a. *Hypertension* (high blood pressure): Several studies show a definite increase in high blood pressure among women taking the pill. (Ref. 8, 9) The effect is more pronounced in older women, and obese women, who *generally* show higher rates of high blood pressure anyway.

To minimize the risk of hypertension while taking the pill, make sure a blood pressure check is done three months after starting the pill and every six months after that. Severe headaches or persistent dizziness at any time may be signs of high blood presure which should be checked.

b. *Eye problems:* Contact-lens wearers have experienced difficulty with the pill because it sometimes causes swelling of the cornea. Other reports suggest that some changes in the retina and optic nerve *may* be caused by the pill; these have not been proved. If any unusual changes in vision or pain in the eyes occur, an examination should be obtained whether the woman is on the pill or not. *Always tell your optician you are taking the pill.*

44. Many medical problems may be aggravated by the pill

The pill affects so many body systems that it should be avoided if at all possible by women who have a disease or a tendency towards a disease.

a. *Diabetes:* The pill decreases the tolerance of some women for carbohydrates—e.g., sugar—making diabetes more difficult to control. Women with severe diabetes have been shown to be at greater risk of coronary thrombosis and should avoid the pill. Those with milder forms of the condition should weigh up the risks of the pill compared with those of accidental pregnancy if using other forms of contraception. Sterilization may well be the best option once the family is complete.

b. *Severe kidney disease* may be aggravated by the pill. The severity must be judged by blood and urine tests.

c. *Heart disease:* If a woman has severe heart disease with shortness of breath and oedema of the ankles, she should avoid the pill. Women with mild or asymptomatic heart disease who feel they must take the pill should only use a low-dose variety. (Ref. 10)

d. *Sydenham's chorea* (usually associated with rheumatic fever) is a nervous disorder affecting the muscles of the face, neck and limbs. It used to be called St Vitus's Dance. It is rare, but may recur when the woman is on the pill. (See p. 368)

e. *Fibroid tumours* (see p. 114): The pill may protect some women against fibroid tumours of the uterus, but *may increase* the growth of fibroids in others. Women who do have fibroids should use low-dose pills and should have an examination every three months to make sure the fibroids are not getting bigger. Women who already have *large* fibroids should *not* use the pill.

f. *Epilepsy* may be more difficult to control in women on the pill. If a woman takes barbiturates, phenytoin or primidone, for treatment of epilepsy, the pill may be rendered less effective: so use a back-up method such as foam. (See No. 50 below)

g. *DES exposure:* There is some early evidence that oral contraceptives may cause changes in the vaginas of women exposed antenatally to DES. (Ref. 11) Because the *original* changes were associated with oestrogens, the pill should be avoided by these women. (See p. 355)

45. Prolonged amenorrhoea and infertility following pill use

About 3 per cent of women who use oral contraceptives experience prolonged cessation (up to two years) of ovulation and menstruation after stopping. This problem is accompanied by a milky discharge from the breasts in one third of the cases. About half the women who develop this problem were not ovulating regularly when they started the pill. For this reason, the pill should not be used by women with irregular cycles (by this we mean women who get their period every two to three months or at wider intervals, not women who vary only slightly in the number of days). The treatment of this problem may be difficult for there is a disturbance in the hypothalamus and pituitary relationship. (See p. 19) If a woman has drainage from the breasts (galactorrhoea) in addition to the loss of periods, she should have studies of prolactin levels (see p. 335) and sometimes skull X-rays, to rule out a coincidental pituitary tumour which might cause similar symptoms in a small number of these patients. (Ref. 12, 13) (See p. 346)

46. The pill and cancer

Probably the biggest worry concerning the pill is as a possible cause or promoter of cancer. (See p. 334 for more extensive discussion of hormones and cancer.) At present, this worry seems to have been justified in regard to the endometrial abnormalities associated with the sequential (variable dose) pills which are not now used. Combined pills and minipills are composed differently from sequentials, however, having a progestogen dominance in most cases. Studies have shown no increase in cervical cancer among women on the pill. (Ref. 14) Watch for more studies on gynaecological cancers.

LOOK AHEAD: The answer on breast cancer will probably not be forthcoming for many years. Initial studies show *lower* rates of *benign* breast disease in pill users: this may be a good sign if these benign diseases are precursors to cancer. However, cancer researchers are generally convinced that female hormones stimulate the growth of pre-existing cancer of the breast (acting as promoters) and strongly urge that women at high risk of breast cancer *not* take the pill. (Ref. 15) There is no hard data on this problem; watch the newspapers for new research; now, you have to judge for yourself and make a decision. Paradoxically, some researchers are using female steroid hormones to treat cancer.

47. The effect of the pill on the foetus

If a woman becomes pregnant while using the pill—usually because she has missed several days without any alternative protection—and then continues taking the pill without knowing she is pregnant, there may be some adverse effect on the foetus. Some studies indicate an increase in limb abnormalities and heart defects among babies whose mothers continued to take the pill before they realized they were pregnant. (Ref. 5)

48. Warning: Wait at least two months after going off the pill before becoming pregnant

Women who become pregnant before two months may have an increased risk of spontaneous abortion, and the foetuses thus aborted sometimes show severe chromosomal abnormalities. (See p. 161) Children born after a woman has stopped the pill have shown no increase in congenital defects. However, an increase in twins has been reported by some researchers.

49. Do not take the pill while breast-feeding

If the pill is started early after a pregnancy, it may inhibit the production of milk. Furthermore, the hormones in the pill can pass into the mother's milk and may have some as yet unknown effect on the child. The ability to become pregnant is naturally diminished during lactation, so another, usually less effective contraceptive method will be very effective now. (See p. 152)

50. Certain drugs may decrease the effectiveness of the pill

In addition to the anti-epilepsy drugs mentioned in No. 44 above, other commonly used drugs *may* decrease the pill's effectiveness. These are phenylbutazone (used for arthritis) and the following antibiotics: ampicillin, neomycin, penicillin V, chloramphenicol, nitrofurantoin and tetracyclin. Isoniazid and rifampicin (used to treat tuberculosis) have been proved to have this effect. (Ref. 16) If the additional drugs are taken for only short periods, use a back-up method such as foam during that cycle. If long-term therapy is needed, check out the advisability of a higher-dose pill or another method or combination of methods.

51. How to evaluate reports on side effects of the pill

A woman must carefully read all published reports in the press and listen to TV discussions of the pros and cons of the method and then make up her own mind. The huge dilemma is that the pill is the most effective and most convenient method of contraception available—but it has the potential for being the most dangerous to the woman's health.

If you are considering stopping the pill, decide on an alternative method of birth control *first*.

Table 2

BRANDS OF PILLS

The following pills were available in the UK in 1981:

Combined pills			Progestogen-only pills (minipills)
Low-dose oestrogen	**Triphasic**	**Medium-dose oestrogen**	
Brevinor	Logynon	Anovlar 21	Femulen
Conova 30	Logynon ED	Demulen 50	Micronor
Eugynon 30	Trinordiol	Eugynon 50	Microval
Microgynon 30		Gynovlar 21	Neogest
Norimin		Minilyn	Norgeston
Ovran 30		Minovlar	Noriday
Ovranette		Minovlar ED	
Ovysmen		Norinyl 1	
		Norinyl 1/28	
		Norlestrin	
		Orlest 21	
		Ortho-Novin 1/50	
		Ovran	
		Ovulen 50	

LONG-ACTING HORMONAL CONTRACEPTIVES

Since 1963, various tests have been conducted with hormonal contraceptives to develop a dosage which would be effective for long periods of time, eliminating the necessity for daily application.

A pill which need be taken only once a month, or a shot which need be given only once in three or six months, is particularly attractive to population planners in underdeveloped countries. In poorer lands, where doctors are so few, and drug supplies and distribution so limited, many families find themselves cut off from medical care for many months by many miles. The side effects of the long-acting contraceptives are often not of prime concern to underdeveloped nations, where deaths from childbearing are so frequent. Research on drugs is now being conducted in many countries. Most long-acting hormonal contraceptives for women are progestogens, for oestrogens are less effective and are associated with major side effects.

52. Depo-Provera, a long-acting progestogen

Depo-Provera is the most widely used of the long-acting hormonal contraceptives. It is over 99 per cent effective. Depo-Provera is an injectable; usually a woman will receive a shot once every three months. The highly sustained doses of Depo-Provera (medroxy-progesterone acetate) block ovulation and in addition change the cervical mucus, thin the endometrium and alter the ability of the Fallopian tubes to move. (Ref. 17)

STOP PRESS: Noristerat (norethisterone oenanthanate) has received a product licence and may be more widely available by 1982 if trials are satisfactory. It is given every eight weeks for three doses, and then every ten weeks. Menstrual cycles are more likely to be regular than on Depo-Provera.

53. Depo-Provera cannot be used for long-term birth control

Depo-Provera is only licensed for use in the United Kingdom as a short-term contraceptive. Doctors may use it for long-term contraception only if the woman has had problems with other methods.

CAUTION: Do not let a doctor persuade you to use this method unless you want to after he or she has explained why it is the method for you.

54. Side effects of Depo-Provera

a. Menstrual disturbances. About a third of women have amenorrhoea (no periods); another third have fairly regular periods (defined by researchers as a cycle length of 18 – 35 days); and the remaining third have completely irregular bleeding. This is usually light, but in a few women may be as heavy as a normal period.

Occasionally women may have amenorrhoea for some time after discontinuing the injection.

b. Mild weight gain, nausea, dysmenorrhoea and decreased libido are minor side effects of Depo-Provera. None of these effects is as pronounced as with some forms of the pill.

c. If Depo-Provera is unwittingly administered during pregnancy it may cause malformations of the fetal heart and limbs.

d. Tests in beagles show that Depo-Provera causes an increase in breast nodules. However, a study in women has shown no increase in breast tumours of any sort. (Ref. 17)

e. Early studies suggested a high risk of carcinoma-in-situ (see p. 352) in Depo-Provera users, but this has not been confirmed by later work.

55. Look ahead: Other sustained-release progestogens for birth control are now being researched

a. Subdermal pellets, implanted under the skin and having an effectiveness against pregnancy of three to five years, are now being tested.

b. Cervical rings which contain time-release progestogen are now being tested. These would be inserted into the vagina like a diaphragm each month after the menstrual period, and left in place until the next period begins.

THE IUD

The IUD (intra-uterine device) is used by about 600,000 women in the UK and many millions throughout the world. It requires little care after insertion and is therefore ideal for use in poorer countries where hospitals and doctors are not readily available. It is cheap.

56. History of the IUD

There are several theories, but little proof about the origins of IUDs. The ancient Greeks are said to have used them, and the Arabs are said to have inserted small stones into the uteruses of their camels to prevent conception during long journeys across the desert.

The forerunners of the modern IUD were cervico-uterine pessaries, first illustrated in the *Lancet* of 1868. They were used for displaced wombs and painful periods. The button-shaped top fitted over the cervix and the stem jutted into the womb. They were made from various materials: gold, silver, wood, ivory and even diamond-studded platinum. But infection proved a serious and frequent side effect. Unexpectedly, women using them were found to conceive less frequently.

The first specifically designed IUD was a ring of silkworm gut and bronze. But it too was associated with infection, and the medical community was so sceptical that it was not widely used. In the 1920s Ernst Graefenberg, a German gynaecologist, developed a silver ring wound round with silkworm gut, and Dr Ota, working in Japan, produced a similar device.

It was not until the population scare of the 1960s that interest in the IUD was revived. Early in 1962, the Population Council convened the first international conference on IUDs in New York. Dr J. Lippes presented a plastic rather than metal loop to the conference. But the addition of copper as a wire or sleeve round a plastic base was found to increase the contraceptive efficacy, and in 1969 copper IUDs were introduced.

Research has now led to hormone-releasing IUDs, in particular IUDs which deliver progestogen at a low and uniform rate.

57. Types of IUD

The Family Planning Association has approved several types of IUDs for use in this country. They should only be inserted by trained medical staff. They are: Lippes Loop, Saf-T-Coil Copper 7, Copper T and Multiload Copper 250. A sixth, Progestasert, is under review for its association with ectopic pregnancies.

58. How the IUD works

The actual mechanism by which the Lippes Loop and the Saf-T-Coil work is still not completely understood. They are made of plastic. They probably create an inflammation (not an infection) in the uterine lining. This local inflammation may destroy the sperm as they pass through the uterus or may inhibit the implantation of the fertilized egg in the uterus. This second theory means that the IUD works by causing repeated abortions before the fertilized egg has implanted. (Ref. 18)

The Copper 7 and Copper T are both made of plastic covered by copper wire. Like the other IUDs, their very presence causes inflammation in the lining of the uterus (endometrium). In addition, the copper wire coating affects the normal metabolism of the endometrium, either killing the sperm or preventing implantation. (Ref. 19) A new mini-Copper 7 may be available soon.

The Multiload Copper 250 is a larger, flatter plastic device. Like the other IUDs it causes inflammation of the endometrium. The copper wire coating affects the normal metabolism of the endometrium, either killing the sperm or preventing implantation. A new mini-Copper 7 may be available soon.

The Multiload Copper 250 is a larger, flatter plastic device. Like the other IUDs it causes inflammation of the endometrium. The copper wire coating affects the normal metabolism of the endometrium, either killing the sperm or preventing implantation.

The Progestasert is a T-shaped plastic device with progesterone in the upright which is released slowly and regularly into the woman's body. Like other IUDs it causes inflammation of the endometrium. In addition, the progesterone works like a minipill (see above), affecting the endometrium and probably the cervical mucus and Fallopian tubes.

59. How effective are IUDs?

All IUDs are 95 to 99 per cent effective. No one of these devices has a better record than any other. For near 100 per cent effectiveness a back-up method such as foam should be used at mid-cycle.

60. How long can the IUD be used?

The plastic IUDs can be used continuously for five years, provided there are no side effects and the device is not rejected and does not fall out. But annual checks are recommended.

The Copper 7, Copper T and Multiload Copper 250 must be replaced every two years, because by that time the copper has become oxidized and disappears, and the safety of the device decreases. However, a recent study suggests that, in practice, they may not need to be changed so frequently. (Ref. 20)

The Progestasert must be changed every year because the progesterone supply runs out.

All IUDs should be removed within six months after menopause.

61. Is there any danger from the copper or the progesterone?

Copper is a naturally occurring element in the body. Women using the Copper 7 and Copper T do not appear to experience any increase in copper levels. The amount of copper released into the body by this device is less than the average intake of copper from food. So there is probably no danger to a woman from the copper itself.

The effects of the progesterone are similar to those of the minipill, except much more localized. Decreased and sometimes irregular menstrual flow is frequently reported. A higher rate of ectopic pregnancy has been found in some studies.

62. When the IUD should be inserted

The IUD should be inserted during a menstrual period or the first week afterwards. It can be inserted immediately after an early abortion. After a late abortion or the delivery of a child it should not be inserted for six to eight weeks. These times should always be respected in order to minimize the risk of perforation of the uterus, which is the most serious complication of IUD insertion.

63. How the IUD is inserted

The IUD must be inserted under antiseptic conditions and only by a doctor or qualified nurse. The cervix and upper vagina are cleansed with an antiseptic solution: sterile instruments and gloves must be used.

Next the cervix is measured with a thin metal instrument called a 'sound' and then dilated with a cervical dilator. The chosen IUD is then loaded into the inserter and pushed out into the opening of the cervix. The inserter and dilator are then removed.

At the time of insertion, a woman should receive instructions in how to feel for the string attached to the IUD that hangs down through the cervix into the vagina (not outside the vagina). She should be able to feel this string if the IUD is properly in place. If she cannot feel the string, or she feels any part of the device besides the string, the insertion should be checked right away.

64. Discomfort during insertion of the IUD

When the IUD is first inserted many women feel severe menstrual cramps. These may start straight away and may last for a few days. In women who have not had a child, pain may come back during the next two or three periods. Take your usual pain-relievers such as soluble aspirin or paracetamol and use a hot-water bottle. In women who have had children, if the pain persists it suggests that the IUD is too large or is being pushed down too low in the uterus.

It is also normal not to feel any discomfort the first time or during subsequent insertions.

65. Routine care of the IUD after insertion

A woman should have an examination six weeks to three months after the IUD has been inserted. The device is more frequently expelled during the first three months if it is expelled at all. Also, during the first few months the woman may not be used to examining herself, so she may miss an expulsion. If you think the device has come out or may be coming out, contact your clinic or doctor. In the meantime use another method of contraception such as the sheath and spermicide.

It is important to make sure you can feel the string, and only the string, two or three times during the first week after insertion, before sexual intercourse and after each menstrual period. Sometimes it is easier to reach the string if you are squatting or sitting on the toilet, or in the bath.

66. Normal side effects after insertion of the IUD

It is perfectly normal not to experience any side effects at all.

There may be sporadic cramps during the first few weeks after the IUD is inserted, and then for two or three days before or during each period.

Some bleeding or spotting between periods may occur during the first two months of use.

The first three periods after insertion may be very heavy and after that heavier than previously.

There may be a mucous discharge the first month or two after insertion. This is normal while the endometrium sets up the inflammation that is the basic birth-control mechanism of the IUD. The discharge is *not* normal if it is foul-smelling and heavy. This could be a sign of infection and should be checked immediately.

67. Satisfaction with IUDs

About 70 per cent of women who have an IUD inserted are still using it a year later. But this means that 30 per cent don't continue with it, so be prepared for possible failure.

The major reasons for discontinuation usually occur during the first year of use. During the first year, about 10 per cent of the IUDs inserted are expelled, but half these women will be able to retain a different shape or size of IUD; about 20 per cent of women using it stop because of pain, bleeding, infection or other problems. Two to five per cent become pregnant, some women not having noticed an expulsion of the IUD.

The skill of the inserter is very important in determining the success of the device, so if you decide to use an IUD, make sure that it is inserted by a gynaecologist or by a doctor or nurse who has done a large number of insertions.

68. Serious side effects of the IUD

    a. Uterine and tubal infections
    b. Increased bleeding
    c. Severe and chronic cramping
    d. Perforation of the uterus

69. Uterine or tubal infections

Uterine or tubal infections from the IUD usually occur in the first few months after insertion and should be treated with antibiotics. The main symptom is a constant, often foul-smelling vaginal discharge, possibly accompanied by fever and pain. If the infection does not improve within a few days, the IUD should be removed and the treatment for the infection continued. Lesser degrees of infection may cause irregular periods which are usually painful.

Women using an IUD are more likely than women using other forms of contraception to develop tubal infections if they catch gonorrhoea.

70. The threat to future fertility after infection

IUDs can heighten the risk of infection, and if an infection goes untreated it can lead to blocked tubes and subsequent infertility. Women with more than one sexual partner are also more likely to become infected and they should therefore avoid using IUDs.

71. Increased bleeding and the risk of anaemia

Women using an IUD lose on average twice as much blood each menstrual period as non-users. This may aggravate an existing anaemic condition and should lead you to seek medical advice if the heavy period is accompanied by general weariness.

Heavier periods are caused by the chronic inflammation in the uterus that makes bleeding start a day or two earlier than usual or by an increase in the amount of prostaglandins released, causing prolonged bleeding and more serious menstrual cramps.

If iron added to your diet does not improve your condition quickly, you should have your IUD removed. Even if it is not causing the condition, it is probably aggravating it. Some women find that switching from the plastic to the copper or progesterone-containing devices helps.

72. Severe and chronic cramping

If the IUD user finds herself suffering from severe or chronic cramps, she should have the device removed. The cramps are probably not a sign of ill health. They may be caused by something as simple as the size or shape being wrong. There are so many other types of birth control available that suffering from cramps with the IUD is simply not necessary.

73. Perforated uterus

In some women, even if the IUD is fitted correctly, and particularly if the uterus is soft (e.g. just after a pregnancy), the

IUD can work its way through the wall of the uterus into the abdominal cavity. This is called perforation and occurs about once in every thousand cases. The symptoms of perforation can be severe one-sided abdominal pain and an inability to feel the strings of the IUD. However, sometimes there are no symptoms and it is not until the woman is pregnant that the perforation is discovered.

74. Length of strings

If the strings of the IUD are too long, they may irritate a man during intercourse. See a doctor, who can cut the strings shorter. If discomfort continues, the device should be removed. Shortly after insertion of the Copper 7 and the Copper T, the strings seem to become longer. Don't worry about this. They can be shortened later. Too-short strings can stub the man during intercourse; in this case the device should be replaced.

75. Lost strings

Usually the string has curled up inside the cervix out of reach and nothing is wrong. Alternatively the IUD has been expelled without your knowing. It may also be a sign of perforation in progress, in which case the menstrual pattern will revert to normal. For whatever reason, an examination is necessary.

76. IUDs lost in the body

If the string is not there, the device must be found. This can be done by X-ray or by ultrasound. Sometimes the IUD can be felt by a thin metal instrument called a sound being passed through the uterus. If not, and the device is not in the uterus, it is in the abdomen and must be removed as soon as possible. Removal is usually achieved by means of a laparoscopy.

77. IUDs and the risk of cancer

It is a common worry that IUDs increase the risk of cancer, but there is no evidence to support this.

78. Warning to diathermy patients

Women using a copper-containing device should not receive diathermy (deep heat treatment for muscle and back problems). The metal in the IUD could become very hot and damage the uterus.

79. Copper allergy

Women who are allergic to copper should not use the copper-containing devices and should mention their condition before any is inserted.

80. Pregnancy when the IUD is present

Some women have died because of septic or infected pregnancies, caused by the IUD being left in position after they became pregnant. The device should be removed immediately the pregnancy is confirmed. If an abortion is chosen, the IUD can be removed at the same time.

81. The Dalkon Shield

The Dalkon Shield is a crab-shaped IUD that was available in this country for a few years. It was withdrawn in 1975 after being associated with numerous cases of infected tubes and septic pregnancies. The Dalkon Shield IUD could remain in place for several years and it is possible that some women still have them inserted. If so, they should check with their doctor or clinic immediately. A Dalkon Shield Association (c/o Anita Bennett, 16B Elvaston Place, London SW7) has recently been set up to help women who have problems after using this device.

82. Ectopic pregnancy

About 10 per cent of the pregnancies that occur when the IUD is in place are ectopic pregnancies, in which the foetus starts to develop in the Fallopian tubes instead of in the uterus. The symptoms are severe abdominal pain and irregular vaginal bleeding. If these occur, see your doctor immediately. He or she can arrange for hospitalization to remove the affected tube and probably also the IUD.

83. When an IUD should not be used

Women with the following conditions or circumstances are advised not to use an IUD device.

a. Women with large fibroid tumours that distort the endometrial cavity.

b. Those with a recent history of venereal or tubal infection or damage should steer clear of the IUD, as it might help to cause a recurrence.

c. Pregnant women must not have the device inserted, otherwise perforation or infection might occur.

d. Those who suffer menstrual cramps and bleeding or who are anaemic might find that the IUD only makes thing worse.

e. Women who have never been pregnant have more problems with the IUD. They can suffer more pain on insertion, higher expulsion rates and heavier bleeding. If you have never had a child or an abortion, but really want an IUD, choose the smaller copper and progesterone-containing devices.

f. Young women who are sexually active with more than one partner should use an alternative method, as the IUD could heighten the risk of infection. This has been shown to be two to five times as high in women using the IUD compared with those using other methods.

DIAPHRAGM (CAP)

The diaphragm is a round rubber dome with a relatively firm edge. It is inserted into the vagina, hooks behind the pubic bone and springs back into shape inside, covering the cervix. It has virtually no serious side effects.

The diaphragm should not be considered a method of birth control in and of itself. It should *always* be combined with a spermicidal cream or jelly. It should be thought of not just as a physical barrier to the sperm, but as a kind of plate which holds in place the medication to kill the sperm.

84. History of the diaphragm

The vulcanization of rubber in 1844 made the development of the diaphragm possible. The first device was developed by Dr. Wilhelm Mensinga, a Dutch anatomy professor, in the 1870s. The Dutch cap or diaphragm is the most commonly used device, but vault, vimule and cervical caps are also available.

The cap was first introduced into Britain in the mid-1880s and until the 1960s, when the pill and the IUD became available, the diaphragm was the most popular method of birth control among women. Now it is regaining popularity as the side effects of IUDs and the pill have become better known.

85. Where to get a cap

It can be prescribed only by a trained doctor or family planning clinic. Spermicidal jelly or cream may be bought at a chemist without prescription, or obtained free from a family planning clinic.

86. How the diaphragm is fitted

The diaphragm must be fitted by a trained doctor or family planning practitioner.

A vaginal examination determines the size required by the individual woman; it should be the largest size that does not give the woman discomfort. A woman should not be aware of the diaphragm within her body. If she can feel it, it is the wrong size. If the diaphragm is too large, it may become painful, especially during the six hours it must be left in place after intercourse. If it is too small, it moves excessively during intercourse—and does not reliably protect the user against pregnancy. Have the size rechecked after a week to make sure the fit is good.

87. A sexually inexperienced woman may find it difficult to have a diaphragm fitted

She may prefer that sheaths be used by the man the first several times she has intercourse. If she uses a diaphragm, then she should have it rechecked for fit several months after she has become sexually active.

88. When should a diaphragm be refitted?
    a. After childbirth or an abortion.
    b. After weight loss or gain (of fourteen pounds or more).
    c. Every six months.

89. It is easy to use a diaphragm correctly

And it *must* be used correctly if it is to give, as it can, excellent protection against pregnancy.

    a. Squeeze the diaphragm into an oblong shape and insert it into the vagina until it hooks behind the pubic bone and snaps in place over the cervix.

Usually the diaphragm is inserted with the dome down; if a woman finds it takes up too much room in the vagina that way, she can insert it with the dome up. For women who have difficulty inserting the diaphragm, inserters are available. These have the additional advantage of not being so messy to use when the diaphragm is covered with spermicide.

    b. Practise inserting the device the first time it is fitted, before leaving the surgery or clinic so that the nurse can check that you know how to insert it properly.

    c. Before inserting the diaphragm, fill it with water or hold it up to the light to check that there are no holes or cracks in it.

    d. Spermicidal cream or jelly must be placed in the centre of the diaphragm on the side which will be closest to the cervix and all around the rim before insertion. *Every time intercourse occurs, a new application of cream, jelly, or foam must be made into the vagina!* The diaphragm should *not* be removed if intercourse has taken place during the previous six hours; rather, it should be left in place and the extra cream, jelly or pessary (see No. 101) inserted.

    e. The diaphragm can be inserted up to three hours before intercourse, but *not longer than that* without adding additional jelly—it can also be inserted immediately before intercourse.

f. The diaphragm must be left in place for six hours or more after intercourse, to give the spermicide time to work.

g. When removing the diaphragm put your index finger over the top edge and separate the diaphragm from the vagina. Wash it with warm water and mild soap, and let it dry. Do not use perfumed soap or talcum powder as these may affect the rubber.

90. Creams and jellies to use with the diaphragm

Most women find creams or jellies easier to use than foam, which makes the diaphragm cumbersome on first insertion. For repeated applications, foam is just as easy as creams and jellies. (See Table 2 below)

Many women use foam *in addition* to the diaphragm and cream, and this makes the method even more effective.

91. Urinary urgency during intercourse with the diaphragm

Some women complain that the diaphragm gives them the feeling that they have to urinate during intercourse. This is because the device is irritating the urethra. You can avoid the feeling by always remembering to empty your bladder before intercourse. If the sensation persists, the size of the diaphragm may be wrong and should be checked. Some women get cystitis (See p. 303) repeatedly with a diaphragm and just have to use another contraceptive method.

92. Difficulty in urinating with the diaphragm in place

Some women find it difficult to urinate or to defaecate with the diaphragm in place. It may help to insert a finger into the vagina and hold the device in place. If a woman finds it continuously difficult to urinate while wearing the diaphragm, the size may be too large; she should have it checked.

93. Many men can feel the diaphragm during intercourse

Some are annoyed by it, or claim it deters sexual drive. If this occurs, have the diaphragm checked for size; neither the man nor the woman should feel irritated by the diaphragm if it fits properly. Sometimes the man's reaction is simply psychological; try and convince him that if you can get used to it, he can too.

94. Psychological blocks about the diaphragm should be overcome

If a woman does not like the idea of the diaphragm, of touching herself repeatedly during insertion, then she should try hard to overcome the feeling. Young girls particularly express this feeling— and they should be told that it will pass in time, that sex without pregnancy is worth the very small cares that must be taken to make the diaphragm effective. The more 'convenient' alternatives, such as the pill, are often preferred by young women for this reason. *They should be aware of all the contra-indications to the pill before choosing it over the side-effect-free diaphragm, or foam and sheaths.*

95. Effectiveness of the diaphragm

If the diaphragm fails to prevent pregnancy, that is almost always because it has not been used properly—usually because the spermicide has not been reapplied properly and in great enough quantity before intercourse or the diaphragm has not been left in place for a full six hours after intercourse.

When used properly, it is estimated that the diaphragm fails 2 – 3 times per 100 woman years. (If a woman used the device for 100 years, she would become pregnant while using it only 2 or 3 times.) (Ref. 21)

If improper use is taken into consideration, the diaphragm is estimated to fail 16 times per 100 woman years. (Ref. 22)

Many women find that the diaphragm slips out of place when the woman is in the superior position during lovemaking. In this case, proper application of the spermicide becomes even more important, or another contraceptive method may be preferable.

96. Watch for news: the collagen sponge diaphragm

The collagen sponge diaphragm is a new type of device now undergoing trials in America. Its advantage is that it is soft and easy to use and is removed only during menstruation. Some of these diaphragms are pre-treated with spermicide, so it may not be necessary to use additional jellies, creams or foam. Watch the newspapers and the media for further news on this innovation.

VAGINAL CHEMICAL CONTRACEPTION
(Foams, Creams and Jellies)

Vaginal chemical contraceptives are often classed with the barrier methods—condom or diaphragm—but act by killing the sperm before they have a chance to meet the egg.

97. History of vaginal chemical contraceptives

For centuries, women have been looking for substances that would turn back or kill the sperm without interfering with intercourse. Egyptian women in the nineteenth century B.C. used plugs of crocodile dung; Indian women used elephant dung. (Ref. 23) In the Middle Ages, rock salt was placed in the vagina—and, in fact, salt is a fairly effective spermicide. In 1885, the first contraceptive suppositories were manufactured from cocoa butter (the medium) and quinine (the active ingredient). Women tried to prevent conception by inserting vaginal sponges soaked with acid substances—for example, citric acid in lemon juice. (Ref. 24)

No one paid much attention to the development of really effective vaginal chemical contraception until use of the diaphragm became widespread. In the 1920s and 1930s, acid and anti-bacterial substances were used in the hope that they would be as effective against sperm as against bacteria.

In the late 1950s, products containing *detergents* were introduced—obviously, not the washing products, but a large number of surface active agents that are very effective spermicides.

98. Contraceptive jellies

The jellies are water-soluble; they tend to become very watery at body temperature. A woman who wants a vaginal lubricant as well as a spermicide may prefer them; for other women, the jellies may be too messy.

99. Contraceptive creams

These are in a water-insoluble base. Some women feel that they tend to be drying or that they do not distribute as well in the vagina as jellies or foam when used without a diaphragm. However, when they are used with a diaphragm—*which is the way they should be used*—they adhere more firmly to the device.

100. Contraceptive foams

The foams are packaged either as tablets or in aerosol cans—the detergent itself is the foaming agent and they come out of the can on the same principle as shaving cream or whipped topping. Sometimes the foam is applied from a syringe.

The advantage of the foams is that they distribute better in the vagina and, without a diaphragm, may have more of a barrier effect for the sperm.

C-film consists of small squares of soluble material which are either inserted into the vagina or stuck to the top of the penis during intercourse. It is less effective than other spermicides.

101. Contraceptive pessaries

A pessary is generally a bullet-shaped wedge which is inserted into the vagina and then dissolves, distributing its active ingredients. This must be inserted at least 10 or 15 minutes before intercourse.

102. Side effects of vaginal chemical contraceptives

So far, no major side effects have been found—and the minor ones occur rarely. These include irritations (*not* infections) either in men or in women. No treatment is usually necessary. Just switch to another product. If chronic irritation persists, see a doctor.

103. How effective are vaginal chemical contraceptives?

When not used with a diaphragm, the chemical contraceptives are not very effective. The foams are probably most effective; failure rates with the foam alone are very low when it is applied carefully before intercourse. Some of the creams are also effective alone with *some* women. RECOMMENDATION: *The best general rule is to use the vaginal chemical contraceptives always in conjunction with a diaphragm, or as an auxiliary method with the IUD or sheath.*

Overall failure rates for foams, jellies and creams when used alone are 10 to 20 per 100 woman years, if the woman always uses the product correctly. The rates of failure taking into account user mistakes are much higher.

104. How to use vaginal chemical contraceptives

a. Women who have just given birth and women who have had many children should use *two applications* of the product rather than one.

b. When using these products with a diaphragm, make sure they are reapplied before each intercourse.

c. Do not remove the contraceptive by bathing for at least six hours after intercourse.

d. Women who are travelling may prefer to use pessaries, which are more compact than foams.

105. Warning: Douching with any substance is not a reliable form of birth control

The sperm pass into the uterus in less than a minute. Thus, no douche can work fast enough to prevent pregnancy. *No woman who is serious about preventing unwanted pregnancy should use this method on its own.*

Table 3

CONTRACEPTIVE PRODUCTS APPROVED BY THE FAMILY PLANNING ASSOCIATION

Barrier Devices
Diaphragms
Durex (flat spring diaphragm
Ortho (coil spring diaphragm)

Caps
Dumas (vault cap)
Prentif Cavity Rim (cervical cap)
Vimule Cap (vimule cap)

Non-Lubricated Sheaths for Use with Spermicide
Durex (teat end, packets of 3)
Durex Allergy (teat end, packets of 3)
Lambutt Latex (teat end, packets of 3)
Lambutt Coral Superfine (teat end, pink, packets of 3)
Transyl (teat & plain end, packets of 12)

Lubricated Sheaths for Use with Spermicide
Atlas (teat end, packets of 12)
Conture (shaped teat end, packets of 3 or 10)
Durex Black Shadow (teat end, black, packets of 3)
Durex Fetherlite (teat end, packets of 3 or 12
Durex Fiesta (teat end, assorted colours, packets of 6)
Durex Gossamer (teat end, packets of 3 or 12)
Durex Nu-Form (plain end, packets of 3)
Durex Nu-Form Extra Safe (teat end, pink, coated with 0.4 g of spermicidal lubricant, packets of 3)
Forget-me-not (teat end, packets of 2 or 10)
Lambutt Ideal (teat end, pink, packets of 3)
Lambutt Safetex (teat end, packets of 3)
Lambutt Tru-shape (shaped teat end, pink, packets of 3)
Tahiti (shaped teat end, various colours, packets of 3 or 10)
Two's Company (teat end with spermicidal pessary, twin packs of 2 or 10 sheaths and pessaries)

Spermicidal Contraceptives
(The FPA recommends that spermicides only be used in conjunction with a barrier method of contraception.)
Foams (supplied in aerosol containers, with or without applicator)
Delfen Foam (Nonoxynol 9, 12.5%, pH 4.5–5.0)
Emko Foam (Benzethonium chloride, 0.2%, Nonoxynol 9, 8%, pH 7.4–7.8)

Creams (supplied in metal tubes)
Duracreme (Nonoxynol 9, 2%, pH 6.0–7.0)
Orthocreme (Ricinoleic acid, sodium lauryl sulphate, Nonoxynol 9, 2%, pH<6.0)
Jellies (supplied in metal tubes)
Duragel (Nonoxynol 9, 2%, pH 6.0–7.0)
Ortho-Gynol Gel (Ricinoleic acid, p-di-isobutyl phenoxy polyethoxy ethanol, 1%, pH 4.5)
Staycept Jelly (Polyoxyethylene octyl phenol, 1%, pH 4.25–4.75)

Pessaries for Use with Sheaths, Diaphragms and Caps
Orthoforms (Nonoxynol 9, 5%, pH 4.0–5.0, packets of 15)
Staycept Pessaries (Nonoxynol 9, 6%, pH 4.25–5.25, containers of 10)
Double Check (Nonoxynol 9, 6%, pH 4.25–5.25, containers of 10)

Pessaries for Use with Sheaths Only (not to be used with diaphragms and caps)
Genexol (Texafor FN11, 0.08 g, fractionated palm kernel oil BP, 1.52 g, pH 5.0–6.0, packets of 12)
Rendells (Nonyl phenol ethylene oxide, 0.08 g, fractionated palm kernel oil BP, 1.52 g, pH 6.0, packets of 12)

POST-COITAL CONTRACEPTION: THE MORNING-AFTER PILLS

106. How the morning-after pill works

Several drugs are effective in preventing pregnancy when taken soon after intercourse. We are not sure how they work. Mainly high-dose oestrogen (plus sometimes progestogen) products, they probably alter the endometrium and movability of the Fallopian tubes. The ratio of oestrogen to progestogen may prevent implantation. These pills must be started within seventy-two hours after intercourse in order to be effective, the earlier the better.

Because of the very high doses of oestrogen needed for this preventive effect, these drugs have a high incidence of side effects such as nausea, vomiting, headache and breast tenderness. Long-term side effects are not yet known. If you have to take them, do so in divided doses, with meals, and have medication on hand to treat nausea. These drugs do not act to bring on a period immediately, and, in fact, the period may be a week late, depending on the time during the cycle that a woman took the pills. A woman who uses this method in an emergency should remember that it only works for one particular incident; she can still become pregnant later in the cycle if she does not use contraception. Recently, a treatment involving two Eugynon-50 pills taken twice daily at 12-hour intervals has been found to be effective. (Ref. 25)

107. Effective post-coital pills
The most widely used post-coital pill treatment is starting ethinyloestradiol (5 mg per day for 5 days) within 36 hours of intercourse. A newer development involves taking two doses of two particular 50-mcg oestrogen pills 12 hours apart within 48 hours of intercourse.

Post-coital progestogens and combined oestrogen/progestogen pills can also be used. Work in South America has shown that taking 100 mcg of levonorgestrol within four hours of intercourse prevents conception in 97 – 100 per cent of women. This may be an alternative method for the older woman who has had sexual intercourse unexpectedly.

108. Insertion of a copper-bearing IUD as a post-coital check on pregnancy
If a copper device is inserted one to five days after intercourse, it is 100 per cent effective against pregnancy. Of course, just as the woman using hormones can anticipate the side effects of a heavy dose of oestrogen, the woman using the device (under circumstances in which she may possibly become pregnant) is risking the side effects of the IUD. (Ref. 26) Once in place, the device will provide ongoing protection, however.

109. Synthetic prostaglandin pessaries
These are being used in Oxford, for very early pregnancy. But the side effects of nausea and vomiting have not been overcome.

VERY EARLY ABORTION

110. Menstrual regulation aspiration or extraction
Menstrual regulation aspiration or extraction is a technique in which a thin plastic tube connected to a syringe is used to suck out the contents of the womb in a conscious woman. It must be done on premises approved for abortions under the 1967 Abortion Act and agreed by two doctors who sign the statutory green form. It is not widely available, but now that pregnancy can be diagnosed before the first missed period by a blood test, it should become a reasonable alternative to later abortion for those women who want it.

ACTION: Women should try to get this service set up in their areas. Menstrual aspiration is half as likely to be followed by bleeding and infection as later abortion and uterine perforation is a tenth as likely.

SHEATHS AND OTHER MALE METHODS OF CONTRACEPTION

The sheath, condom or French letter is an excellent method of contraception. It is relatively cheap, convenient and without side effects. Before the appearance of the pill and IUD, it was widely used by the men in this country. It requires complete participation by the male. Sheaths can be bought over-the-counter or from vending machines, or obtained from a family planning clinic.

Certainly it is vital for the mother of sons to make sure her boys are familiar with sheaths as a primary lesson towards making them sexually responsible people.

111. History of the sheath

The sheath is a pliable casing which fits over the penis and prevents the sperm from entering the vagina. It was originally conceived not as a method of birth control but as a device to prevent venereal disease and other infectious diseases. Primitive people who otherwise wore very little often wore sheaths to protect the man against infectious tropical diseases. In the Middle Ages, workers in slaughter-houses found that animal intestines could be used as sheaths. Fallopio, discoverer of the Fallopian tubes, advised men to wear linen sheaths in a publication of 1564. The most effective proponent of the device, however, was Casanova, the legendary Italian lover of the eighteenth century who used animal-intestine sheaths for his own protection. At this time sheaths were widely sold in brothels to protect customers against the almost certain venereal disease of prostitutes. Since use of the sheath began to decline in the 1960s with the advent of the pill and the IUD, there has been a rise in venereal disease.

112. When to ask a man to use a sheath

a. A woman who is otherwise unprotected against pregnancy should be forthright in asking a man to use a sheath.

b. A woman who may otherwise be protected against pregnancy but who has some doubt about the health of the man she is with should ask him to use a sheath.

113. Sheaths available

Most sheaths are mass-produced of thin latex rubber. Standards for tensile strength and to guard against holes are laid down by the

British Standard Institute. These sheaths will carry a 'kitemark'. Always look for this when buying.

Many shapes, colours and brands are available, lubricated and non-lubricated, coated and textured. Trials will show which best suits you and your partner. There are non-rubber sheaths for those allergic to rubber.

114. Effectiveness of sheaths

The sheath is effective and the Oxford Family Planning Association study showed a failure rate of only 4 per 100 woman years. However, it must be used every time intercourse is attempted and other studies have shown failure rates as high as 15 – 20 per 100 woman years. The use of a spermicide will increase the effectiveness of the method and will provide additional lubrication if needed.

115. Important: There are virtually no side effects from sheaths for men or women

116. The few disadvantages of the sheath are procedural

A man does not have to have an erection to put on a sheath—but many men find it much easier if they do. If this is the case, just putting on the sheath requires an interruption in lovemaking which is very annoying to some people. Sometimes a woman can put it on, which helps. But the sheath must be rolled on to the penis before it becomes hard and before intercourse begins for effective protection. Some couples report that it decreases sexual sensation. Whether this is actual or a psychological reaction is impossible to prove.

117. Sheaths are useful in preventing premature ejaculation

Some men ejaculate too quickly for their own and their partner's satisfaction; this usually is an emotional—sometimes a physical—condition. For such men, sheaths tend to be helpful in maintaining an erection longer. (See p. 98)

118. The pill for men

It is well known that androgens, oestrogens, or progestogens can be used to limit sperm production by the testicles; therefore, it is entirely possible that a hormonal compound pill could be produced for men.

119. Why the development of the male pill is moving slowly; the value of hindsight.

Researchers today have the advantage of hindsight on side effects of the pill. With so many side effects for women, surely there would be as many or more side effects for men. For example, progestogens and oestrogens can cause decreased *libido* (sex drive) and cause breast enlargement; testosterone may cause increased incidence of heart attacks and cancer of the prostate. It has taken the scientific community years to minimize the risk of pill side effects in women, and many women have been adversely affected in the meantime. This in itself is enough to deter a similar outlay of time, money and risk in developing a male pill. There are other factors involved as well:

a. The original pill development was for women because it was assumed that women were more interested in birth control than men (since women had to bear and care for the babies) and that women would therefore be more reliable, conscientious users of the pill. Although many people may reject this assumption, it certainly holds true for most people in the world. Only a very few women can trust men to protect them against pregnancy. Obviously, it is unfair for women to have to bear the whole responsibility in this matter—a woman should insist that the men in her life participate and cooperate.

However, before governments donate huge amounts of money for research in this particular area, they need the assurance that it will be a widely used method, once developed. This may not be the case, especially in developing countries.

b. Finally we must recognize that men control all the funding agencies which might contribute to this research, and may be feeling a bit apprehensive about the whole area of research. (Ref. 27)

120. New methods of male contraception

Even now, male contraceptive methods are not very successful, the main difficulties being loss of libido and the problem of trust on the part of the female partner. Most hope lies in the area of easily reversible sterilization techniques.

At London's King's College, pills containing testosterone and a progestogen which stop sperm production are on trial. Tests on gossypol pills, made from an extract of cotton seeds, are confined to China and are known to have discovered some serious side effects.

A naturally occurring hormone, Inhibin, has just been discovered and is being developed into a pill. Another male pill affects the mature sperm, although there are worries that some sperm may 'escape' and cause abnormal embryos.

Other new techniques include the insertion of a gold tap in the vas, immunization to stop sperm production and the development of dissolvable sheath devices.

121. Other methods of male contraception

a. *Withdrawal* of the penis before ejaculation (coitus interruptus) is probably the oldest and most widely used method of contraception in the world. It is a difficult and distressing method for most couples and should be used only in birth-control emergencies. The man must be able to recognize when he is going to ejaculate and withdraw before that. However, even this is not completely safe, because before ejaculation the lining of the man's urethra contracts along with the vas and seminal vesicles and the contents of the urethra go into the vagina. Sperm are frequently present in these drops of fluid, so pregnancy may result.

Other problems with the method are the fact that intercourse cannot occur again until the man urinates, which may be up to several hours. Also under these circumstances a woman may not achieve orgasm and may thus be short-changed sexually by a method that may leave her pregnant in the end—20 – 30 failures per 100 woman years. Ultimately withdrawal places a great strain on both partners which is unjustified when there are so many other methods of birth control.

b. *Heat and ultrasound to decrease sperm count*

Under some carefully controlled experimental conditions, heat and ultrasound waves applied to the testicles before intercourse have been shown to cause *reversible* decreases in sperm count, thereby decreasing the chance of pregnancy. Whether these methods are applicable to widespread use remains to be proved. (Ref. 28, 29)

RHYTHM OR SAFE PERIOD

The rhythm or 'natural' method of birth control depends on the rhythmic cycles of fertility and sterility within a woman's menstrual cycle, and allows her to protect herself somewhat against unwanted pregnancy by having sexual relations only during her non-fertile period.

Of course, the great difficulty lies in determining exactly *when* the non-fertile period occurs. For this reason, rhythm is not a reliably effective method of preventing pregnancy for large numbers of women.

122. History of the rhythm method

The cyclical nature of fertility has been understood for thousands of years—yet it was understood *wrongly* until 1930.

Soranus of Ephesus, a Greek physician who lived in the second century A.D., suggested that the most fertile days of the cycle were the two days immediately after menstrual bleeding ended. He believed that pregnancy occurred when the sperm implanted itself in the uterus, that menstruation prevented this implantation and that, therefore, the best time for implantation—the most fertile time—was just after menstrual bleeding ended.

The trouble with Soranus's theory was that he simply did not know of the existence of eggs; he thought the sperm did all the work. So as far as he and his cohorts for the next sixteen centuries were concerned, a woman's body produced nothing that was necessary to conception except the locale.

In 1827, the eggs of the female were discovered. However, for a long time scientists believed that menstruation produced ovulation in women as it does in animals, and so continued to say that the most fertile period was immediately after menstruation.

Only in the 1930s was the time of ovulation—the most fertile time—correctly placed at the middle of the menstrual cycle. This new knowledge for the first time made rhythm a viable method of birth control. (Ref. 30)

123. Basic methods of rhythm

There are three basic methods of testing when ovulation occurs and a woman is fertile: the calendar method, the temperature method, and the cervical mucus method. These can be used separately or in combination. Many couples use rhythm in conjunction with mechanical contraception.

124. Why rhythm is not reliably effective

Sperm usually live in the female reproductive tract for at least three and sometimes five or six days. Therefore, people practising rhythm must correctly calculate the time of ovulation so that they can cease having unprotected sexual intercourse *at least three days before ovulation occurs*. Virtually no woman can rely on complete regularity in her menstrual cycle, so any judgement as to when ovulation will occur is fraught with risk. (See p. 17) The calculation is complex and the safe days are relatively few.

125. When rhythm is most effective

a. Rhythm is most effective as birth control among women who are *extremely* regular in their menstrual cycles. Even for them, it is not as effective in preventing pregnancy as other forms of contraception.

b. Rhythm is most effective when used with mechanical birth-control devices, such as diaphragms or sheaths. (Rhythm without a diaphragm is like a diaphragm without spermicide—very, very risky.)

126. The calendar method

With the calendar method of rhythm, a woman must record the dates of six to twelve successive menstrual periods, and from these, calculate the range of possible ovulation days. Then she adds three or four days at each end of the range, and abstains from sexual intercourse during that entire time.

For example:

For one year, a woman has menstrual cycles from twenty-seven to thirty days long, counting from the first day of menstrual bleeding to the next onset of bleeding.

She can calculate, therefore, that ovulation will probably occur on days thirteen, fourteen, fifteen or sixteen of her menstrual cycle. She adds four to each end of the ovulatory period. And she abstains from sexual intercourse (or uses a mechanical method) on days nine to twenty of *each* cycle. (Ovulation is most likely to occur thirteen to fifteen days *before* the next period.)

127. Difficulties with the calendar method

The calendar method becomes unreliable when a woman experiences menstrual irregularity and especially when she experiences a shorter cycle wherein the 'risk days' are more numerous than she had anticipated. *These eventualities are not predictable.*

128. The temperature method

The appearance of progesterone in the second half of the menstrual cycle often causes a slight rise in the basal body temperature of a woman. The temperature method of rhythm works by the woman recording her temperature until she detects the rise (sometimes preceded by a slight drop), at which time her ovulatory period is probably over, and she can return to sexual intercourse shortly thereafter.

A woman takes her temperature each morning while she is still in bed, after five or more hours of sleep. She uses a regular thermometer or a basal body thermometer; she can take her temperature rectally or orally. When progesterone becomes dominant, her temperature will rise between 0.5 and 1.0 degree. She waits for this temperature rise to repeat itself *three days in a row*. Then she can probably safely return to unprotected sexual intercourse.

129. Difficulties with the temperature method

If all other conditions are controlled, the temperature method has a failure rate of only 2 – 6 times per 100 woman years. (Ref. 29) However, body temperature is indicative of so many other factors in a woman's health that the margin for error in ascertaining when the 'safe days' have arrived is relatively great.

a. The temperature method requires that couples abstain from sexual intercourse until *after* ovulation—for roughly the first twenty days of the cycle. This leaves relatively little time for sexual intercourse unless mechanical methods are used as well.

b. Often the rise in temperature is not abrupt and is difficult to detect.

c. Ovulation *can* occasionally occur without a rise in temperature, foiling the method completely.

d. Any external factor—a common cold, a bad night's sleep—can be enough to throw off the temperature method.

130. Combining the calendar and the temperature methods

Since many couples find it difficult to abstain from sexual intercourse during the days of probable risk both before and after ovulation, the temperature and calendar methods may be combined with good effect. The calendar method determines when the earliest possible ovulation can occur, allowing couples some safe days beforehand. The temperature method determines when ovulation is probably over, allowing couples some days afterwards.

131. The cervical mucus method

A more recent proposal for rhythm is the cervical mucus method, which depends on a woman recognizing the changes in her cervical mucus that normally occur during the menstrual cycle. A viscometer has been developed to assist this.

The cervical mucus goes through five phases:

Phase 1: right after menstruation. At this time, there is very little cervical mucus. A woman will find her vagina and cervix rather dry.

Phase 2: prior to ovulation. At this time, a woman will detect a cloudy, white, sticky mucus.

Phase 3: around ovulation. At this time, a woman will notice a feeling of wetness, usually for three or four days.

Phase 4: after ovulation. There will be a decrease in the amount of mucus, and that which is detected will be cloudy and sticky.

Phase 5: before menstruation. At this time, a woman will notice that the cervical mucus is thin, watery and clear.

The unsafe period is roughly from the beginning of Phase 2 through to the first four days of Phase 4. (Ref. 30, 31)

132. Difficulties with the cervical mucus method

a. The entire method is predicated on the woman being able to recognize the changes in her cervical mucus. *But an estimated 30 per cent of women do not have a regular mucus flow,* which means that they cannot detect the changes as they occur.

b. Like body temperature, the cervical mucus is responsive to many outside factors. For example, a minor case of vaginitis can alter the mucus completely, foiling the method. Thus the failure rate is very high—an estimated 25 times in 100 woman years. (Ref. 45)

133. Experiments in rhythm

Other means of predicting the time when ovulation begins have been tried in recent years, *without success.* These including testing for sugar in the saliva and chloride in the cervical mucus by means of specially treated paper strips. Tests are currently being performed on a tampon-like device which is placed in the vagina and which, by a chemical change depending on the state of the cervical mucus, can determine the phase of the cycle.

134. The rhythm method and fetal abnormalities

The assumption that the rhythm method has no side effects has been challenged recently by some highly suggestive evidence that *conceptions occurring when rhythm is used are subject to higher rates of fetal abnormality—miscarriage and mental retardation.*

It is theorized that this may be due to the "overripeness" of the egg. Since failures in the rhythm method often occur at the very end of the ovulatory period, an egg fertilized at this time has been in the tube for a relatively long while. There is no definite proof that this causes higher fetal abnormality rates—but the evidence to that effect is disturbing. (Ref. 30)

135. Experimental methods of birth control for women

Numerous types of new birth control devices are being tested, mainly in Scandinavia and America. Some of these experiments might lead eventually to safe and convenient methods, others will enter the annals of science fiction.

Vaginal rings made from silicon containing slow-release progestogen are currently only effective for a week or two, but there is hope that this can be extended. Vaginal sponges are impregnated with spermicide and are used similarly to a diaphragm. Work is also being carried out on intracervical devices, which contain either hormonal or spermicidal substances.

Tests in Brazil on silastic implants are quite promising. These are plastic rods which contain slow-release hormones and are placed beneath the skin. So far they have been found to be effective for up to six years. Removable silicon plugs, placed in the Fallopian tubes, are an offshoot of Patrick Steptoe's work (see p. 110) and, if successful, mean easily reversible sterilization.

In the United States, immunization techniques are being developed. Two types of vaccine have been tried—one that produces antibodies against human chorionic gonadotropin (HCG), another that produces antibodies to a particular male's sperm. Other injectables are also being tested which avoid the side effects of Depo-Provera.

In Edinburgh, nasal sprays which allow hormones to reach the pituitary quickly are being tried.

Research on more natural methods includes the development of dipsticks which indicate the presence of LH in urine; and ultrasound tests to detect rupturing follicles in the ovary.

VOLUNTARY STERILIZATION

136. Recommendation: Tubal surgery (cutting or clipping) is the most acceptable sterilization procedure for most women

A woman who of her own free will wishes to end her childbearing days through permanent sterilization should consider surgery on her Fallopian tubes. There are several rather simple operations by which the tubes are cut and sealed off so that the sperm and egg do not meet. Other methods such as hysterectomy are now totally unnecessary.

137. History of female sterilization

For almost all of recorded history, a woman who was unable to bear children felt herself cursed. She would never seek sterility therefore, and sterilization was generally something that men mandated for a woman who had no way of resisting.

In the fourth century B.C., the Greek physician Hippocrates, known as the Father of Medicine, recommended sterilization of women to prevent inherited insanity. Some Middle Eastern peoples, eager to protect men from dishonour by women who might sleep with someone not duly authorized, created methods of "temporary" sterilization whereby the lips of the vagina were sewn together, or a ring was placed through the labia. During the Crusades, wives were locked into metal and leather girdles known as "chastity belts". The only key was left with someone more trusted than the wife—or taken off by the husband to the Crusades!

Eventually the world progressed so that sterilization was recognized as a procedure more related to the health of the woman than the honour of the man. The first tubal ligation was performed in 1880 at the same time as a Caesarean section delivery. (Ref. 32) For the next eighty years, tubal ligation was almost always performed immediately postnatally—by doctors who were convinced the woman's health would be endangered by further child-bearing.

138. Voluntary sterilization

Although Dugald Baird in Aberdeen began to sterilize women with five or more children in 1935, it is really only since the 1967 Abortion Act forced gynaecologists to look at the whole problem of fertility control that elective sterilization has become available to women. Free vasectomy did not become available until the mid-1970s.

139. Procedure before sterilization

Initially, you should tell your general practitioner, or family planning clinic that you want a sterilization. You should then receive expert counselling to ensure that you understand the procedures and are not making the decision for the wrong reasons. Both partners should attend the counselling sessions. Although doctors like the consent of your spouse, it is not legally necessary. Once the forms have been signed, you may have to wait several months for an NHS operation in some areas. It can be performed the same day if done privately, so ask your GP what the local situation is like.

140. Make sure you are not pregnant when you go for a tubal sterilization

As the risk of post-operative thrombosis is higher in women on the pill, many doctors ask you to stop taking it four to six weeks before the operation. Make sure you use an alternative method of contraception or abstain.

It is a terrible shock indeed for a woman who thinks she cannot become pregnant to become so after tubal sterilization. So take every possible precaution to guarantee that you are not pregnant at the time of the operation. Have a pregnancy test—*even if you have just completed what appeared to be a normal period.* Some doctors suggest a D & C (dilatation and curettage) be performed at the time of the sterilization to see that any pre-existing pregnancy will be ended. This is a simple operation (see p. 330) that does not add substantially to recovery time.

141. Methods of performing tubal sterilization

There are various methods of entering the abdomen to look at the tubes and to operate on them:

a. Laparotomy
b. Laparoscopy
c. Colpotomy
d. Culdoscopy

142. Laparotomy

Laparotomy means that an incision is made in the abdominal wall and the tubes are *directly* visualized as they are operated on. The size of the scar determines the recovery period needed. If performed immediately after delivery, a very small scar below the navel is all that is needed. If performed when the woman has not recently been pregnant, a larger incision will usually be needed and this will be placed at the top of the pubic hairline.

There is now a procedure called *mini-laparotomy,* which many surgeons are using, which needs only a small incision (one to two inches). For mini-lap, a small tube called a cannula is placed in the uterus so that the tubes can be brought up to the abdominal wall and grasped with a clamp. Then the tubes are tied and cut as with ordinary tubal ligation.

143. Some methods of tying the tubes at laparotomy

Once the belly has been opened, there are various procedures which can be done on the tubes. The most common is the *Pomeroy tubal ligation* in which a loop of the midsection of the tube is elevated, tied and cut. A section is removed and sent to the pathologist to check that the right anatomical structure (and not the round ligament, which looks like the Fallopian tube) has been removed. This is the most easily performed method, and can be done with a very small incision in the belly. Between one woman in

200 and one in 500 have been reported as having become pregnant after this operation.

The Irving method of tubal sterilization involves burying the cut ends of the tube into the tissue around the tube. This method is almost 100 per cent effective but has the disadvantage of needing a larger scar and a longer operating time with general anaestheia.

144. Routine procedures before laparotomy

a. The hospital should perform routine lab tests several days before the surgery. These include blood tests, urinanalysis, and a chest X-ray, if the woman has not had one recently.

b. The woman will be asked not to eat or drink anything eight hours before the operation.

c. The abdomen will be shaved, and then scrubbed in the operating room.

d. A catheter will usually be placed to keep the bladder from interfering with the surgery, but this is removed immediately after the procedure.

145. Routine procedure after laparotomy

The recovery and post-operative pain are directly related to the size of the surgical scar. If performed immediately after delivery, the area is sore but does not require any extra days in the hospital than the usual three to four postnatal. If a laparotomy is performed at any other time, the woman will have to stay one to five days depending on the size of the scar. In some places, the mini-lap is being performed as an out-patient procedure, but this is difficult except on thin women, when a very small incision can be used.

As with all surgical procedures, there are risks of infection in the wound or excess bleeding but these are very minimal in tubal sterilization procedures. The only restricted activity would be on heavy lifting for the first three to four weeks after surgery.

146. Laparoscopy

A laparoscope is an instrument, known for almost seventy years, which allows a physician to see the Fallopian tubes. Until recently, it was used only as a diagnostic instrument to examine the contents of the abdomen in case of disease, and to determine what, if anything, was blocking the tube and preventing conception. (See p. 94) Now it is also being used to extract eggs from women in the very new test-tube fertilization (See p. 110)

As a method of sterilization, laparoscopy is the most popular, for it is fast and relatively easy, requires little recovery time, and leaves only one or two scars which are usually buried in the folds of the navel and lower abdomen (depending on the type of equipment).

A small needle is placed into the abdomen just below the navel. Two to three litres of CO_2 (carbon dioxide) are allowed into the abdomen through this needle, expanding the abdomen. A cut, 1.5 cm long or less, is made under the umbilicus (belly button/navel) and a trocar is inserted into the abdomen. The sharp, triangular inner part of this is removed and the laparoscope passed into the abdomen so that the doctor can see the tubes. Another small instrument is passed into the abdomen, either through the scope itself or through another small incision. The tubes are either cauterized (electrically burnt) for a length of 3–4 millimetres, and the ends sealed shut, or clips are placed over the middle sections of the tubes.

The whole procedure takes less than an hour in the operating room. The woman is left with several stitches in her navel which are removed after the wound has healed, about one week later. Some stitches are absorbed. A general anaesthetic is usual, and this means that a patient will spend a couple of days in hospital recovering. Local anaesthetics, which can be used in day care clinics, are becoming more popular.

147. Procedures before laparoscopy

These are essentially the same as before laparotomy. (See No. 144 above)

148. What to expect after laparoscopy

a. Mild abdominal pain that should not last longer than a day or two.

b. Some shoulder pain, a result of the CO_2 that was injected into the abdomen. It can be fairly severe, but mild analgesics will control it.

c. A woman should be up on her feet the day after the procedure, but should try to take it easy for a day or two.

d. The two or three stitches may cause mild discomfort; they usually dissolve themselves or are removed in about five to seven days.

e. There should be no fever, bleeding or severe pain after the operation. If there is, see a doctor immediately.

f. There will usually be no noticeable scar.

149. Possible complications of laparoscopy

a. Burns of the skin and internal organs, particularly the bladder, stomach, or bowel. New instruments have considerably reduced the risk of this side effect—which occurs in less than 1 per cent of cases.

b. Bleeding from the tube or other organs sometimes occurs during the operation. It usually can be easily controlled, but may require a large incision.

c. Pelvic infection may occur. It is always a risk with any abdominal surgery.

d. The total incidence of major complications (burns, tubal bleeding, pelvic infection) from laparoscopy is 0.7 per cent. (Ref. 33)

e. The failure rate is somewhat higher than with laparotomy, varying from 0.1–2.0 per cent. As more and more doctors are becoming more experienced with the device, the complications and failures will decrease.

f. After tubal sterilization by cautery, there may be an increase in irregular menstrual bleeding. For this reason, tubal clips are becoming more popular.

150. Who should not have laparoscopy?

a. Women with heart or lung disease
b. Women with pelvic infection or scarring
c. Women with hernia from the umbilicus
d. Women with abdominal scars which may limit the pathways of necessary incisions
e. Severely obese women

For women with these contra-indications, one of the other tubal sterilization procedures is preferable.

151. Laparoscopy with tubal clips or rings: an alternative to cautery

Since the most severe adverse side effect of laparoscopy with cauterization of the tubes is accidental burning of the bowel or other pelvic organs, some doctors recommend the use of tubal clips or rings to do the same job as cauterization.

The clips or silicone rings are placed over the mid-section of the tubes, using specially adapted laparoscopy equipment. The process can be done under local anaesthestic in a day clinic.

While the clips are safer than the cautery method, the failure rate is higher, up to three per cent. Early data on the silicone rings (Fallope rings) show a better success rate. (Ref. 33)

There is a higher chance of reversing clipping than cauterization, but if you have reversal in mind you should not be sterilized.

152. Tubal ligation through the vagina: colpotomy and culdoscopy

The Fallopian tubes may be visualized by making an incision in the top of the vagina, between the uterus and the rectum. The tubes can be grasped with instruments and either a Pomeroy procedure or *fimbriectomy* can be performed. A fimbriectomy is the removal of the entire distal end of the tube, including the fimbria (the fringed ends).

Although colpotomy incision is a simple procedure in most cases, bleeding may be heavier and the incidence of infection is higher, since the vagina is a relatively non-sterile place to operate through. In most of the reported studies, severe infection has occurred in between one in a hundred and one in 300 women, and has led to women having the uterus and tubes removed. Prophylactic antibiotics and careful post-operative care should prevent this occurring. Post-operative discomforts are minor—there is no abdominal scar. Intercourse must be avoided for four to six weeks, to give the vagina a chance to heal. (Ref. 34)

A culdoscope is an instrument similar to the laparoscope except that it is inserted, as with a colpotomy incision (see above) into the top of the vagina. The tubes are caught, pulled out through the vagina, tied and cut. The procedure has the same advantages and disadvantages of the vaginal colpotomy.

153. Other methods of tubal sterilization

Various procedures are being tried using a hysteroscope (an instrument for viewing the inner surface of the uterus through the cervix.) These methods involve inserting plugs into the Fallopian tubes or injecting caustic substances which cause the tubes to seal off. These methods are still experimental but, if perfected, would offer simple procedures for out-patient sterilization. Early studies have shown *very* high failure rates. (Ref. 35)

154. Tubal sterilizations are neither 100 per cent effective nor 100 per cent reversible

None of the procedures described above is 100 per cent effective *even if performed correctly*. There are many reports of tubes developing new channels or coming "untied". (For some reason, the risk of this is somewhat greater if sterilization is performed right after a pregnancy—either after delivery or abortion.) However, the vast majority of women who have surgical sterilization will never again become pregnant (98 per cent at least). One should always approach sterilization with that in mind. Failures are most likely to be dangerous ectopic pregnancies in 10–20 per cent of women.

Although some doctors occasionally claim that one or another sterilization procedure is reversible, it is not something that a woman should count on. Sterilization is for good, and although we can never fully anticipate our lives, it should only be sought by women who are mature and completely convinced that they will never want another child and, even if they change their minds at a later date, will be willing to accept the fact of their sterility.

Tubal sterilization does not affect a woman's normal level of hormones, so there should be no loss of sex drive or any other hormone-related reaction.

WARNING: Women sterilized at the time of abortion are the most likely to regret the operation. Do not accept an abortion on condition that you are sterilized at the same time. This is more dangerous, as well as it being the wrong time psychologically. No less than 15 per cent of women who had NHS abortions in 1977 were sterilized at the same time, whereas only two per cent of women who paid for their abortions had this done.

155. Vasectomy: the recommended method of voluntary sterilization for men

In recent years, as men have finally come to see that birth control is their responsibility too, vasectomy (vas-ECK-toe-me) has become increasingly popular. It is a much simpler procedure than any form of tubal sterilization. Although it has been available for many years, it has been passionately resisted because men are generally traumatized about any surgery on the genitals, because most doctors are men, and because women too are very frightened about possible emasculation. As public information has increased, the general fear of all groups has subsided. About 50,000–100,000 vasectomies are now performed each year in the United Kingdom. In other countries, like India, where the population crush is desperate, mass campaigns have been successful.

For a mature man who knows his own mind, who is content that he has brought enough children into the world and wants no more, vasectomy is an ideal form of birth control.

156. The vasectomy procedure

The vas is a muscular tube inside the scrotum that carries the sperm. If it is cut, the sperm count eventually drops to zero, leaving the man sterile. In the vasectomy procedure, the patient comes to an out-patients' or day clinic. The pubic and genital hair is shaved. The genital area is cleansed with an antiseptic solution and local anaesthesia is given. Either one incision is made down the centre of the scrotum or two incisions are made, one on each side. The vas is isolated and clipped, or tied and cauterized. The incisions are small. The patient can walk out an hour later, with little discomfort.

157. Routine care after vasectomy

Normal activities can be resumed a few hours after the procedure, but driving a car or operating machinery should be avoided for 24 hours. Heavy lifting should also be avoided. Some doctors suggest avoiding intercourse for five to ten days afterwards.

158. A man is not immediately sterile after vasectomy

Sperm that are already in the vas are capable of fertilizing the egg for some time after a vasectomy. It may take several months until all the sperm are gone. Therefore at eight and twelve weeks semen samples should be checked for sperm and, if it is still present, again a month later. When two consecutive sperm checks come up negative, then the man is considered sterile, but until this point another method of birth control must be used.

159. Who should not have a vasectomy

The only medical contra-indications to vasectomy are local infection of the genital area or previous scarring that may complicate the incisions and healing. Of course, a young man who may one day want to have some or more children should think very carefully before having this procedure.

160. Complications of vasectomy

Haematoma (he-ma-TOE-ma—blood collecting under the skin) and infection occur in less than 4 per cent of vasectomies; these are the major complications and are unlikely with an experienced doctor working under sterile conditions. Some men develop sperm antibodies after vasectomy and the notion that these would cause everything from thrombophlebitis to arthritis has created considerable hysteria. *There is no scientific evidence at all to substantiate these reports at this time.* (Ref. 36, 37)

161. Will vasectomy affect potency?

No. Vasectomy affects no known male function. Erection and ejaculation occur normally as before—except that there are no sperm in the semen, five-sixths of which is produced in the seminal vesicles close to the penis. Psychological changes may affect potency, however.

162. Vasectomy should not be considered reversible

Although some vasectomies have been reversed and the man rendered fertile again, this is a chancy supposition. *No man having a vasectomy should anticipate that the operation will be reversible.* Like tubal sterilization, vasectomy is for good.

163. Sperm banks

There are some private sperm banks which allow a man to store his sperm before a vasectomy. Should another child be wanted, the sperm is used to artificially inseminate the mother. For patients who have NHS sterilizations voluntarily, no sperm banks are available.

164. Abstinence: an alternative for free people

Because birth control is today so readily available, and so reliable, many women feel they no longer have an excuse to say "no" to sexual intercourse. A woman may sleep with men she neither knows well nor likes much just because saying "no" is unfashionable.

Nothing prevents sexual fulfilment more thoroughly than sex under pressure. *Social pressure is not a valid reason to have sex.* Sex is for individual people, not social trends. It should be an emotional event, not the fulfilment of a social obligation.

So consider abstinence. It keeps you from getting pregnant. But just as important, it can keep you from becoming uninterested in sex; it can keep you free.

Table 4
ORAL CONTRACEPTIVES
APPROVED BY THE FAMILY PLANNING ASSOCIATION

	Oestrogen	Progestogen
Low oestrogen dose preparations		
Microgynon 30	0.03 mg ethinyloestradiol	0.15 mg levonorgestrel
Ovranette	0.03 mg ethinyloestradiol	0.15 mg levonorgestrel
Eugynon 30	0.03 mg ethinyloestradiol	0.25 mg levonorgestrel
Ovran 30	0.03 mg ethinyloestradiol	0.25 mg levonorgestrel
Conova 30	0.03 mg ethinyloestradiol	2.00 mg ethynodiol diacetate
Brevinor	0.035 mg ethinyloestradiol	0.50 mg norethisterone
Ovysmen	0.035 mg ethinyloestradiol	0.50 mg norethisterone
Norimin	0.035 mg ethinyloestradiol	1.00 mg norethisterone

	Oestrogen	**Progestrogen**

Tri-phasic low oestrogen, low progestogen combination

	ethinyloestradiol	levonorgestrel
Logynon	0.03/0.04/0.03 mg	0.05/0.075/0.125 mg
Trinordiol	0.03/0.04/0.03 mg	0.05/0.075/0.125 mg
Logynon ED	0.03/0.04/0.03 mg	0.05/0.075/0.125 mg

Medium oestrogen dose preparations

Demulen 50	0.05 mg ethinyloestradiol	0.50 ethynodiol diacetate
Ovulen 50	0.05 mg ethinyloestradiol	1.00 mg ethynodiol diacetate
Eugynon 50	0.05 mg ethinyloestradiol	0.50 mg DL-norgestrel
Ovran	0.05 mg ethinyloestradiol	0.50 mg DL-norgestrel
Minilyn	0.05 mg ethinyloestradiol	2.5 mg lynestrenol
Orlest 21	0.05 mg ethinyloestradiol	1.00 mg norethisterone acetate
Minovlar	0.05 mg ethinyloestradiol	1.00 mg norethisterone acetate
Minovlar ED	0.05 mg ethinyloestradiol	1.00 mg norethisterone acetate
Norlestrin	0.05 mg ethinyloestradiol	2.50 mg norethisterone acetate
Gynovlar 21	0.05 mg ethinyloestradiol	3.00 mg norethisterone acetate
Anovlar 21	0.05 mg ethinyloestradiol	4.00 mg norethisterone acetate
Ortho-Novin 1/50	0.05 mg mestranol	1.00 mg norethisterone
Norinyl 1	0.05 mg mestranol	1.00 mg norethisterone
Norinyl 1/28	0.05 mg mestranol	1.00 mg norethisterone

Progestogen-only oral contraceptives

Norgeston	0.03 mg levonorgestrel
Microval	0.03 mg levonorgestrel
Neogest	0.075 mg DL-norgestrel
Micronor	0.35 mg norethisterone
Noriday	0.35 mg norethisterone
Femulen	0.5 mg ethynodiol acetate

4

INFERTILITY

It takes two to be fertile. Whether or not a couple can have a child is an abstract concern before a child is wanted. If they are healthy, they usually assume that they are fertile, and spend early years of sexual activity trying to *control* fertility—trying *not* to become mothers and fathers.

But when two people want a child, their concern is no longer abstract but deeply personal. They become—for some of the rarest moments in life—completely committed to each other: to each other's health, each other's ancestors, each other's continuation. If people with that kind of commitment are unable to have a child together, they face an emotional, a historical, crisis that can break the strongest heart and shake the strongest relationship.

About one in ten couples who want children face difficulty in having them. At one time, little help was available. If investigations into the woman's fertility provided no answers, the matter was often dropped. Today, since it has been recognized that men are equally responsible for the fertility of a couple, the possible causes—and possible cures—for infertility have more than doubled. The infertile couple can try many possible solutions before abandoning hope of having children naturally. And even after infertility has proved an insurmountable problem, there are solutions—from the adoption agencies and artificial insemination, for example—that can still give some couples, who want them so desperately, the joys and agonies of parenthood.

While a single woman is treated as a married woman as far as fertility is concerned, if the woman does not have a steady partner or is a lesbian, it may be difficult to find a gynaecologist who is sympathetic to her dilemma. Keep looking.

1. Why are women infertile?
Because of:
a. Hormonal imbalance and menstrual irregularity
b. Ovarian abnormality, or corpus luteum abnormality
c. Tubal abnormality
d. Uterine abnormality
e. Cervical mucus abnormality
f. Habitual abortion

2. Why are men infertile?
Because of:
a. Low sperm production, which can be caused by:
   1. Hormonal imbalance
   2. Genital abnormalities
   3. Autoimmunity (antisperm antibodies)
b. Block in the transport of sperm from the testicles to the vagina.
c. Sexual dysfunction—impotence or premature ejaculation.

3. Why are couples infertile?
In about 85 per cent of all cases, the problem of infertility can be traced to one of the partners. However, several causes of infertility affect *couples,* and such problems are especially hard to solve because generally they pertain to the *immunology of conception,* about which little is known at present. Somehow, the woman's body rejects the sperm, most often at one of three critical junctures:
a. If the cervical mucus and the sperm are not compatible.
b. If capacitation (see No. 18) does not occur properly as the sperm pass through the uterus.
c. If incompatibility occurs during the actual fertilization process in the tubes.

In all of these processes, the *compatibility* of the two partners is absolutely essential to fertility.

In one in ten cases, no reason is found for infertility.

CAUSES OF INFERTILITY IN WOMEN

4. Hormonal imbalance as a cause of infertility in women
Any hitch in the menstrual cycle may be enough to prevent fertility. (See p.16)

If the hypothalamus does not produce the releasing factors for follicle-stimulating hormone or luteinizing hormone, then the pituitary is not stimulated to release them. Too much or too little oestrogen or progestogen production can alter fertility as well.

Since the menstrual cycle is very sensitive to problems affecting the woman's general health, anything affecting general health can affect fertility. For example, a serious illness and a high fever can alter the cycle; when the illness is cured, the cycle may return to normal and fertility be restored. A severe psychological shock may alter the cycle and cause infertility; when the trauma is ended, fertility may be restored.

Another cause of irregularity may be an abnormally high level of prolactin (see p. 335). Women with this condition may have no periods at all and may notice a secretion of breast milk. About a third of such women have small pituitary tumours.

5. Ovarian abnormality as a cause of infertility

If a woman cannot ovulate, she cannot become pregnant. Therefore, any disease of the ovary which prevents ovulation causes infertility.

a. *Congenital abnormalities,* in which a woman is born without ovaries or with malformed ovaries, prevent fertility absolutely. Most of these causes will be detected before or at puberty. An example is Turner's Syndrome, in which a girl is born without one X chromosome, which is essential for complete female development. (See p. 26)

b. *Polycystic ovaries* is a more common condition in which the ovaries develop a thick coating that prevents ovulation. Many small follicle cysts develop, and the ovaries enlarge. The syndrome may be related to an imbalance between the hormones from the ovaries and those from the adrenal gland, or it may be caused by abnormality in the hypothalamus.

Women suffering from infertility due to polycystic ovaries frequently begin to ovulate in response to Clomid or as a result of surgery in which a wedge of ovary is removed. (See Nos. 37 and 40 below)

c. *Infections of the ovaries* by gonorrhoea or mumps can cause infertility. (See pp. 97, 299)

d. *Premature menopause* (See p. 21)

6. Abnormality of the corpus luteum as a cause of infertility

In some women, the second half of the menstrual cycle (from ovulation to menstruation) is abnormally short, because the glandular tissue in the ovary known as the corpus luteum (see p.114) begins to degenerate after four to five days rather than after the normal fourteen days. This is called luteal insufficiency. The normal amounts of progesterone and oestrogen are not produced, leaving the endometrium inadequately prepared for implantation of the fertilized egg. Luteal insufficiency can also cause recurrent abortion (see No. 10 below), but it is very rare.

Progesterone therapy is a frequently suggested treatment which may possibly help—but it has its limitations. (See No. 38 below)

7. Tubal abnormality as a cause of infertility in women

After ovulation, the egg must be picked up by the fimbriated (or fringed) end of the Fallopian tube. Then the egg must move freely along the tube to the ampulla, a wider portion of the tube which is lined with secretory cells. It is here that fertilization of the egg by the sperm takes place. After fertilization, the fertilized egg must move down the tube at just the proper speed to arrive in the uterus at the right time for implantation.

The Fallopian tube is a muscular organ; the power the muscles have to move spontaneously is known as motility. Scarring or blockage will prevent the muscle from moving spontaneously, carrying the egg to the womb. *The motility of the tube is crucial to fertility.* Similarly, any scarring or blockage of the fimbriated end of the tube which prevents the egg from being picked up in the first place can cause infertility.

Abnormalities in the tubes can be caused by:

a. *Pelvic infection* that blocks or scars the tube, usually caused by gonorrhoea, non-specific genital infection or by infection after abortion or delivery. *A ruptured appendix* may also cause damage to the pelvic organs if pus is discharged into the pelvic area. (See pp. 60, 301)

b. *Endometriosis*, a condition in which some endometrial tissue gets out into the pelvic cavity (see p. 331), is associated with infertility, probably because tubal motility is disturbed.

c. *Adhesions* (bands of connective tissue) can form after inflammation or local tissue reaction, which then hold down the Fallopian tubes, so not allowing free movement.

8. Uterine abnormality as a cause of infertility among women

Once fertilization occurs, and the fertilized egg (conceptus—con-SEPP-tus) is released into the uterus, the uterus must be in good enough shape to receive it for implantation. If something has gone wrong in the hormonal cycle, if the egg arrives too soon or too late, if the lining of the uterus is not ready for implantation, or a physiological defect in the lining of the uterus makes implantation impossible, the conceptus will not take hold and infertility may result.

For example, scarring from previous disease or injury that makes the endometrium rough or alters the even blood supply to it can prevent implantation.

a. An infection or inflammation, for example from venereal disease or tuberculosis, can prevent implantation, causing infertility.

b. Fibroids may distort the shape of the uterine cavity so that implantation is difficult. Malformation, such as a double uterus or a uterus with a septum, can have the same effect. (These abnormalities are more likely to cause habitual abortion, usually in the mid-trimester of pregnancy.) (See No. 10 below)

9. Abnormality of the cervical mucus as a cause of infertility

The sperm cannot penetrate the cervix unless there is enough cervical mucus at a proper thinness, with a welcoming chemical balance.

a. Infection or inflammation of the cervix can cause the mucus to be filled with white blood cells that keep the sperm out, causing infertility.

b. Hormonal imbalance may leave the cervical mucus too thick for the sperm to penetrate, causing infertility.

c. Sometimes the cervical mucus is the site of an immunological reaction between individuals that prevents fertility. This is an interaction between the partners. (See No. 3 above, and Nos. 17 and 46 below)

10. Habitual abortion as a cause of infertility in women

In this rather special form of infertility, the woman has no difficulty in conceiving but repeatedly (more than twice) loses the pregnancy. There are several possible causes:

a. Genetic abnormality of the fetus (if this is suspected, both partners should be evaluated genetically. (See Chapter Seven)

b. Medical problems of the mother, such as thyroid disease or severe heart disease

c. An abnormality of the uterus, such as fibroids or a deformed cavity with a septum (usually causing late abortions)

d. Corpus luteum insufficiency

e. Exposure to environmental pollution. The following substances have been shown to increase the rates of miscarriage if women are exposed in early pregnancy: fumes from heavy metals such as lead or mercury, hydrocarbons such as polychlorinated biphenyls (PCBs), anaesthetics such as halothane and methoxyfluorane and high doses of X-rays. If a woman works in a plant or in an operating room she should avoid exposure to such substances.

f. Infections such as mycoplasma and toxoplasmosis. These infections can now be detected in a culture taken from the cervix, or by blood tests. (See p. 293)

g. Incompetent cervix, when the cervix is unable to hold the developing fetus.

About 80 per cent of women who have suffered from habitual abortion eventually have normal pregnancies.

CAUSES OF INFERTILITY IN MEN

11. Abnormal sperm production due to hormonal imbalance

Hormone production in men is controlled by the hypothalamus and pituitary just as in women—but it is a more constant, non-cyclical process. Millions of sperm are produced each day. Follicle-stimulating hormone (FSH) and luteinizing hormone (LH) must be present together, all the time, for adequate sperm production to occur. Diseases of the hypothalamus or pituitary, such as brain tumours, can block production of FSH and LH, causing the testicles to atrophy and become incapable of producing sperm, thus leading to infertility.

12. Abnormalities of the testicles causing low sperm production and infertility

a. Some men have congenital absence or deformity of the testicles which renders them infertile. As with Turner's Syndrome in women (See No. 5a above), such a condition is usually noticed early in life and is usually accompanied by other deficiencies in masculine development. Hormone treatments can normalize the man's life—but infertility will probably persist.

b. Undescended testicles: Sometimes, a testicle will not grow in the scrotum but will remain up in the abdominal cavity. This condition, usually detected in young boys, can be corrected by surgery.

Unless the testicle is moved into the scrotum, it will not produce sperm. This is because the testicles in the scrotum have a slightly lower temperature than the rest of the body.

13. Body temperature is critical to sperm production

Conditions which elevate the temperature of the environment in which sperm are produced will inhibit sperm production and may lead to infertility. Men with varicosities in the spermatic vein may have a low sperm count because of the increased blood flow and increased heat to the testicles. This condition can often be corrected by surgery, rendering the man more fertile. For the same reason, men who wear jock-straps or tight jeans a lot tend to show lower sperm counts than those who don't. (In fact, some researchers have suggested applying heat to the scrotal area as a means of birth control.) (See p. 75) Prolonged sauna bathing may have the same effect.

14. Other causes of decreased sperm count

a. Certain infections—*mumps* is a prime example—can render a man permanently sterile by stopping sperm production. Mumps causes sterility only when it infects the testicles. Other acute infections, such as gonorrhoea, can cause temporary sterility.

b. Various medications—*corticosteroids* particularly—may inhibit sperm production.

c. Exposure to some industrial chemicals—notably those used in some pesticides—can cause decreased sperm count. For this reason, pesticide manufacturers might suggest that only older people who have completed their families should work with these chemicals.

d. Excessive use of drugs, such as marijuana, nicotine or alcohol can lower sperm count.

e. Sperm production usually decreases with age—but this is by no means a reliable event. It depends on individual make-up, and should never be assumed in decisions about birth control.

f. Some men have an autoimmune reaction to their own sperm. Antisperm antibodies circulate in their blood, preventing the production of strong sperm in sufficient quantities for fertility.

Frequently, men suffering from sperm autoimmunity have had previous infection or obstruction of the vas deferens (see No. 15 below), which caused the sperm to leak into the tissue around the genitals and set up an immune response in the blood stream. Since research into the immunology of conception is only now coming into its own, this remains the most baffling source of male infertility. Every breakthrough in such far-flung fields as organ transplants and the immunological reactions that accompany them brings us closer to a solution to the autoimmunity problem.

15. Abnormality in transport of the sperm from testicles to the woman's vagina as a cause of infertility.

Sperm have to travel a long way from the site of production in the testicles to the ejaculation through the man's urethra; any obstruction along the path can cause infertility.

After production in the testicles, mature sperm are stored in the *epididymis* (ep-ih-DID-dee-mis), eighteen feet of coiled tube, which must be navigated by the sperm before they reach the vas deferens. This is the tube which leads from the epididymis to the area of the prostate. It is the tube which is sealed off in a vasectomy. (See p. 87) In the area of the prostate, the sperm are mixed with the fluid of this gland and the other sex organs, and this entire mixture of sperm and fluids is ejaculated through the man's urethra into the vagina. Any blockage in any of these sites, or any lack in quantity of fluid to carry the sperm out during ejaculation, can cause infertility.

Inflammations or infections are most frequent causes of blockage; scar tissue from previous disease can alter the motility of the sperm passages in much the same way as it can alter the motility of the Fallopian tube through which the egg must pass. (See No. 7 above)

16. Abnormalities in sexual function as a cause of infertility in men

a. *Impotence,* the inability to have an erection and ejaculation, will, of course, render a man infertile even if sperm production is normal. Other men who suffer from low testosterone (male hormone) production are impotent and sterile as well.

b. *Premature ejaculation* (ejaculation before entering the vagina) may be a cause of infertility if no sperm ever get to the vagina. Other men with neurological damage suffer from *retrograde ejaculation* in which the sperm and seminal fluid are ejaculated into their bladder rather than into the vagina. This also renders them infertile. (See p. 73)

c. Sperm should be deposited *high* in the vagina for fertilization. Anything which prevents this—for example, injuries that make it hard for a couple to position themselves during intercourse—can cause infertility. For example, if a man's penis is abnormal in structure (*hypospadias*) and the hole that is usually at the tip is in an abnormal position, sperm is often deposited in the wrong part of the vagina so that an insufficient amount of sperm is delivered which cannot reach the cervix.

CAUSES OF INFERTILITY IN COUPLES

17. Immunological reaction of woman to man's sperm as a cause of infertility

Some women, for unknown reasons, develop antisperm antibodies to their partner's sperm. These can be detected in the blood stream and are also secreted into the cervical mucus. At the level of the cervix, these antibodies may act to block the passage of the sperm into the uterus. The post-coital test screens for this problem. (See No. 26 below)

18. Problems with capacitation and fertilization as causes of infertility

There is a theory, which has gained support in the United States, that once the sperm gets through the cervical mucus it is altered in some manner not completely understood by substances in the endometrium and by tubal secretions. This alteration is known as *capacitation* and must occur if the sperm is to be able to penetrate the coat of the egg and fertilize it.

Although the exact mechanism of capacitation and fertilization remains mysterious, abnormalities in these functions may cause infertility among couples in which no other cause seems pertinent. Immunological interactions, for example, may have a role in blocking the processes.

FERTILITY TESTING

19. The fertility investigation

There is now a series of tests for men and women which can determine the cause of the infertility and lead to measures to overcome it. *It is very important not to expect miracles from a fertility investigation.* Too little is known about some of the causes of infertility—especially the immunological causes—to provide clear answers for all couples.

One thing is certain: fertility investigation is worthwhile. In two out of three couples who undergo it, the investigation provides an answer—and even if the answer is that there is no hope for the particular couple to have a child naturally together, it is an answer, an end to worry and conjecture and the beginning of a new plan of action that can lead to parenthood.

20. When to seek investigation

When you have tried unprotected intercourse, at least two times weekly, for at least a year without a resulting pregnancy, explain the problem to your GP, who will refer you to an infertility clinic. Other couples should seek evaluation earlier. This would include couples who are over age 35 and couples who know that they have a problem which would make infertility very likely, such as very irregular or no menstrual periods or low sperm count.

21. Preliminary questions

a. Complete family and medical histories should be taken on both partners. Questions which must be answered include: Are there others in either of your families with similar infertility problems? Have either of you had children with other people before? Do either of you have any past or present medical problems?

b. The pattern of sexual activity between you must be determined. You will be asked how often you have sexual intercourse, what position you assume most frequently (the woman inferior position is usually suggested to couples having difficulty conceiving). You will get some advice on how to improve chances of conception, for example that the woman should remain in bed twenty to thirty minutes after intercourse; that she should not use lubricating jelly, and should not take a bath or shower after intercourse; that the couple should watch the calendar and determine by the woman's menstrual cycle which are her most fertile days (see p. 20) and the couple should attempt to have intercourse at least every other day from days ten to twenty of a twenty-eight-day cycle.

Try to attend these preliminary interviews together; it will save you and your doctor a lot of time. Men are often shy about discussing these matters; they may feel threatened by the possibility that the infertility is their problem. It may therefore be no easy task to get your man to cooperate with the investigation from the beginning. Don't give up; if he is the man you want for the father of your children, then it's a worthwhile struggle.

FERTILITY INVESTIGATION IN WOMEN

22. Basic tests for infertility in women

These include:

a. A pelvic examination with cervical smear and tests for venereal disease

b. Basal body temperature testing

c. Endometrial biopsy

d. Postcoital test

e. Hysterosalpingogram

f. Laparoscopy and dye test

g. Tubal insufflation

23. Pelvic examination with cervical smear and tests for venereal disease

A pelvic examination may suggest a number of simple physiological reasons for infertility which must be ruled out before further tests are done; the same goes for the cervical smear to rule out cancer of the cervix, and tests for venereal disease, which may prevent conception. If vaginitis or cervicitis are present, these should be treated, for they likewise may decrease fertility. (See p. 287)

24. Basal body temperature testing

The first step is to see if you are ovulating. The best way to test for this is by taking basal body temperature.

Every day before getting up, you should take your temperature and record it. If you are ovulating your temperature will rise in the second half of the cycle. (See p. 114) If the second half of the cycle is shorter than normal (six to eight days instead of fourteen, for example), then insufficiency of the corpus luteum must be suspected as a cause of infertility. (See No. 6 above) Do this test for several months before seeing the doctor. It will save time.

25. Endometrial biopsy

In this test a small scraping is taken from the lining of the uterus during the second half of the cycle. The procedure is performed in the clinic, takes only a short amount of time and involves some cramping pain, not usually severe. The tissue sample is then sent to the pathologist, who can tell several things upon examining it:

a. Whether the woman has ovulated during that cycle;

b. Whether the endometrium has developed to the point it should have for that day in the cycle. After ovulation, there is a day-by-day change in the endometrium, and if the changes have not occurred in orderly progression, something is probably awry in the development and degeneration of the corpus luteum, indicating a hitch in the hormonal cycle. If the endometrium is out of phase with the cycle, the test will often be repeated during another menstrual cycle—to verify the suspected hormonal imbalance.

c. Whether infection or inflammation is present in the endometrium, preventing successful implantation of the fertilized egg. White blood cells are signs of infection; they will be seen by the pathologist from the biopsy. If infection is detected, the woman can receive antibiotics or other drugs to cure the infection or inflammation and restore the endometrium to a healthy state in which implantation is possible.

26. Post-coital test for couples

If a woman is ovulating normally, another cause of infertility may be abnormal cervical mucus or incompatibility of the man's sperm with the mucus.

The couple is asked to have intercourse at mid-cycle; the woman comes to the clinic for an examination two to six hours afterwards. At this time some cervical mucus is extracted and examined under the microscope. If the cervical mucus is not thin and stringy, if it is too thick for the sperm to penetrate—that may be causing infertility. Or it may just be the wrong day of the cycle. The number of motile (moving) sperm will also show up on the test. Too few indicates a problem in sperm production, or infection or immunological reaction that has made the cervical mucus hostile to the sperm. *This test may be repeated several times to get an accurate evaluation.* It is painless.

27. Hysterosalpingogram (HISS-ter-o-sal-pin-go-gram)

This is an X-ray of the uterus and the tubes. A special thick liquid is injected into the cervix which outlines the uterine cavity and the tubes in the X-ray picture. A woman may feel some discomfort in the lower abdomen while the liquid is being injected. Sometimes it contains iodine, and you will be asked about iodine allergy first.

Hysterosalpingography shows several things immediately. Are the tubes open? Are they normal? Is the uterine cavity outline triangular and smooth? Fibroids or anything else distorting the shape or surface of the uterus will show up on the X-ray; so will any blockage or scarring of the tubes.

The hysterosalpingogram is usually performed in a hospital X-ray department. Afterwards, a pad will have to be worn to keep the liquid from staining your clothes. This procedure should be done early in the cycle to avoid the possibility that the woman may already be pregnant.

28. Laparoscopy and dye test

Laparoscopy (lap-ar-OSS-copy) is a surgical procedure by which the tubes and uterus are visualized directly through a telescopic instrument. (See p. 83) Some doctors believe that they get more information from this procedure and do not do hystero-salpingo-grams. Others perform laparoscopy if there is an abnormality noted in the tubes on the X-ray study.

The procedure has two parts. The laparoscope is inserted into the abdomen and the tubes are observed for any abnormalities. After a general anaesthetic, the abdomen is expanded with carbon dioxide gas and the laparoscope is inserted through the abdominal wall just under the belly button. At the same time another surgeon injects a coloured dye through the cervix into the uterus and tubes in the same way as for hysterosalpingography. The surgeon using the laparoscope can see directly whether the dye is coming out of the tubes in a normal way. The blockage, if there is one, can be identified; endometriosis can be identified; and pelvic scarring or other pelvic pathology can be identified. Surgery may be performed at the same time or at a later date, depending on what condition appears.

29. Insufflation

Insufflation is a process by which carbon dioxide gas is allowed into the abdomen through the cervix and the pressure needed for passage of the gas recorded on an attached electronic device. For years before the hysterosalpingogram and laparoscopy were available, this test was used to see if the tubes were blocked.

It still is used occasionally. If the tubes are blocked, the gas cannot get through; the machine registers a low gas intake and high pressure; the woman feels only mild cramping. If the tubes are open, she will experience fairly severe shoulder pain due to passage of the gas upward in her body. Although this test tells whether the tubes are open, it does not detect scarring and adhesions which might be interfering with fertility.

FERTILITY INVESTIGATION OF MEN

30. Basic tests for infertility in men
These include:
   a. Semen analysis
   b. Testicular biopsy
   c. Urological examination

31. Semen analysis
Semen analysis is an absolutely essential test to determine if low sperm production or other abnormality is responsible for the infertility of the couple.

Usually, the man is asked to masturbate and ejaculate into a clean jar which has been kept at room temperature. For couples whose religion prohibits masturbation, *coitus interruptus* may be the only way. Under no circumstances should the man submit for testing semen ejaculated into a normal sheath for these contain material which immobilizes sperm and will render the test inaccurate. The man is asked to avoid ejaculation two to three days before the test; he brings the semen to the lab immediately, no later than one to two hours after ejaculation.

The test can tell several things:

a. The total sperm count per cubic centimetre of semen.

b. Whether enough of the sperm are motile.

c. Whether the sperm are the right size and shape. If the test shows any abnormality in sperm production, motion or character, the man will probably be tested again to verify a diagnosis.

d. Whether the volume is normal (both too much and too little fluid may cause infertility) and whether the viscosity (stickiness) is normal.

32. Testicular biopsy

This is a simple procedure, done under local anaesthetic, and is indicated if semen analysis has revealed that the sperm count is low or nil or if the sperm are abnormal.

33. Urological examination

A complete urological examination, to determine if any disease or abnormality is causing infertility, is routine in America and should be more widely done here. It is comparable to the pelvic examination of the woman—*and every bit as important.*

34. Other tests for infertility in couples

If tests on the individual man and woman show no clear reason for infertility, then other tests should be done. These include blood tests for diabetes and thyroid problems, and X-ray of the pituitary gland if there is a hormonal imbalance. If hormonal abnormalities are suspected in either partner, more specific tests on blood and urine can be done for oestrogen, androgen and progesterone.

35. The psychological aspects of infertility

If your doctor, having tested you and your partner completely, says your problem is psychological, react with healthy disbelief. Few doctors would dare to give this as the only diagnosis today; too much is suspected, and too little actually known, about the interchange of endocrine function and mental state. It is far wiser to believe that the source of your infertility as a couple is still beyond the ken of medical understanding and hope that, as with so many conditions, your kind of infertility will be soluble for couples in the not-too-distant future.

The most pressing psychological aspect of infertility is not as cause but rather as effect. Testing, surgery, drugs, endless visits to doctors who have no answers, all this can wear a person down emotionally so that the search for fertility actually becomes counter-productive.

Men are particularly sensitive to fertility testing; often, they confuse fertility with sexual health, and the testing is so distressing to them that it just isn't worth the trouble.

If you find yourself and/or your partner growing hysterical over childlessness, if the tests are beginning to make you anxious and depressed, seek counselling.

Many couples try private treatment after NHS investigation has proved fruitless. Ask your doctor what the reputation and practice of the hospital is before embarking on expensive and repeat tests.

INFERTILITY TREATMENT

36. Treatments for infertility

A number of treatments are now available that may help certain infertile couples. These include:

a. Fertility drugs—Clomid; the gonadotropins and bromocriptine

b. Progesterone treatment for luteal insufficiency

c. Surgery to correct endometriosis, tubal scarring or adhesions in women or blockage in the male genital tract

d. Artificial insemination

e. Psychological counselling may make an infertile marriage happier and, in a few cases, may help to establish pregnancy.

37. Fertility drugs

WARNING: *These drugs are only for infertile women who are not ovulating, or infertile men who had a pituitary problem.* Most women to whom the drugs are recommended have infrequent periods spaced far apart. A few may be menstruating regularly but have found, through the basal body temperature testing method or endometrial biopsy, that they are not ovulating. Polycystic ovaries are also treatable with the infertility drugs. The drugs fall into three basic categories:

a. *Clomiphene citrate (Clomid):* Most women who are not ovulating regularly still have some follicle-stimulating hormone (FSH) and oestrogen. What they are missing is the mid-cycle spurt of luteinizing hormone (LH) which triggers ovulation. Clomid is an anti-oestrogen; that is, it tricks the hypothalamus into thinking that the body's oestrogen levels are too low. This causes an increased production of FSH-releasing factor and FSH and therefore increases body oestrogen. When the oestrogen gets to a certain level, the hypothalamus puts out LH-releasing factor which in turn stimulates LH release and ovulation occurs.

Generally, a woman will take Clomid once a day for five days following a period (which may have to be induced with progesterone). She takes her basal body temperature daily to see if ovulation has occurred. If ovulation does not occur after three months of treatment, the dose is doubled. When used for the appropriate cases, the results for fertility have been excellent. There is a 5–10 per cent incidence of twins from this therapy, but not the multiple gestations as with Pergonal (see below).

b. *The gonadotropins—HCG (Pregnyl), HMG (Pergonal):* Some women are infertile because of damage to the hypothalamus or the pituitary that cuts down or eliminates gonadotropin production. Follicle-stimulating hormones (FSH) and luteinizing hormone (LH) are two gonadotropins vital for fertility. A woman suffering from the lack of these can take HMG—human menopausal gonadotropin—which is a mixture of FSH and LH extracted from the urine of menopausal women. HCG—human chorionic gonadotropin—is very similar to LH and an additional dose may be given at mid-cycle to simulate the spurt of LH.

A woman undergoing gonadotropin treatment for infertility needs to be closely followed with daily tests for oestrogen levels in blood or urine. At a certain level of oestrogen in the blood, the gonadotropins should be stopped. These drugs have been associated with multiple births. However, methods for determining the right dosages of gonadotropins are much improved, so that the risk of multiple births is now much lower—*if an expert is administering the drugs.*

c. *Bromocriptine (Parlodel):* This is a relatively new drug which is used to treat women with elevated prolactin levels causing infertility. (See No. 4 above) Again, this should be administered by an infertility expert.

In some women high prolactin levels can be due to a pituitary tumour which can enlarge during pregnancy. It is therefore essential that the woman should be investigated and the tumour removed surgically or destroyed by X-rays or lasers or is treated with bromocriptine, prior to embarking on pregnancy.

38. Progesterone as a treatment of corpus luteum insufficiency

If the endometrial biopsy and the basal body temperature charts suggest that luteal insufficiency (see No. 6 above) is causing infertility or habitual abortion (see No. 10 above), progesterone treatments may be tried. Vaginal suppositories containing progesterone can be administered or injections can be given through the second half of the cycle and during the first three months of pregnancy to correct the deficiency. WARNING: *synthetic progestogens such as norethisterone should not be used in early pregnancy because of the possibility of fetal damage.* An auxiliary treatment used by some doctors is a low dose of HCG or Clomid to maintain the corpus luteum.

39. Danol and other hormones may be used to treat endometriosis

Endometriosis may be treated with high doses of hormones to keep symptoms such as pain under control. (See p. 331) However, these treatments result in making a woman infertile for six to nine months. For this reason, surgery (see No. 41 below) is more appropriate for older couples immediately interested in pregnancy.

40. Ovarian wedge resection: a surgical treatment for polycystic ovaries

Many women who do not ovulate and are infertile because of polycystic ovaries have this corrected by the surgical procedure of removing a wedge of tissue from each ovary. This is treatment of last resort; it should be done only if the woman does not respond to Clomid. (See No. 37a above)

41. Surgery to correct tubal scarring, adhesions or endometriosis

If a hysterosalpingogram shows that tubal scarring, adhesions or endometriosis are causing infertility, a laparoscopy is essential to get at the *exact* nature of the problem. It should be done by the same surgeon who will do any further corrective surgery if this proves necessary. *Be very careful which doctor performs these procedures.*

Occasionally a small amount of tubal scarring can be corrected during laparoscopy. Sometimes a laparotomy for fertility is necessary thereafter. An infertility laparotomy has many varieties, depending on what the problem is. If adhesions are found these are removed and the uterus is often suspended from the front wall of the pelvis so that the adhesions will not re-form. If endometriosis is the problem, then it can be removed from the walls of the uterus, tubes and pelvis.

42. Surgery to correct tubal blockage or ligation

If the tubes have been tied, or if a blocked section of tube needs to be cut out, the surgeon can try to sew the two ends of tube back together. Microsurgery must be used for this procedure, for the tubes are so thin that they can only be seen to be sewn using a microscope. A plastic "splint" is usually inserted into the tube and the uterus to keep channels open until healing is complete. This can be removed at a later date through the cervix.

If the tubes are blocked at the fimbriated end, then a two-stage operation called a tuboplasty may be suggested. In stage one, the blockage at the fimbriated end of the tubes is cleared away and small plastic hoods are placed over the tubes. They stay there for three to six months. Then in stage two the hoods are removed. Essentially, the tubes are being forcibly kept open in the hope that they will reconstruct themselves over time and *stay* open. It doesn't always work. Only about 20–30 per cent of the women who undergo tuboplasty conceive and bear a living child. These are pretty bad odds, considering the strain and risk of two major operations. However, if the tubes are closed, this is the only option unless *in vitro* fertilization becomes widely available. (See No. 50 below)

Microsurgery to reverse vasectomy has a higher success rate.

43. Ectopic pregnancy is one danger of tubal surgery.

A woman who has had tubal surgery is more likely to experience a tubal (ectopic) pregnancy. (See p. 164) Women who have had severe infection may experience a recurrence of pelvic inflammatory disease (PID).

44. Treatments for infertility due to failure of implantation

Any uterine infection that is preventing implantation of the fertilized egg can be treated and very often cured with antibiotics. If large fibroids are preventing implantation, these can be removed surgically by myomectomy. (See p. 327) If there is a septum in the uterus, this can be removed surgically by a specialist.

45. Treatment of infertility due to abnormal cervical mucus

Some women do not develop the normal stringy mucus (spinnbarkeit) at mid-cycle. Oestrogen treatments up to mid-cycle may help to make the mucus thinner. If the cause of mucus abnormality is infection of the cervix, cyrosurgery (surgery by freezing, see p. 294) and antibiotic treatment are often effective. Male partners must be checked for NSU (non-specific urethritis).

46. Treatments for immunological reactions causing infertility among couples

a. If you are one of the few women who has an immunological reaction against your husband's sperm—that is, if you have antisperm antibodies in your blood—you can try a relatively simple treatment. Use sheaths during intercourse so that no sperm passes into your body. Blood tests may show that the number of antibodies in your blood will gradually decrease. Antibodies form expressly in response to the challenge of the presence of their specific enemy—in this case, the sperm. Take away the sperm, and the antibodies will have no reason to form.

Once the antibody count in the woman's blood stream is down, the sperm may be able to enter without adverse reaction. Therefore, the use of the condom should be continued except at mid-cycle, on the days most likely for ovulation. This is a way of sneaking the sperm past the antibodies before they have a chance to array themselves against it. If the day is right, and the immune reaction is mild enough to respond to this treatment, pregnancy may result. Other treatments may be forthcoming.

b. Autoimmunity in the man (when he reacts against his own sperm) is a more difficult problem. One treatment that has been tried is testosterone, a male hormone which is taken by the man until the sperm count goes way down and the antibodies in the man's blood that form against the sperm have no reason to form. In some men, the supression of sperm production leads to the complete elimination of the immune reaction. Testosterone treatment is then stopped, and, it is hoped, the autoimmune reaction will have stopped as well. Short-term high doses of corticosteroids are being used as well. Keep your eyes open for many discoveries in this area of the immunology of conception in the next few years. Many doctors do not believe these treatments are of any value.

47. Treatments for infertility due to low sperm count in the man

a. Abstinence during the first half of the cycle, up to the woman's most fertile days (days ten to twenty), may help to build up the man's sperm count so that he can make the woman pregnant. Clomid (see No. 37a above) may help some men with low sperm counts.

b. If the man has no sperm at all, or a very low sperm count, then *artificial insemination* is a possibility. The basic procedure is that for five days at mid-cycle a woman visits the doctor daily or every other day and semen is placed either directly in the cervix or in a cap which fits over the cervix. There are several sources of semen for the procedure:

1. A man with some sperm but not enough to father children may have his semen mixed with that of a sperm donor, so that the resulting pregnancy has *some* chance of being his;

2. A man who chronically ejaculates prematurely can collect samples of semen to be used in artificial insemination so the baby will be his;

3. Women whose partners have no sperm at all may have to be inseminated entirely with donor semen.

48. Artificial insemination is an important option for couples carrying traits for genetic disease

If both the man and the woman carry the trait for Tay-Sachs, for example, or sickle-cell disease, then artificial insemination with the sperm of a non-carrier would insure a normal baby without the need for amniocentesis and possible abortion. (See p. 214)

This is also possible for a woman with Rh sensitization. (See p. 177) If inseminated by an Rh negative donor she will have no Rh problems with the pregnancy.

49. Sperm banks and sperm donors

Men who serve as donors for artificial insemination are very carefully screened for illness, infection, blood type and Rh and genetic problems. Attempts are made to match physical and intellectual characteristics with the woman's partner. Ideally the semen is donated on the day of the insemination, but this is not always possible. If not, the semen is fast-frozen and kept for short periods of time.

50. Test-tube babies

In 1978, Mr. Patrick Steptoe and Dr. Robert Edwards achieved what they and many other doctors had been trying to achieve for years: the birth of a living, healthy "test-tube baby". The child's mother had been unable to conceive naturally because of blocked tubes. The doctors extracted an egg from the mother which was fertilized by sperm from the father *in vitro* (in the laboratory), grown to the eight-to-sixteen-cell stage and then reimplanted into the uterus of the mother, where it grew normally. Couples seeking to solve their infertility problem by resorting to this procedure should be aware that it is very, very difficult, not yet widely available and that the failure rate is high. However, the success with Lesley Brown's daughter is reason to rejoice. It is important to note that these doctors did *not* create life. They simply replicated in the laboratory a process which could not, for a wide variety of reasons, occur in the mother's body, thereby giving a childless couple the baby they so desired. Steptoe and Edwards have set up a clinic for this work in Cambridge, and other countries are now also having "test-tube baby" successes.

51. Cloning

Cloning is asexual, single-parent reproduction. It is a way of making cells reproduce themselves on their own, so that the child is an exact reproduction of the parent. Scientists have managed so far to make it work with frogs and rabbits. But despite the hold that such a process has on the imagination of novelists and philosophers, doctors and scientists have not yet attempted to go to the great trouble necessary to make the process work on humans. Let us hope that their restraint continues.

52. Adoption

Adoption is a legal, not a medical matter, and should be considered by infertile couples before the final blow of learning that they cannot produce children of their own. Unfortunately, it is not as easy as it once was. The availability of birth control and the legalization of abortion have drastically reduced the number of babies given up for adoption.

Children available for adoption nowadays are likely to be older, from an ethnic minority, handicapped, or in family groups. Adopting these children is no less rewarding. And if you cannot adopt a child, consider fostering. There are literally thousands of children in local authority homes waiting to be offered family life.

5

HAVING CHILDREN

Pregnancy is one of nature's greatest challenges to a woman, and if this were a different time or society, she would have no choice but to accept it. Today we are separated by only a few decades from the countless generations of women who had little choice but to bear children as often as their bodies allowed; often, until their bodies gave out. However, just because birth control has allowed freedom to plan and limit families, we're not free of the natural processes that cause women to become pregnant; nor are we free of the political and social forces that conspire to make pregnancy seem a preferred state. Much of the world, and many of us (if we examine our feelings truthfully), still measure a woman's worldly success and status by whether anyone calls her "Mother".

Although it is unlikely that women in the western world would ever want to return to the "natural" state in which they could not help but be pregnant, there is a lot to be said for sustaining "natural" *emotional* reasons for becoming pregnant. Today a woman may become pregnant (or not) for political reasons; financial reasons; religious reasons; she may begin to feel that having a baby, or not having one, is equivalent to making a *social* statement.

All this has bearing on the decision about pregnancy—but it is not enough to *support* the decision. There is still only one good, basic reason for a woman to become pregnant—and that is because she wishes to have a child and feels emotionally and socially ready to rear this child—even in the absence of the father.

Pregnancy, with all its trouble, may feel like something a woman does alone, for herself. In fact, some of the great mistakes in mothering are made by women who somehow forget that the end product is a *separate* human being, who will probably not care about being a "social statement" but will concentrate rather on living his or her own life.

Pregnancy is a complex process physiologically, and although it works well for the majority of cases, there are some natural dangers at various stages. Initially, for a woman to become pregnant, an enormous number of circumstances must be perfectly synchronized. (See Chapter 4, Infertility) Many problems can arise between conception and delivery. For a woman to deliver a child safely, without injury to herself or her baby, is a difficult and miraculous occurrence; doctors and midwives, and electronic devices can watch over the pregnancy, labour and delivery, but they cannot guarantee the results. For a baby to be born alive and well requires good personal health care, good medical care and good luck—and it happens over 95 per cent of the time.

Once a woman makes a decision to be pregnant (ideally, a mutual decision with the father), she must take her pregnancy seriously and seek help for the rigorous challenge her body is about to accept. Medical advice is essential at this time; self-esteem, self-care and a loving partner, family or friends are *crucial*.

CONCEPTION AND DEVELOPMENT OF PREGNANCY

1. The moment of conception

Conception occurs when a particular sperm meets and fertilizes the egg in the ampulla (a slightly dilated portion of the Fallopian tube). The sperm must then penetrate the thick, clear coating that covers the egg—the *zona pellucida* (pell-OO-sidda). The zona is made up of some protein substances, and in order to get through it the sperm releases a protein-digesting enzyme from its head.

Once it has penetrated the zona pellucida, the sperm drops its tail, rather like a rocket separating from its propulsion gear after lift-off. The head of the sperm combines with the egg; the fertilized egg then begins to divide and multiply into a many-celled structure.

2. The fertilized egg reaches the uterus: implantation

It takes about three days for the fertilized egg to move through the tube into the uterus. All the while it is dividing and multiplying; it has about eight cells by the time it reaches the uterus. Once there, it floats through the uterus for another three days, seeking a suitable place for implantation. Having found the right spot, it burrows into the endometrium—the rich, nutrient-filled lining of the uterus, where it will grow through pregnancy.

At the time of implantation it has been about seven days since ovulation and six days since fertilization.

3. The egg differentiates into fetus and placenta

By the time the fertilized egg burrows into the endometrium, it has two distinct sections—the section that will grow into the infant, and the section that will form the *placenta*. The placenta (pla-SEN-ta; derived from the Latin word for cake) is the flat, cake-shaped mass of vascular tissue that filters the substances passing between the metabolism of the mother and the metabolism of the child. *There is no direct contact between the blood stream of the mother and the blood stream of the child*—nutrients and oxygen from the mother's blood reach the fetus through the medium of the placenta; the fetal blood is cleaned of carbon dioxide, nitrogens, and other wastes through the placenta. (See below) The placenta has, in microcosm, the functions of the air and the environment, allowing separate organisms to live together without poisoning each other.

4. Corpus luteum functions are vital in initial stages of pregnancy

Six to seven days past ovulation is the time of peak strength of the corpus luteum in the ovary during the normal cycle. (See p. 18) The corpus luteum ensures that the endometrium is thick and rich enough to house the conceptus (the fertilized egg) in early pregnancy. If implantation occurs, the corpus luteum in the ovary continues to grow (it would degenerate if there were no pregnancy) and produce high levels of hormones to support the life of the pregnancy in the first few weeks. The corpus luteum is working so hard to fulfil this support function that the ovary may become enlarged and cystic during the first three months of pregnancy. A routine pelvic examination may detect the ovarian enlargement, which generally reverses by the fourth month. Unless other symptoms arise, it is nothing to worry about.

5. Differentiation: the formation of the fetus' vital organs

When the conceptus burrows into the endometrium, the endometrium actually covers it up. Then the placenta starts to spread out; the conceptus starts to grow an *amniotic* (am-nee-OTT-ik) *sac* around it. This is a thin-skinned bag full of fluid that will provide the growth medium for the embryo.

From the moment of fertilization until the twelfth to fourteenth weeks of gestation, the cells of the embryo are undergoing *differentiation*—that is, the cells are differentiating themselves into those that will form the heart, those that will form the brain, the eyes, ears, etc. *These first twelve to fourteen weeks of pregnancy, during which differentiation of organs is taking place, is the time when the embryo is most sensitive to damage by drugs, environmental*

114

chemicals, infections and radiation. A woman should be very careful to avoid such dangers at this time. (See pp. 210-11 for more discussion.)

6. When are the basic organs of the embryo formed?

During the first twelve weeks of pregnancy a woman is likely not to *look* pregnant to herself or to the world—but the most critical developments are occurring within her: she is more *delicately* pregnant, her child is in relatively greater danger, than at any other time during the pregnancy.

The following organs form at these times after ovulation:

Brain: 2–5 weeks
Heart: 3–6 weeks
Legs and arms: 4–8 weeks
Eyes: 4–8 weeks
Ears: 6–12 weeks
Mouth, teeth, and palate: 7–12 weeks
Genitals and urinary system: 7–16 weeks

Formation does not automatically lead directly to proper *function.* After the cells differentiate and the organs are formed, they get bigger and stronger continually during the last six months of pregnancy. With all the advanced current technology of neonatology (nee-oh-na-TOL-ogy)—medical speciality dealing with the fetus and newborn—it is still not possible to tell how well a new human being's body will function after it is born.

7. How a pregnant woman feels is not necessarily an indication of how her baby feels

What is good for a fully grown woman may be destructive for an embryo composed of a few hundred cells. Remember, you are pregnant from the minute of conception.

Thus, during the first twelve to fourteen weeks of pregnancy, when a woman still has not lost her shape and may feel quite unburdened with the weight and pressure of the child, the embryo itself is going through its most difficult stages. Miscarriage is most frequent during this early period, when a woman may feel at her strongest and the embryo is at its weakest and is due mainly to "design" faults in the fetus.

8. How the fetus is nourished in the uterus

The placenta grows towards the blood vessels of the mother which are lodged in the endometrium. The blood of the fetus flows to the placenta through the umbilical cord. A thin membrane separates the two blood systems. This membrane (the *placental barrier*) allows the waste materials of the baby to flow into the mother's system so that she may eliminate them, and the nutritional donations of the mother to flow into the baby's body so that the baby can grow.

The amniotic sac around the fetus enlarges constantly through the first three months, and does not fill the entire uterine cavity until three months is over.

9. Oxygen from the mother's blood is the vital nutrient for the growing fetus

The growing fetus depends *totally* on oxygen from the mother's blood supply. This is a major nutrient drawn from the blood vessels of the endometrium through the placental barrier to be picked up by the umbilical cord. The mother's blood count must be high enough to carry a good oxygen supply to the infant. Iron is very important in the formation of *haemoglobin* (HEEM-oh-glo-bin), the blood substance that carries oxygen, and most pregnant women will need an iron supplement. (See p. 120)

10. Complications in the flow of oxygen from mother to child

Anything decreasing the oxygen supply in the mother's blood endangers the child, as does anything that decreases the blood flow to the uterus. Usually these conditions only accompany severe diseases—heart disease, high blood pressure, and severe anaemia. However, smoking may decrease the oxygen supply as well. Good antenatal care is important to detect these medical problems early, and women should stop smoking during pregnancy.

In late pregnancy, when the uterus is very big, it may press on the *vena cava* (veena CAVE-a), the large vein that carries blood back to the heart from the lower extremities, and this may decrease the flow of blood to the uterus. RECOMMENDATION: One way to alleviate the loss of oxygen flow from pressure on the vena cava is to avoid sleeping flat on your back in late pregnancy; sleep on your side instead, preferably the left side.

Other nutrients beside oxygen that are carried by the mother's blood to the placenta are sugar, amino acids and all the other substances needed for human growth. (See Nos. 17–19 below)

11. The corpus luteum and then the placenta produce hormones needed to sustain pregnancy

When a woman does not become pregnant, the hormone buildup that triggers the enrichment of the endometrium stops and menstruation occurs. But when a woman becomes pregnant, the hormones must stay at a high level to keep the endometrium rich and sustain the flow of nutrients to the growing fetus.

The maintenance of this hormone supply is critical to the continuation of the pregnancy; if there are not enough hormones, miscarriage may result. (See p. 114)

Early in pregnancy, the corpus luteum supplies the oestrogen and progesterone in large quantities. Later, the placenta produces the majority of the required hormones—oestrogen, progesterone and *human chorionic gonadotropin* (HCG), a close relative of luteinizing hormone. Production of HCG begins right after implantation, increases steadily for the next fifty to seventy days, then decreases steadily toward the end of pregnancy.

HCG is believed to maintain the corpus luteum during the early weeks of pregnancy until the placenta takes over the production of oestrogen and progesterone.

12. Detection of HCG is the basis of current pregnancy tests

Most pregnancy tests now in use depend on the detection of an immunologic (antigen-antibody) reaction to the presence of HCG in the urine. This includes the pregnancy test kits which are now available for home use. The instructions in these kits should be followed exactly. *No test is 100 per cent accurate!* Any woman with symptoms of pregnancy should see a doctor even if her home test is negative.

WARNING: An ectopic or tubal pregnancy, which is a serious development (see p. 164), may produce a negative urine test, so always double-check with a doctor.

Older pregnancy tests involved injecting samples of the woman's urine into the abdomens of lab animals, particularly rabbits. If HCG were present, the animal ovaries would swell and begin to haemorrhage. When they were examined a day or two after the injection when the animals were killed, the woman's pregnancy could be verified

More sensitive blood tests that will determine the presence of HCG in the blood stream even before the first period is missed are now available in London from Technical Laboratory Services Ltd, 48–50 Bartholomew Close, London EC1 (01-606 0361), price £7.50.

13. Normal signs of early pregnancy

a. Breasts may enlarge and be tender with frequent burning or tingling sensations.

b. Fatigue is natural during the first few months followed by the opposite, a surge of energy and feelings of great good health and well-being.

c. Frequently the vagina and cervix will have a bluish look during early pregnancy (called "Chadwick's Sign" after James Chadwick, the American gynaecologist who first detected them). The blueness is caused by general congestion of blood in the pelvic region.

d. Nausea and vomiting are very frequent. "Morning sickness" is a misnomer, because the nausea can occur at any hour of the day or night.

e. Urinary frequency, common in early pregnancy, is caused by pressure of the growing uterus on the bladder.

ANTENATAL CARE

14. Recommended care

One "unnatural" thing about having children in our time is that most British women can expect, and must ask for, regular medical care during pregnancy. For healthy women, antenatal care is preventive medicine—routine weight and blood pressure checks, and blood testing, all of which verify that the correct nutritional exchange is being made and the fetus is growing normally while the woman maintains good health.

15. Select a doctor early in pregnancy

If you don't hit it off with your doctor, it's best to change to another early. Pregnancy involves a year of care, and it should be with someone you like.

If your own GP is not on the obstetric list, you can ask him or her to recommend, or you can choose, a doctor for GP obstetric care. Look at the medical list in the post office. "M" signifies that the doctor is specially trained and willing to do antenatal care. Some also do deliveries in GP units in hospitals or at home.

If you are going to a private physician, check out the cost of the *total* pregnancy at the first visit. Try to make sure that you are covered by your insurance *before* you become pregnant; many insurance companies will not cover a pregnancy which has already begun.

The actual medical care involved in a pregnancy may be routine, but the emotional care is not. Make sure the doctor or the midwife you are going to is interested *in you*. Are they pleasant? Do they ask how you are feeling? Do they answer your questions readily, or do you feel intimidated, too intimidated even to ask the questions you want to ask? If so, get yourself to another doctor or clinic. Accessibility is a vital barometer of antenatal care. Can you reach your doctor quickly? Is your doctor responsive, even when you ring between visits? Are surgery or clinic hours convenient for you?

16. Routine medical care during pregnancy

The first visit to the doctor or clinic should be made before the third month. The initial visit should include:

a. A complete medical history of the patient (and her family and forbears) and a complete physical examination

b. Pelvic examination

c. Blood pressure

d. Various blood tests: a test to determine blood count and detect anaemia; a serological test for syphilis; blood typing to determine whether the mother is Rh-negative; a cervical smear; a smear for gonorrhoea; and an optional test for rubella (German measles). Jewish women should be tested for Tay-Sachs disease, black women for sickle-cell anaemia; people from the eastern Mediterranean and Asians for thalassaemia (see pp. 214-19)

Visits for a healthy woman without special problems are usually monthly up to the seventh month; every two weeks during the eighth month; every week during the ninth month.

Blood pressure is checked at each visit to detect any sign of pre-eclampsia (pre-eck-CLAMP-see-a; high blood pressure of pregnancy, see No. 149 below) which may also cause protein in the urine and swelling of the ankles. Urine will be checked at each visit for the presence of protein or sugar. Sugar may be a sign of diabetes (see No. 157 below). Weight will be checked. After about the twentieth week (sometimes earlier), the fetal heartbeat is audible; the new ultrasound devices now make for easy, exciting listening for mother as well as doctor. The uterus may be measured with a tape measure to make sure that the growth is at a steady normal rate.

There should be time at every visit for the woman to ask questions and receive advice, especially on diet and nutrition. *Write down your questions beforehand so you don't forget to ask them.*

17. How much weight should you gain during pregnancy?

The general opinion is that bigger babies are healthier and brighter, so optimal maternal weight gain is believed to be between 1st 10lb (10.9 kilos) to 2st 2lb (13.6 kilos).

Essentially, a woman should watch her weight gain if she is fat to begin with, and worry less about it if she is thin to begin with. Excess weight gain may complicate the pregnancy, because it gives a woman a tendency towards hypertension, diabetes and general fatigue; it may complicate the delivery, by putting excess strain on her body in addition to the strain of the swollen uterus; and it may leave her with a weight problem. Too little weight gain may result in a small infant, more susceptible to ill health.

18. Diet during pregnancy

a. It is logical and normal for a woman to experience increased appetite during pregnancy (it is also normal for her not to).

b. A pregnancy diet should be exceedingly well balanced and nutritious; lots of vegetables are a must for vitamins. To satisfy the enormous protein needs of the growing fetus, eat milk, meat, fish, eggs or dried beans in increased amounts. Milk and milk products like cheese and yoghurt supply protein, carbohydrate and calcium. (See p. 116)

Often, a woman's body will instruct her which foods to choose; a confirmed coffee drinker may find coffee intolerable during pregnancy; a woman who hardly ever touches cooked vegetables may find they are exactly what she wants above everything; a woman who has always loved fruit will find that oranges give her heartburn. Follow your instincts; *eat what makes you feel good, but keep your dietary choices within the realm of the nutritious.*

c. *Junk food is not good for you when you are not pregnant; when you are pregnant, it is not good for you and your baby.*

d. Vitamin supplements in moderation may be helpful for pregnant women, excess supplies do you no good.

e. In pregnancy folic acid supplementation is advisable.

f. Calcium supplements may be needed by women who are not getting the equivalent of a pint of milk per day.

g. The need for protein escalates gently; about 2½ to 3 oz (70–80 g) per day is suggested.

19. Women need extra iron during pregnancy

As the fetus produces blood cells and the woman's blood volume increases, the diet requires extra iron. An average diet contains 5–15 mg of iron and a pregnant woman must have 18 mg or more. Most obstetricians recommend iron supplements for all pregnant women; usually in the form of 300–600 mg of ferrous sulfate or ferrous gluconate per day. If a woman is anaemic to begin with or if she has had a pregnancy within the last two years, more iron may be required. (See Anaemia, p. 356) Even if a woman is not anaemic, her bone-marrow stores of iron may become very low if extra iron is not given. Iron should be started in the second half of pregnancy as some women find it makes them constipated.

20. Don't go on a weight-reduction diet while you are pregnant

Whatever problems you may be having with your weight, don't try to solve them just before or during pregnancy. Every nutritious thing you don't eat is being denied to the fetus as well, and the fetus is *not* overweight. A woman cannot in good conscience make her unborn child pay for her own dietary excesses before she became pregnant. So gain at least 1st 7lb to 1st 10½lb (9–11.3 kilos), and if that leaves you fat, diet after delivery. Some obese women may be given a high-protein reducing diet.

21. Pica: outlandish food cravings during pregnancy

Some women develop fairly outlandish cravings for various foods during pregnancy—this is probably related to the signals transmitted from the gastrointestinal tract to the "appestat" (the appetite control centre in the brain) and the sense of taste. When the foods you crave are healthy (pickles, ice cream), then you can indulge yourself. But some "unnatural " foods, frequently craved by pregnant women, are very dangerous to them and their unborn children; laundry starch, clay from the soil, coal, even kitchen cleansers. These substances irritate the stomach and can cause severe anaemia. Avoid them at all costs.

22. What to wear during pregnancy

During pregnancy women frequently perspire more heavily, therefore choose comfortable, absorbent clothing and try to avoid synthetic material. Wear comfortable shoes that give you support; high heels or clogs which distort the alignment of your spine or throw your body forward generally only contribute to any back discomfort you may have from the forward-pull of the baby. For breast tenderness in early pregnancy, a slightly padded brassiere may help. If you feel pressure in your lower back, a girdle ay help. Maternity shops carry special girdles that make room for the bulging baby but give extra support in the back. If you feel excess pressure or experience swelling in your legs in late pregnancy, take the pressure off by every device available—wear a pregnancy girdle; wear sturdy, low-heeled shoes; wear stockings or support tights and elevate your legs frequently. Your breasts will enlarge gradually during the pregnancy. Even if you don't normally wear a brassiere, you may find that you want one now. Make sure it isn't too tight or too flimsy; the breasts are filling up with milk in late pregnancy and need support. If you plan to breast-feed your baby, start wearing a nursing brassiere in your last month.

23. Loss of balance is common in late pregnancy

By the seventh month, a woman may be carrying around over a stone (9 kilos) of extra weight, much of which is the body and environment of another human being. It is common under these circumstances to experience a loss of balance that is akin to but is not actually dizziness. A woman may, for example, take a step and find that the floor is not exactly where she expected it to be; she may sit down and find that the chair is actually higher, or lower, than she expected it to be. This is normal. Wear low shoes at this time to minimize the chance of twisting an ankle and actually falling. Stick to a pattern of exercise in which loss of balance cannot result in injury. Make sure someone helps you in and out of the bath or shower in late pregnancy.

When riding in a car, do not place the seat belt across the fetus. The lap strap should be pulled across your pelvis *below* the fetus. Use the shoulder strap. This helps avoid injury to the fetus in case of an accident or sudden stop or sharp collision with the car behind you.

24. Exercise during pregnancy

Exercise is important during pregnancy for all women (unless specifically restricted for medical reasons); it improves circulation and minimizes many ordinary discomforts, such as swelling of the legs and back pain due to pressure on weakened muscles. Sports which were standard before pregnancy should be continued as long as there is no danger of losing balance and falling in the later months.

Every pregnant woman should begin a programme of exercise early in pregnancy, especially if she wasn't in good shape when she started. Try walking or swimming every day for thirty minutes, at least. Exercises given in natural childbirth classes are helpful, especially sit-ups and straight-leg raising with one knee bent to strengthen the abdominal muscles. Remember that the pull you feel when doing leg lowering exercises, for example, is *not* a pull on the fetus; it is a pull on the abdominal muscles, which will need to be strong for delivery.

25. Sexual intercourse is perfectly all right all through pregnancy

The old-fashioned practice of limiting intercourse after the seventh month is senselessly punitive to both man and woman, and in fact, drives them away from each other at a time when they need to be especially close.

For both partners, there are frequently many changes in sexual drive during pregnancy—with both a psychological and physiological basis. During early pregnancy a woman may feel less interested in sex, especially if she is suffering from fatigue and other minor discomforts. (See No. 27 below) Interest in sex frequently increases during the middle three months, sometimes more than before the pregnancy. In late pregnancy, because of increasing discomfort, interest in coitus may decrease. Changing position may help.

The pain of an episiotomy (see No. 93 below) may interfere with sex for several weeks after delivery. If a woman is breast-feeding, her vagina may be dry with some resultant burning or pain during intercourse. Lubricating jelly (*not* vaseline) can be used. In addition, the great emotional involvement which the mother has with the child after delivery may decrease her interest in sex temporarily. This should normally return after a few weeks.

A man may experience a wide range of sexual feelings during the pregnancy. He may unjustifiably fear injuring mother or baby during intercourse. He may not find the woman sexually attractive in late pregnancy, but this feeling should pass. Most men take great pride in their potency; and this makes them feel sexually even closer to the mother of the child.

After the delivery both partners must make adjustments. A new human being is around, demanding a huge amount of attention and usually disturbing the parents' sleep. Both partners may feel quite exhausted for the first few weeks; therefore, sexual activity may decrease.

Certain adjustments in sexual technique will be necessary as the pregnancy advances. The male-superior position may become more uncomfortable than other positions. The man may find that he cannot thrust so deeply in later months, no matter what the position is. Many couples use alternate forms of sexual expression such as oral sex and mutual masturbation if intercourse isn't feasible.

If a woman is experiencing a leakage of fluid or bleeding during late pregnancy, she should avoid intercourse until she is examined by a doctor.

26. Orgasm and premature labour

Some doctors believe that orgasm experienced by a woman in late pregnancy may initiate labour. Orgasm does cause uterine contractions, but there is no evidence that these lead to the onset of labour either prematurely or at term.

DISCOMFORTS OF PREGNANCY

27. Minor discomforts in pregnancy

These include:

a. Nausea and vomiting
b. Constipation
c. Increased salivation
d. Heartburn and belching
e. Increased heart rate
f. Nosebleeds
g. Light-headedness and dizziness
h. Varicose veins and piles
i. Shortness of breath
j. Urinary frequency
k. Skin changes
l. Breast changes
m. Vaginal discharge
n. Mild abdominal pains and spotting
o. Orthopaedic problems
p. Leg cramps and pains
q. Oedema (swelling of ankles)
r. Insomnia
s. Eye problems
t. Psychological changes

All of the above are usually normal, easily anticipated and nothing at all to worry about. They can almost invariably be lived through without resorting to drugs.

Most pregnant women experience a couple of these discomforts. Some experience none at all. Even if you experience every single one, and feel absolutely miserable, you can still assume that you and your baby are healthy.

Medical treatment will do little to help the woman suffering the normal discomforts of pregnancy. The advice of other women will serve just as well. However, if a symptom persists or worsens, seek a medical opinion to assure yourself that nothing serious is happening.

28. Nausea and vomiting

Nausea and vomiting in pregnancy is probably a gastrointestinal reaction to hormonal changes. Although many women feel sick in the morning, many will feel sick at any time of day. Usually, the condition starts about the fifth week of gestation and ends by the twelfth week; but some women experience it (and are still healthy) throughout the pregnancy.

Treatments to try include:

a. Sipping soda water
b. Nibbling a dry biscuit or a piece of dry toast
c. Eating frequent small meals

Nausea occurs most often with an empty stomach (that's why it occurs so frequently in the morning). So keep plain biscuits or crackers in your bag for munching on during the business day, or in other circumstances when you're away from home. The cracker often works because it absorbs the saliva and thereby rids the palate of the nauseating taste. Avoid dreadful smells that make you feel sick.

Nausea may be related to the taste in your mouth. Some women find that it is relieved by a morsel of sharp, taste-changing food such as a strong peppermint or a stick of cinnamon.

Some doctors believe that nausea and vomiting come from vitamin B-6 (pyridoxine) deficiency. Pyridoxine tablets may help and are harmless. If you are vomiting all the time and losing weight, drugs must be used if natural remedies have failed. (Also see pernicious vomiting, No. 143 below). But be careful. Some anti-nausea drugs have been suspected of causing fetal damage in humans and have been shown to cause it in rats and rabbits.

29. Constipation

Constipation is very common, especially in later pregnancy, when the swelling uterus presses on the descending colon. It may also be related to decreased muscle tone in the intestinal tract due to high hormone levels. It is a major side effect of the iron pills often prescribed.

Try adding fresh fruits, bulky vegetables and bran to the diet. Drink more fluids. If all this doesn't work, try bulk stool softeners such as psyllium seed or cellulose. Do not expect a bowel movement every day, even when you are not pregnant. Constipation occurs when stools are hard and when you have been unable to move your bowels for *several* days. Once a woman has moved her bowels and broken the cycle of constipation, she should attempt to defaecate without additional aid as always, while adjusting her diet appropriately.

If the iron pills you are taking cause constipation, ask your doctor to prescribe stool softeners.

Avoid laxatives. Stool softeners are much better. If you must have a laxative, use milk of magnesia or Senokot. Mineral oil may inhibit absorption of vitamins from the intestinal tract, and other laxatives contain substances which have not been proven safe for use in pregnancy. (See p. 234)

30. Increase in salivation

Women who are severely affected find they must carry tissues and spit frequently. Increased salivation often accompanies other digestive problems of pregnancy. No treatment is effective. Delivery ends the problem.

31. Heartburn and belching

Heartburn and belching, extremely common effects of pregnancy, are caused by the lessening capacity of the cramped stomach to hold down food. Increased pressure on the abdomen as the fetus grows leads to a kind of backup of the stomach juices into the lower part of the oesophagus (e-SOFF-a-gus), the muscular tube leading from the throat to the stomach, with concurrent irritation from the acid. Also, during pregnancy progesterone relaxes the valve at the upper end of the stomach which allows regurgitation of the stomach contents into the oesophagus. The causes of heartburn are related to those that cause nausea; the food you eat does not pass smoothly into the lower stomach; you taste it long after you have eaten it; you may experience a rising bitterness in your throat, a feeling that you have incompletely digested what you have just eaten. Certain foods may increase heartburn: coffee, citrus fruits, vegetables like cabbage and marrow. Avoid the particular foods that seem related to the problem; try the same treatments recommended for nausea (see No. 28 above); try over-the-counter antacids; don't lie down after eating because this will further hamper digestion. Some women find it possible to "walk off" heartburn.

32. Dental problems

Pregnancy in itself does not trigger increased tooth decay, but it is important that routine dental care continues during pregnancy. Dental work is free during pregnancy and for 12 months afterwards. The old taboo against dental care and extractions during pregnancy is no longer medically valid. If X-rays are absolutely needed, the abdomen can be shielded to protect the fetus. However, *do not have major dental work requiring general anaesthesia during pregnancy.* The work should be done under local anaesthesia, because the risks of general anaesthesia involve decreasing the oxygen supply to the fetus.

Two conditions of the gums seem to be peculiar to pregnancy.

a. *Gingivitis* (jin-ji-VY-tis), an inflammation of the gums, is common in non-pregnant women as well, but one particular type gets much worse during pregnancy and then dramatically subsides after delivery.

b. Small *"pregnancy tumours"* may grow on the gums during pregnancy. They are benign, but should be removed by the dentist because they will probably grow again during the next pregnancy. The "pregnancy tumour" looks like a small red polyp on the gum, and is related to gingivitis.

33. The volume of blood in a woman's cardiovascular system grows steadily throughout pregnancy, causing several minor side effects

By the time a woman is nine months pregnant, the volume of blood in her body is about 1½ times that of her normal non-pregnant state. This occurs in response to the nutritional requirements of the fetus. The increased blood volume may cause accelerated heart rate and/or nosebleeds. These are *minor* side effects—uncomfortable, but no danger to general health.

34. Increased heart rate

To pump the greater volume of blood, the heart must beat faster, and occasionally, this will cause palpitations—a feeling that the heart is racing. Anaemia, a deficiency of red blood cells, aggravates palpitations. Iron is an important dietary supplement to avoid this side effect. (See No. 144 below)

35. Nosebleeds

Nosebleeds are common during pregnancy because the increased volume of blood makes the little blood vessels in the nose break more easily. The high hormone levels in pregnancy may also have this effect. The nosebleeds are nothing to worry about and will usually stop of their own accord after a few minutes.

36. Light-headedness and dizziness

"Postural hypotension" is the name given to the dizziness that pregnant women sometimes experience when they change their position suddenly—get up or sit down quickly. It is probably related to a momentary lag in circulation, when the large uterus presses on the vena cava (the major abdominal vein) and the larger volume of blood is trapped below the waist, unable for a second or two to get to the brain. As a result, a woman may feel dizzy—or experience a stabbing headache that disappears almost immediately. *This is nothing to worry about.* Lie down on your side, so the blood supply can even out through your body; then get up again, slowly. Postural hypotension is one major reason that many ordinarily athletic women find it hard to continue active sports later in pregnancy. If this happens to you, substitute slower, more controlled exercise like calisthenics or yoga. If a woman actually faints, she should be examined by a doctor. But this may also be due just to changes in circulation.

37. Varicose veins and haemorrhoids

As pregnancy progresses, women may notice that the veins of their hands and arms as well as the legs become more prominent. This is caused in general by increased blood volume. Because there is greater pressure on the body's lower area, varicose veins of the legs are a very common complaint at this time, as are haemorrhoids or piles—varicose veins of the anus. "Varicose" implies that the veins have stretched and expanded abnormally. Take care to wear supportive clothing and tights for varicose veins, and avoid constipation which will aggravate haemorrhoids. (See p. 125)

Varicose veins may also appear on the vulva or the labia majora, the large outer lips of the vagina. These can be very uncomfortable. Alleviate the pressure that causes them by wearing special elastic briefs, available from maternity shops.

38. Shortness of breath

In late pregnancy, the growing fetus may push the diaphragm (the major breathing muscle) upward, causing pressure on the lungs and shortness of breath. There is little to be done about this except to lie down on your side with your head elevated so that the weight of the baby falls away from the diaphragm. The symptom may disappear in very late pregnancy, when the baby drops in preparation for birth. Women who report shortness of breath in *early* pregnancy are probably responding to the increased fetal need for oxygen. Sit down; breathe deeply. WARNING: If shortness of breath occurs at night or is persistent or severe, consult your doctor.

39. Urinary frequency

In the first three months, urinary frequency is so common a complaint that it can be taken as a *sign* of pregnancy. It is caused by pressure of the uterus on the bladder. *It requires no treatment. Do not limit intake of liquids—these keep the bowel functioning well;* just stay within range of a toilet. The symptom may be alleviated in the middle months and may reappear in late pregnancy, when the baby's head—in preparation for birth—sinks down and puts new pressure on the bladder. WARNING: If frequency is accompanied by pain or fever, this may be a sign of kidney or bladder infection. (See p. 307) See a doctor.

128

40. Increased skin pigmentation and chloasma

It is quite common for a dark pigment to be deposited around the nipples, in the genital region and/or in a straight line down the middle of the abdomen during pregnancy. Some women will be annoyed by a brownish discoloration over the face, called chloasma (klo-AZ-ma) or the mask of pregnancy. These changes occur because, due to the higher levels of oestrogen, the pituitary is producing higher levels of melanocyte-stimulating hormone, which spurs the growth of cells containing *melanin* (MEL-a-nin), a skin pigment. Exposure to sun aggravates these changes. There is nothing to be done about them; they are almost never very serious; and usually, when the pregnancy is over, they remain, although they may fade a good deal. Oral contraceptives can cause the same problem in some women. (See p. 45)

41. Stretch marks

Overweight people, or people who have been overweight and have dieted, sometimes acquire stretch marks, light-coloured striations. Very often, in men, they appear on the upper arm; in women, on arms, hips and breasts. During pregnancy, a woman may experience stretch marks on her breasts and abdomen.

Increased amounts of steroid hormones are produced in pregnancy. These corticosteroids (from the adrenal glands) are thought to change the consistency of the elastic tissue in the deeper layers of the skin, which then tear rather than stretch, leaving red purplish marks known as *striae gravidarum*. They may appear in the fifth and sixth months of pregnancy, and after delivery they fade to a whitish colour and may be quite inconspicuous.

Home remedies, such as application of olive oil or expensive creams, do no good. *It may help to keep the body weight under control before and after delivery.*

42. Increased perspiration and body odour

This is perfectly natural for the pregnant woman. Use normal hygiene: frequent bathing, deodorants if you feel the need and absorbent cotton clothes.

43. Changes in hair distribution and quality

Hormonal changes may cause some increase in facial and abdominal hair and some hair loss around the temples and throughout the head. Hair that held a curl well before pregnancy may straighten out and become limp. After delivery, hair will return to normal. WARNING: *Avoid colouring your hair during pregnancy.* Although it is unlikely, you may be allergic to chemicals in the hair colour that never affected you at all before. (See p. 229) Also, some hair dyes have been suspected of causing cancer in experimental animals.

44. Itching and dryness of the skin

During pregnancy the skin of the abdomen is severely stretched and may become dry and itchy as a result, especially over the hip bones and belly. Frequent bathing to control increased perspiration may aggravate the dryness. Most women find that oil or a dry-skin cream (*not a hormone cream!*) applied to affected areas controls the problem.

Very severe itching and dryness may indicate that liver functions are changing in reaction to the increased oestrogen levels of pregnancy; it will end with delivery, but should be reported to your doctor so that liver problems can be ruled out.

45. Breast changes

Early in pregnancy the nipples may be very sore and the breasts very tender. This usually stops by the third or fourth month, as the body adjusts to the new hormone levels. Expect your breasts to enlarge continually through to term. Small amounts of watery fluid leak from time to time. The little bumps around the areola (dark area), called Montgomery Tubercles, will also tend to enlarge and occasionally drain. All this is normal and nothing to worry about. Wash the nipples daily and remove any dried secretion.

46. Vaginal discharge

As hormone levels increase during pregnancy, a woman normally experiences increased vaginal discharge, generally watery, whitish in colour, not foul-smelling and not irritating to the vulva. (If these latter signs occur, suspect vaginal infection and have yourself checked.) Don't be alarmed if your underwear seems rather wet all the time; cotton pants are recommended for their absorbency. Vaginal infections, with the exception of candidiasis or thrush (see p. 288), do not increase unduly during pregnancy.

47. Abdominal pains, cramps and spotting

Throughout her pregnancy a woman may experience a multitude of various aches and pains which suggest nothing except the reaction of her body to the demands of housing a different body within her. Sometimes, in early pregnancy, a woman may feel cramps that would normally make her think she was about to get her period. When the uterus grows out of the pelvis, this usually stops. If bleeding accompanies the cramps, that may be a sign of something more serious.

Bleeding is very common in early pregnancy. A day or two of spotting with a small amount of cramping may occur at the time of implantation of the conceptus into the endometrium (about a week earlier than the normal menstrual period). Between 20 and 25 per cent of the women who carry to term report bleeding during the first three months. Only rarely is the bleeding as heavy as that of a normal period, although if a woman has lost track of her menstrual schedule, the bleeding can confuse her sufficiently so that she actually doesn't realize she is pregnant. Slight bleeding or spotting during the first three months is usually nothing to worry about; if it is continuing or heavy, or accompanied by severe pain, it probably constitutes the beginnings of a spontaneous abortion (or miscarriage) and the doctor should be contacted immediately. (See No. 118 below)

Later in pregnancy, wind is frequent and often severe. It can usually be relieved by a diet heavy on fruit, bran and other whole grain cereals; to prevent constipation, avoid wind-producing foods.

Between four and six months, a woman may experience sharp, distinct pains in the lower abdomen or on either side of the uterus, especially when she changes position and the uterus moves. These are *round ligament* pains: the round ligaments attach each side of the uterus to the pelvis, and when they are stretched and the uterus moves, there is a corresponding pain on the pulled side. This should be considered a normal abdominal pain.

In the second half of pregnancy, the baby itself is moving. If the baby kicks and hits a woman's liver, she will feel a very sharp pain, It will not persist, but it may recur, and nothing can relieve it except possibly a change of position and ultimately the delivery of the baby.

Abnormal abdominal pain during pregnancy has these features:

a. It persists for hours;

b. It is unrelieved by a change in position that allows the uterus to move;

c. It is unrelieved by a bowel movement.

d. The uterus is tender to the touch. The organ itself should not be hurting.

e. Fever or bleeding accompanies the pain.

48. How a moving baby feels

Nothing can be told about a fetus from the way it moves. Some seem to be slumbering in the womb, and occasionally stir a little;

some seem to be wrestling with the womb—a woman's stomach can actually be seen moving suddenly and violently this way and that way—it bulges and bumps and has, literally, a life of its own.

WARNING: *Do not take anything to calm the baby down*, and do not be offended if people seem to be staring at your stomach. Old wives' tales that predict the sex and/or personality of the child from the way it moves in the womb are all nonsense; movements in the womb are quite involuntary, and are not connected with sex or personality.

In late pregnancy the baby gradually moves less because the space becomes more cramped. A sudden cessation of movement should send you to your doctor, who can listen to the baby's heart or perform a stress test (see No. 174 below) to see if the fetus and placenta are well.

49. Backache

This can be a nagging problem, especially in late pregnancy, and is due to the change in posture created by the pull of the growing child. Many women tend to arch their backs and lean backward to counter the forward pull of the abdomen. *Backache can be largely prevented* by a programme of exercise begun in early pregnancy —sit-ups and leg-raising exercises strengthen the abdominal muscles so that they are better equipped to carry the weight of the baby and take the pressure off the back. A pregnancy girdle can help. (See References for information on exercises.)

50. Relaxation of the pelvic joints

In some women, the sacroiliac and the pubic joints relax excessively during pregnancy, causing backache and a nagging ache in the pubic area that can become very aggravating if you stand on your feet too long. The problem, if it occurs, usually starts in the seventh month. A pregnancy girdle is helpful, but sometimes nothing will help except resting and putting your feet up.

If these symptoms are so severe as to be crippling, ask your doctor for referral to an orthopaedic specialist.

51. Problems with the joints of the legs and hips

In late pregnancy, when the weight build up is relatively great and loss of balance (see No. 23 above) can distort a woman's sense of just how and where her legs are carrying her, there may be pain in the hips or knees. Occasionally, the knee joints may give out—the leg will just collapse. This is not a problem unless a woman injures herself in the fall. Try to walk with someone when you get really big; make sure you've got something, or someone, to hold on to when you get in and out of the bath.

52. Women with pre-existing orthopaedic problems should take special care when they are pregnant

Some orthopaedic problems, such as *scoliosis*—a twisting of the spine—are aggravated by pregnancy. If a woman has a weak back, weak hips or legs, she should consult her orthopaedic specialist before she becomes pregnant, and allot a great deal of time during the pregnancy to lying and sitting down, or to physiotherapy if indicated.

In the case of arthritis, pregnancy can be a blessing as well as a danger; the increased weight that must be borne by the inflamed joint may make the condition more painful; on the other hand, the higher hormone levels of pregnancy may relieve the pain considerably. *No woman with a chronic disease should become pregnant without fully understanding the conditions and complications that might surround the pregnancy and delivery.* (See No. 156 below)

53. Leg cramps

In the second half of pregnancy, severe muscle spasms (cramps) in the calf muscles of the legs are very common. Some say this is caused by a lack of calcium or lack of salt.

Frequently, leg cramps occur at night. Try these treatments: pull the toes up forcefully with the leg extended straight; this will stretch the muscle that is in spasm and help relax it. Or have someone massage the muscle very briskly. Or place a pillow at the foot of the bed at night to prevent the legs from straightening out completely during sleep.

54. Pinched nerves and numbness in the legs

Toward the end of pregnancy, as the uterus enlarges, and the head of the baby settles into the pelvis, the nerves of the upper legs may be pinched by the pressure. In some women this causes numbness in the legs; in other women, the simple act of walking may complicate the pressure and cause pinching of the nerves in the thigh. Shake your leg; change position; get off your feet. The pinching will stop after delivery.

55. Oedema (swelling) of the feet and ankles is extremely common in late pregnancy

It is a rare woman who gets through a pregnancy without experiencing oedema (ed-EE-ma) of the feet and ankles, usually most pronounced at the end of the day. It is primarily due to increased pressure on the veins of the legs because of slowed circulation as the blood must flow around the enlarged uterus: some fluid that is normally cleared just stays in the lower extremities.

Varicose veins aggravate the problem. Tight clothing, excessive salt intake (salt causes water retention), and a lot of standing during the day, will also aggravate the oedema.

Try putting your feet up often. Whenever you sit down, put your feet up on a stool, another chair, whatever is handy. Do not cut down on salt intake too much, because this will lead to sodium deficiency, which is not good for pregnancy. Cut down a little but *do not use salt substitutes routinely*. If you have varicose veins or must be on your feet continually, wear elastic stockings, and *always* avoid tight clothing. WARNING: If oedema spreads to the hands and face and is as bad in the morning as it is at night, this may be a sign of toxaemia. (See No. 149 below) Have your blood pressure and urine protein checked.

Diuretics should not be prescribed for uncomplicated oedema of pregnancy. They may be dangerous to the fetus.

56. Headache and fatigue

These two complaints are almost universal among pregnant women, especially in the first and last trimesters. Fatigue is due to the extra metabolic needs of the baby and the sheer weight of the pregnancy. Rest when you need to.

Headaches are generally mild.

WARNING: *Do not take anything for them if possible until the fourth month, and then take only mild pain-killers.*

Avoid aspirin in the last three months because excess aspirin intake has been associated with bleeding tendencies in babies.

57. Insomnia

In late pregnancy, it is sometimes very difficult to find any comfortable position in which to sleep. A woman may have to be satisfied with napping for short periods during the day; if she has been sleepless the night before, her household will just have to adjust to her irritation and fatigue the day after. WARNING: *Do not take any sedatives in early pregnancy. This includes over-the-counter drugs.* Avoid any but the mildest sedatives recommended only by your doctor in late pregnancy, and use them only if you are wild from sleeplessness and have tried every sleeping position, including sitting up in a chair, with your feet elevated, and lying on your side (this position allows for maximized blood flow to the uterus by avoiding pressure on the vena cava by the uterus).

58. Eye problems

Some women experience relatively great changes in their eyes during pregnancy, perhaps because the extra fluid they are retaining is altering the shape of the eyeballs. If at all possible, do not invest in new glasses while you are pregnant, because you will probably need your old ones back again soon after you deliver the baby.

59. Psychological changes

Hormones have enormous influence on the mood of the individual, and a pregnant woman is undergoing an upheaval in hormone levels.

Anticipate mood changes; don't attach too much importance to them; make sure those around you are likewise prepared. Remember: you are just as likely to feel elated as you are to feel depressed.

a. *The emotional circumstances under which a woman becomes pregnant in the first place have as much to do with her mood as hormone levels.* If she wants the baby and cares about the father, she is likely to have a happier time being pregnant than if she is having her fourth or fifth child, accidently conceived by a man she no longer likes.

b. *Depression is frequent during pregnancy. Never treat it without medical advice.* It is absolutely normal when you have been throwing up and running to the bathroom every half hour to feel furious with the man who got you into this predicament and also very down about life in general. If your depression is severe and unceasing, seek reliable professional help.

c. *If this is your first child, it is natural to fear the pain of labour.* Don't talk to older women about this, talk to your contemporaries, to women at your clinic, discuss pain relievers with your doctor and attend childbirth classes. (See No. 66 below)

d. *If you are worried about genetic defects in the child, try to think things through carefully. Unless there is a specific genetic disease in your family, you have a greater than 95 per cent chance of bearing a perfectly normal child once past the third month of pregnancy.* Many familial diseases can now be detected by amniocentesis. (See p. 214) If you are over thirty-five, you could ask for

e. *The last thing a pregnant woman needs is an internal crisis about the loss of her looks. So before you become pregnant, make*

135

peace with the fact that you will soon lose your shape. Apart from your waistline, there is no reason to believe that you will lose any feature that makes you attractive. In fact, most pregnant women look better in many ways. Your skin may have more tone, your mood may be better, and the father of your child may think you are more wonderful than ever before. Few women bulging with child can get through their pregnancy without feeling their vanity assaulted. But now is not the time to be vain. Now is the time to be healthy.

f. *Dependency on the doctor* is a common phenomenon among pregnant women and certainly is encouraged to varying degrees by doctors who, like most people, love to be loved. It happens mainly to women who mistakenly discount their own ability to control their situation.

Remember, in the majority of cases, that the presence or absence of your particular doctor is not critical to the outcome of the delivery. *You* are having the baby and the most important determinant of successful delivery is generally your health and preparedness. 80 per cent of deliveries in Britain are performed or supervised by a midwife. Of course, in case of emergency, the doctor's skill is important, but most deliveries do not end in emergencies.

g. *Changes in libido*—sexual responsiveness and desire—often occur during pregnancy. (See No. 25 above)

NORMAL LABOUR AND DELIVERY

60. Labour and delivery

Most women can expect normal labour and delivery. Don't expect emergencies or complications, but provide for them in the back of your mind and in your plans for where you are having your baby.

61. Preliminary contractions and "false labour"

Small uterine contractions occur from time to time throughout pregnancy; they are not usually painful or even noticeable. In the last month or two, many women begin to *feel* preliminary contractions which are sometimes so strong that they are hard to differentiate from true labour. These Braxton Hicks contractions (named after John Braxton Hicks, the gynaecologist who discovered them) are more prominent in women who have had children already. They probably help to soften the cervix and stretch it for labour. Try not to feel too disappointed if the labour you thought you were having turns out to be false. The real thing will start soon enough.

62. Lightening: engagement of the baby's head in the lower pelvis

Lightening occurs typically about two to four weeks before labour, *in white women having their first child*. Suddenly, the baby seems to drop; a woman will feel less pressure under her heart; she will be able to breathe better; she will feel "lighter" and will also experience urinary urgency, for the baby has now pushed its head between the bones of the pelvis and is probably pressing on the bladder too.

Lightening is a good sign. First, it signals that the pregnancy (which may feel by now as though it has lasted ten years) is soon to be over. Second, it signals that the pelvis is probably wide enough for the baby to get through. Observers may notice that the baby is pushing the stomach outward in more pronounced fashion.

If lightening doesn't happen, there is nothing to worry about; it will usually occur closer to actual labour. *Women who have previously borne children should not expect it. Many black and Asian women find that the head remains high until the onset of labour.*

63. Bloody show and loss of the mucus plug

For some weeks prior to labour, the cervix is effacing (thinning) and dilating (stretching). A few days before labour, there may be a little bleeding and/or loss of the plug of mucus that has served as a cervical barrier throughout the pregnancy. This may happen naturally, or it may be brought on by a pelvic examination close to term, or it may not happen at all. Bleeding, if it does occur, may be only a tiny spot or as much as can be trapped on one sanitary towel. If there is more, notify your doctor right away.

64. Rupture of the membranes

The rupture of the membranes and escape of the amniotic fluid may occur as an immediate prelude to labour, which will begin right away or in a few hours. Most women do not experience it until labour is in progress.

But some women who haven't had a labour pain yet will suddenly experience the gushing release of the fluid. This may feel like a constant slow leak or it will come pouring down your legs in a relatively heavy stream. Call your medical adviser or the hospital.

Labour should start within twelve hours after the rupture of the amniotic sac. If it does not, labour should be induced, because once the membranes have broken, there is some danger of infection. Do not wait at home alone for labour to start; by doing so, you are running unnecessary risks. Temperature and heart tones must be monitored. If the fetus is not term size when the membranes burst, then the birth may be more complicated. (See No. 132 below)

65. Labour

There are two points of view in the delivery room: that of the woman giving birth and that of the medical people attending her. They *see* the labour, she *feels* it.

Medical people observe a birth by palpating (examining by touch) the cervix and measuring the stages of labour by its *dilation*—the widening of the opening of the cervix—and its *effacement*—the thinning of the cervical wall as it stretches. As labour continues, the cervix becomes progressively wider, until it is wide enough to allow the infant through.

To a doctor or midwife the stages of labour look like this:

Stage 1-A: Called *the latent phase,* this is the first half of the first stage of labour. The cervix is dilating rather slowly, and the woman says that her contractions are rather far apart. When the cervix is 5–6 centimetres dilated, the first half of the first stage is ending. During this stage, the woman is normally happy to walk around.

Stage 1-B: The second part of the first stage usually starts when the cervix has opened to about 5–6 centimetres in width. This is actually the shorter part of the first stage, and is called the *dilatation (or accelerated) phase.* The contractions become stronger and closer together, thus bringing about the stretching of the cervix until it is fully dilated to about 10 cm. During this stage, the woman will probably want to lie down.

The first stage in its entirety can last a variable length of time: sometimes more than twenty-four hours, sometimes only an hour.

Stage 2: The second stage starts when the cervix has dilated completely, and lasts until the baby is delivered. It should not last more than two to three hours (see below).

Many medical people will say that "true" labour only starts when the cervix begins to dilate at a steady rate. Women, however, tend to measure labour from the first pain to the last; thus the process may seem much longer to a woman that it does to those attending her.

To the woman, the stages of labour feel like this:

Stage 1: She feels distinct, separate cramps which at first feel the same as the occasional Braxton Hicks contractions she may have had before. (See No. 61 above). They may start in the back and pass around to the front of the abdomen. (The difference from the Braxton Hicks contractions is that contractions of labour gradually become more regular and last longer. They may start at thirty minutes apart, but then a pattern develops and they get closer and closer together.)

By the time the contractions are five to seven minutes apart, you should have called the ambulance or midwife or be on your way to the place where you are having your baby. (Start out earlier, or later, depending on how many children you've had and how far you live from the hospital. Discuss this with your doctor ahead of time.)

A labour pain is caused by the movement of the uterus, as it contracts to help push the baby towards the birth canal. In the latent phase of labour (Stage 1-A above) these contractions are relatively weak, and the pain should be relatively easy to take. Depending on a woman's personal pain threshold and the particular circumstances of her labour, the pain may be bad or not—but there is time between the contractions to recover from one and prepare for the next.

Stage 2: The second half of labour has three parts: dilatation, transition and expulsion.

During dilation, the contractions are three to five minutes apart and becoming more forceful. Most of the work in dilating the cervix is done at this time.

During transition, the cervix reaches 8 to 9 centimetres of dilatation, the contractions begin to come very close together and the woman may feel severe pressure on her rectum and an urge to push, although it is too early to do so. (See No. 67). This is the most difficult part of labour because the contractions are so close together that it is almost impossible to recover from one before another starts. Luckily, it doesn't last too long.

When the second stage is reached, observers report that the cervix is completely dilated and the woman can push with her contractions. This is a great relief: it means the end is near; the pain is about to be over; many women report a kind of euphoric feeling.

Don't ever imagine that you should have your baby alone!

Both points of view are needed if a birth is to be handled properly. A woman who is trying to deal with the labour needs another voice besides the voice of her own nervous system to reassure her; the doctor, midwife or husband trying to assist her delivery needs to be told by the woman how she feels, how bad the pain is, how frequently it is coming. There should be a lot of communication in the labour room and the delivery room.

Pain, of course, is relative. Some women will swear they had an easy time in labour, some will say afterwards that it was absolutely dreadful. No woman can really know what her labour will be like, even if she has had children already. Assume then that labour will be hard (it may surprise you and be easy); prepare for it by exercising regularly during pregnancy; seek instruction from groups that will teach you breathing exercises which are extremely helpful in ameliorating labour pains. And when you are in labour, keep your mind firmly fixed on one idea—that the stronger the pain is, the closer you probably are to giving birth to your baby.

66. Where to seek training for labour

Hospital antenatal clinics and departments of obstetrics and gynaecology provide their maternity patients with exercise and training classes. The National Childbirth Trust in your locality will provide information and training for both mother and father to prepare for childbirth. Even if you are not planning to go through labour without anaesthesia, these classes will improve your muscle tone, help eradicate anxiety about labour and teach you invaluable aids for dealing with the pain.

67. When to "push" during labour

By the time the cervix is dilated 8–9 cm, the emerging baby will be pressing, quite often, on the rectum, and the woman will feel a strong urge to push as though she were defaecating. This is what makes transition, the stage immediately before expulsion and birth, so difficult. Resist the urge and listen to the advice of your medical attendants. If you start pushing too soon, before the cervix is completely dilated, you may cause it to tear and complicate the delivery. Wait until the people with you say the cervix is completely dilated. *Then* push or bear down along with the contractions. Since there is usually extreme rectal pressure at this point, you probably wouldn't be able to resist pushing even if you wanted to. For a lot of women, the signal that the cervix is sufficiently dilated for them to bear down is a joyous moment. When you can push with the contractions, a lot of the pain may be relieved. Some women experience a feeling at this juncture akin to orgasm. Whatever your physical reaction, you know now that the labour is about to end—and that's enough to make anybody happy. Childbirth classes and books on natural childbirth (see References) will give a woman a good idea of efficient methods of pushing.

68. Try not to lie flat on your back during labour

Blood flow to the uterus is best if you lie on your side, and this strengthens contractions. Many women find that if they sit up, the pains are easier. If your pains are far apart, try walking around between them. Good circulation is vital to the labour process.

69. Yelling does not strengthen contractions

Some women believe that if you yell during a labour pain, the contraction is stronger and labour progresses more quickly. This is an old wives' tale. If you need to cry out during labour, go ahead; but don't make a philosophy of it. It may waste your strength, diverts the people around you from their job, which is to watch over the delivery, and won't do anything at all for your contraction.

70. Episiotomy

An episiotomy (eh-PEEZ-ee-otomy) is an incision in the bottom of the vagina, made at the time of the delivery of the head of the baby, to give it more room to get through. A local anaesthetic should be given before the cut is made. At best, it prevents *random* tearing of the vagina and the rectum by the emerging baby; at worst, it is unnecessary. If your doctor thinks it is necessary, he or she should *tell* you on the spot; it is no fun to be surprised by a surgical incision, with stitches, that may hurt a lot after you've given birth. The stitches will be absorbed. (See No. 93 below) Episiotomies *may* be overused. Make sure that your hospital does not expect to do one on you as a matter of routine, but only if the birth requires it. Women who have had children are much less likely to need an episiotomy than those who are delivering for the first time.

71. Delivery of the placenta, or "after-birth", by the Brandt-Andrews method—Stage 3

After the baby is born an injection of syntometrine (a mixture of oxytocin and ergometrine which stimulates contractions) is given and the midwife delivers the placenta by pulling on the cord with one hand and pushing the uterus up with the other, once she is sure separation has occurred. This is called the Brandt–Andrews method. Most hospitals in Britain no longer allow a natural third stage where the placenta separates and the woman pushes it out on her own, because there is a higher risk of bleeding.

72. Shrinking of the uterus after delivery

The uterus will begin to shrink naturally after delivery, getting back to a size it has not been for many months. This causes minor "after-birth" pains for a few days. If the infant feeds immediately at the breast, this will help contract the uterus as well. The uterus is back to normal size by six weeks after delivery.

73. Many women prefer to have some anaesthetic during labour

Natural childbirth is much praised in our time, and for many women, it is everything they hoped for. However, if you happen to feel the need during your labour, remember that there are a number of analgesics and anaesthetics which can ease your pain and still not interfere with the baby's well-being or your own enjoyment of the birth. *If you find you cannot go through childbirth totally unsedated, don't feel ashamed or guilty.* Your pain threshold is yours alone, and only you know what you are going through. Don't stand for your partner (who feels expert since he came along to all your natural childbirth classes) saying "Your friend Millicent had natural childbirth; what's the matter with *you*?" There's nothing the matter with you. There is something the matter with people who think all women are alike.

74. Pain relief during labour

a. *Recommendation: General anaesthetics should not be used during a normal delivery.* First, when a woman is asleep, she cannot push when she needs to and otherwise help her labour along. Second, general anaesthesia puts the baby to sleep too, may depress its breathing after birth, or slow down its heart rate, decreasing the oxygen supply to the brain during birth. Third, a sleeping baby and a sleeping woman can prolong labour unnecessarily, increasing the risk of unnecessary complications, requiring the use of unnecessary outside aids, such as forceps. Finally, if you are asleep when the baby is born, you are cutting yourself off from one of life's more indescribable joys. General anaesthesia should be reserved for emergencies.

b. *Analgesics:* Early in the first phase of labour, a woman who needs pain relief can receive a narcotic by injection. Tranquillizers such as Valium are only used if the woman has high blood pressure or is very anxious, as they pass to the baby and may interfere with feeding for as long as ten days after birth. The narcotic makes it possible to relax or even doze off between contractions without actually going to sleep. Too much sedation can lengthen the latent phase, so bear with the early labour if possible. If given too close to the time of delivery, narcotics may cause a baby to have a low Apgar score. (See No. 88 below)

c. *Epidural anaesthesia* (eh-pee-DUR-ral) is an option for woman entering the active (dilation) phase of labour. (Stage 1-B, No. 65 above) A needle is inserted into her back, *near the spinal canal but not into it.* Then a small plastic catheter is inserted into the epidural space, and the anaesthetic is injected through it. It will make a woman feel numb from the waist down and should almost completely relieve the pain of labour and delivery. Epidural anaesthesia should not be confused with a spinal block, in which anaesthetic is injected into the fluid of the spine, causing a temporary paralysis. With epidural anaesthetic, a woman can usually still move.

Epidural anaesthesia is a technique which requires a lot of training and is not always successful. Some obstetricians can handle it, but in most places, an anaesthetist will be needed. When the anaesthetic is being given, great care must be taken that the catheter is not inserted in the spinal fluid; for this reason, a test dose is inserted first, to make sure the right area has been located.

WARNING: *The anaesthetics injected through the catheter are in the xylocaine or lignocaine family, so if you know from your experience with the dentist that you are allergic to this type, tell your doctor first. A substitute anaesthetic material can be found.*

As the lower extremities become numb, blood pressure may decrease. To guard against this possibility, a woman will have fluid running intravenously into her arm throughout the procedure, maintaining volume in her blood vessels. She should not lie flat on her back, and foam wedges are used to tilt the body.

One relatively frequent problem with epidural anaesthesia is a definite increase in the number of patients who require forceps delivery; lacking feeling below the waist, they can't bear down and push the baby out as well. Episiotomy is also more frequently needed with epidural anaesthetic. A woman should remember that even though she will feel no pain, she will feel a pulling sensation when the baby is delivered.

d. *Caudal anaesthesia* is essentially the same as epidural anaesthesia, except that it is administered lower in the back in the region of the tailbone. It is useful for delivery but not for the first stage of labour.

e. *Gas* can be given to a woman in light doses in the second stage of labour, to lessen the pain without putting her out. This is given by the woman herself who places a mask periodically over her own mouth and nose. The gas used is Entonox which is 70 per cent nitrous oxide and 30 per cent oxygen.

f. *Saddle block* is an injection of anaesthetic into the spinal canal which numbs only those areas of the pelvis that would touch the saddle if you were riding a horse. It is usually given when a woman goes out of the labour room into the delivery room. Low blood pressure is a risk here as well, and intravenous fluid must be used to prevent it.

g. *Pudendal block* (pew-DEN-dal): The pudendal nerve supplies sensation to the perineum (per-ee-NEE-um), the area around the vagina and the vulva. A pudendal block is a series of two injections given just prior to delivery, just inside the vagina into the pudendal nerve on each side. This numbs the lower third of the vagina and the external genitals. For forceps deliveries and for episiotomy, it provides excellent relief.

75. In the labour ward

If you are going to have your baby in hospital, take a look at the delivery room while you are pregnant. Most of the time, unfortunately, it will be a bare and spiritless place—blank walls, nothing to divert the eye; a large clock, ticking loudly, which guarantees that time is your primary companion. Some hospitals have begun to realize that this is the worst environment for labour—silent, lonely, and starkly oppressive—and have actually built bright new wings for maternity care.

If your hospital has not already made an effort to warm up the room, bring your own diversions. Bring magazines to look through between contractions; bring a radio with earpiece and set it on the all-music (not the all-news) station; bring your partner and make sure he knows when he should talk to you. Bring a crossword puzzle or a deck of cards. Diversions make the time go faster. If you just lie there, timing your contractions, listening to the clock ticking, the time—and the pain—will be unnecessarily burdensome.

Talk to the midwives and doctors who come to check you periodically so that you know what your progress is. If they are cold or uncommunicative or pleasant and helpful, inform the hospital administrators when you go home with your newborn baby. Like other institutions that serve the public, hospitals are sensitive to what they hear. It will certainly improve the environment of maternity wards if you take the trouble to criticize a bad performance by hospital staff and heap praise on a good one. A thank-you letter is appreciated more than a box of chocolates.

76. Back labour

Some women feel the pain of labour most acutely in the lower back; this may mean that the baby's head is coming into the pelvis in a posterior position (with the baby facing forwards instead of backwards). This is nothing to worry about. The position of the head will rotate, usually by the latter part of the first stage.

77. Recommendation: It is a good idea to involve men in labour and in delivery

At one time, husbands were virtually never invited into the delivery room. Now they are often included in the birth process at the request of the mother. If your hospital refuses to allow men to attend the birth of their children, find this out early in pregnancy, when there is time to choose another hospital. Likewise, if your doctor refuses to allow your man to be with you, and you disagree, thrash out the issue early in pregnancy so, if you must, you have time to find another doctor.

A man needs some preparation for labour. Almost all natural childbirth classes encourage the presence of the man as well. If you expect your partner to be with you, make sure he knows generally what to expect; it will be something of a surprise to him anyway. Try to be understanding if he cannot stand to see you in pain and runs away when the going gets rough. And don't let your man, high on a little bit of knowledge, become the "expert" on your labour. He is part of the supporting cast. *You* are the star.

78. Fetal monitoring with ultrasound is a must for high-risk pregnancies; but its use for all pregnancies is highly debatable

A fetal monitor is a relatively new electronic device which monitors the strength and frequency of contractions as well as the fetal heart beat. Two "receivers" are strapped around the mother's abdomen and transmit to heated pens which record on special paper what is going on inside the belly. Newer machines may have a small screen. One measures the contractions and the other the fetal heart rate. It gives hospital personnel added information about the baby's heartbeat and general progress during labour. For the woman, it is a rather cumbersome device and can be annoying during labour. Later on in labour, part of the device can be replaced by a small clip that can be attached to the baby's scalp, and this is more comfortable for the woman. A new device (a telemetry unit) allows the woman to walk around once the scalp clip is applied. Recording takes place on a machine up to 400 yards (360 metres) away. At other times a pressure transducer is placed inside the uterus to measure the intensity of the contractions. The fetal monitor shows two patterns:

   a. the fetal heart rate and

   b. the frequency and strength of the contractions of the uterus.

Certain patterns in the baby's heart rate may suggest that not enough blood and oxygen are getting to the brain. In these cases, if oxygen administration and change of the mother's position do not work, a Caesarean section would be advisable.

Fetal monitoring is necessary for women who have high-risk pregnancies—such as diabetics, or women with hypertension. (See No. 156 below) Women who are having induction of labour with Syntocinon (oxytocin) should be monitored to make sure the contractions are not too strong or too close together. If you have any complications of pregnancy, it would be best to have monitoring in labour. If your labour is normal, there is no good evidence that fetal monitoring is better than using the fetal stethoscope.

As far as the safety of ultrasound, which is used to monitor the heart rate, most experts say that it is very safe; others question whether routine use is really acceptable. There are rare reports of minor scalp infections from the clips. *Watch for reports* on the pros and cons of routine fetal monitoring.

79. Fetal blood sampling

If mild irregularities in heart rate are noted on the monitor, a tiny sample of blood may be taken from the scalp of the baby and tested for acidity and oxygen content. If the baby's blood is too acid or too low in oxygen, the diagnosis is fetal distress—and a Caesarean section should be performed to avert the possibility of brain damage, which might occur if the decreased oxygen flow were allowed to continue.

80. Artificial rupture of the membranes (bag of waters)

Sometimes during labour, a quantity of amniotic fluid collects in front of the baby's head and, rarely, prevents the head from descending into the pelvis. In these cases the obstetrician or midwife may rupture the membranes with a sterile instrument. This procedure does not have to be done routinely, for in most cases the membranes will break naturally. Some doctors even believe that the routine practice is dangerous and may increase the chances of fetal distress (Ref. 1). However, it may accelerate contractions that have slowed late in labour. Also, if there is any fetal distress it is useful to see if the fluid is clear and apply a monitoring scalp clip.

81. Labour should not be induced for the sake of convenience

Labour can be induced by the administration intravenously (through a vein in the arm) of oxytocin, which stimulates contractions. This is the same preparation used to stimulate stronger contractions when a woman has been in labour a long time with irregular contractions.

This procedure should be saved for special circumstances, and

146

avoided otherwise.

Elective induction is when the mother wants to have her baby on a specific day. Make sure that doctors do not suggest induction because it is more convenient for them. This kind of reordering of the priorities of life is not recommended, since induction may involve a certain amount of extra risk to the fetus. One of the major risks of elective induction is prematurity: if someone has miscalculated the dates, labour may be induced too early. Also, induction may fail and the woman may have to be delivered by Caesarean section.

Medically indicated inductions may occur when the risk for continuing the pregnancy to term is too great either for mother or child. Induction might also be indicated for a woman with a history of very fast deliveries who suspects she might not make it to the hospital in time, or when a woman is two or more weeks late.

82. Forceps are for special cases only

Every effort should be made to allow the mother to deliver the child naturally, without any outside assistance. However, in some cases, forceps—various instruments which help pull the baby's head further into the birth canal—are helpful and necessary.

If a woman has epidural or general anaesthesia, her body may be too relaxed to bear down in the final stage of labour and push the baby out. A doctor may have to assist the baby by pulling its head an inch or two lower with forceps. This should only be resorted to when the baby's head is very low in the pelvis.

When the baby's head is still up in the mid-pelvic area, the forceps should only be used in special or emergency cases—for example, if the fetal heart rate becomes suddenly irregular, indicating that the baby is in distress and the birth process must be speeded up right away. Another situation requiring forceps would be a prolonged second stage of labour. Generally, it is considered dangerous to the infant if labour continues for more than two to three hours after the cervix is completely dilated.

Forceps may leave red marks or swellings on the cheeks of the baby, which should disappear in a few days.

83. Anxiety may complicate labour

It seems that the higher the woman's level of anxiety during labour, the more likely she is to have an abnormal labour. It is a relatively simple matter to avoid extreme anxiety during labour; use the nine months you are given to prepare for it by reading and learning relaxation exercises for labour.

84. The baby's environment immediately after delivery

Doctors should not slap a baby's bottom when it is born. If the mother is awake, she can hold the baby immediately. If the baby wishes to breast-feed immediately, that is fine; it will help contract the uterus. The baby may make a loud cry after it is born, or a small noise, or no noise; medical supporters will check the baby's vital signs in all cases, and make sure that it is all right. If a woman has had general anaesthesia, the baby may be asleep when delivered—and in that case, the midwife or doctor may go to some lengths to wake the baby up, to make sure that it does not "forget" to breathe.

RECOMMENDATION: *Discuss Leboyer's theories with your obstetrician.* (Ref. 2) The French obstetrician Leboyer has brought forth a whole set of theories on how to calm the environment in which the baby is born; to create a pleasant, tensionless atmosphere in which there is no loud noise, no extreme of temperature, no machinery, no forceps. As long as neither baby nor mother has a problem, this or a modification of it is the recommended method of delivery. (It remains to be proved, however, that this type of delivery makes the child grow stronger and healthier, as Leboyer contends.)

On the other hand, if there is a problem, the machinery—such as fetal monitoring and forceps—may be critical to the baby's well-being, and should be available just in case.

85. Home delivery is usually safe, but not always so

If a woman wants to have her baby at home, she should make sure there is hospital backup within minutes of her house. Some of the major risks in pregnancy occur just at the time of delivery—for example, postnatal haemorrhage or fetal distress—and *they cannot be adequately handled outside a hospital.* Obviously, there are excellent reasons for wanting to have a baby at home, where everybody loves you and the environment is warm and welcoming. But for the occasional woman and the occasional baby who gets into trouble, home delivery can be dangerous. Discuss this with your doctor. In general, it may be more productive for women to press for hospitals to be made more like home.

86. Midwives

For generations, the people who helped women deliver their babies were midwives—other women skilled and experienced in childbirth. In Britain, 80 per cent of deliveries are still supervised by midwives, although antenatal care now centres on doctors and hospitals. Some midwives work in the community and do home deliveries. They may be attached to a group family doctor practice. Some are based in the hospital where they may deliver the woman and take her home six hours later. If your own doctor and local hospital are unhelpful about home or short hospital stay delivery, contact your district community physician's office. In Britain there is a group called Radical Midwives who fight for the right of women to decide when and how they want to give birth. A few midwives practise privately and will supervise home deliveries.

All midwives work in collaboration with a doctor or medical team, although they differ from other nurses in being practitioners in their own right. They are able to prescribe drugs and carry out procedures without reference to a doctor.

87. Emergency delivery

Sometimes a woman goes into labour very quickly, and the labour is so rapid she simply has no time to get to the hospital and the physician or midwife who was supposed to help her with the delivery is unable to get to her quickly enough. In these cases dial 999. The ambulance will come immediately. Any ambulance attendant and almost any police officer have emergency training sufficient to assist at the delivery of a baby.

In most areas, there is a flying squad which will come out from the local hospital. This consists of an obstetrician, midwife, paediatrician, incubator, delivery pack and supplies of blood. If you are bleeding profusely at home, it is important that the squad should come to you. Do not try to travel, but tell the ambulance controller that you are pregnant and bleeding.

If no one can get to you fast enough, and you are alone when your baby is born, *don't panic*. The swiftness of the labour and delivery probably indicates that things are going *well*.

If you can, find a clean sheet and put it under you, so that the baby is born onto a clean surface. You can reach over and catch the child as it comes out.

Make sure the baby is breathing. Rub its back and/or throat and try to keep the baby's head down. This will help free the mucus secretions from nose and mouth so the baby can breathe easily.

If the child is not breathing, put your mouth over his nose and mouth and suck inward. This will help clear mucus. Then give the baby the kiss of life, about twenty to thirty puffs per minute.

Wrap the baby in something warm.

If you have time, tie the cord in the middle with any material available. This is not absolutely necessary, for the vessels in the cord will close off themselves after a few minutes. Usually the placenta will deliver itself within five to ten minutes. This can be assisted if the baby nurses at your breast. If the placenta seems slow in coming out, try bearing down; it may be in the vagina.

Also, it is important to rub your uterus through the abdomen so that it will contract and make the bleeding minimal. Don't pull on the cord or you may break it and cause more difficulty delivering the placenta.

By this time, help should have arrived. Even if everything went well and your baby is fine, make sure you and the baby see a doctor afterwards.

Lightning-fast emergency births of this kind are frightening, but they can be handled if you keep your cool and remember throughout that *a fast delivery is usually a sign of good health* in both mother and child.

88. The Apgar score

Named after Virginia Apgar, the noted anaesthetist, this score is a way of evaluating the general health of infants immediately after birth. It scores an infant on heart rate, colour, cry, muscle tone and reflexes. The test is made one minute after birth and again five minutes after birth. A perfect score is 10; a fine healthy baby usually scores between 7 and 10. Babies born under general anaesthesia often score lower, and in fact, it was the application of this test which placed general anaesthesia into such discredit for routine deliveries. If a baby scores lower than 7 on the Apgar score, it may need some added treatment (oxygen)—but this only means that the baby is not in peak health at the time this is made; it does not necessarily forebode future ill health and should not be used for prognosis unless there is later evidence that the baby is not well. The baby will be watched more closely by paediatric staff if the Apgar score was low.

NORMAL POSTNATAL COURSE

89. Normal postnatal care

The postnatal period begins after delivery of the placenta and lasts six to eight weeks. The care that a woman gives herself at this time, when her body is gradually returning to its non-pregnant state, is vital for her general health in the future.

90. Two to eight days in the hospital is the normal stay

Most women who have had normal first deliveries remain in hospital for seven or eight days afterwards. For subsequent births,

150

a stay of 48 hours is often all that is required.

Walk as soon as you feel well enough, to improve circulation and speed healing.

Urinate and move your bowels as soon as possible. It is normal to need a laxative in the first few days, for the pressure of the baby's head on the rectum during delivery may have left rectal muscles sore and stretched. If you have had an episiotomy, you may be afraid to defaecate, for fear of tearing the stitches. Usually, this fear is groundless, for the incision does not extend into the rectum except in rare instances. (If it does, your doctor should tell you.)

Follow your own preference when deciding how long to stay in the hospital. Keep these considerations in mind:

a. Is the baby strong enough to go home, away from the surveillance of the medical staff? Do you feel able to cope? Community midwives call daily for the first ten days.

b. The baby must have a blood test on the second or third day of life. Midwives will take blood from the baby's heel at home if you are discharged earlier. (This test is to check for the disease phenylketonuria, which causes mental retardation. It is called the Guthrie test.)

c. Will you have assistance at home if you leave earlier than three days?

d. Are there other children at home who are unlikely to understand that their mother needs extra rest at this point? Many women find that they need the breather away from busy family life.

91. Recommendation: "Rooming in" is the best postnatal arrangement

"Rooming in" means that the baby stays with the mother after delivery, and usually that the father can visit at any time. The alternative is to keep the babies separate from the mothers, to bring them to the mothers only at "feeding time", every four hours, and requires that fathers observe strict visiting hours. While you are pregnant, check which method is used in your hospital. A woman who has had a baby is not sick; she should not be separated from her baby as though she were sick; a well father should not be separated from his baby. "Rooming in" satisfies family emotional needs and dissipates the feeling that the postnatal days are somehow post-operative days. Most hospitals do allow rooming in now, but if you want your baby with you all night, you may have to argue about it.

92. Lochia: postnatal bleeding

Lochia (LOW-key-a) is a normal postnatal bleeding. For the first two to three days after delivery it is quite red: small clots are normal; large clots are not. The amount of flow may increase when a woman nurses her baby, for the uterus usually contracts during breast-feeding. (See No. 98 below) From one to two weeks, the bleeding becomes thin and pinkish; this then changes to a whitish-tan discharge (still a form of lochia) which generally lasts no more than another two weeks. The first menstrual period should occur six to eight weeks postnatal, unless a woman is breast-feeding. (Breast-feeding may delay the renewal of menstruation. (See No. 101 below) Lochia should not smell foul; it has a distinct odour, like that of menstrual blood. But if it smells really bad, this may signify infection. See a doctor.

93. Care after episiotomy

The pain of an episiotomy depends on the size and location of the incision and the number of stitches that were taken. The stitches will either absorb themselves or may fall out fifteen to twenty-one days after delivery. The pain will let up in two or three days, and the best way to relieve it is with hot water; try salt water baths, or stand in the shower, spread your buttocks and let the water run on the stitches. Perineal tightening exercises help the healing. (See No. 96 below)

It is also a good idea to take a look at your episiotomy with a hand mirror. First of all, this reassures you that it is healing. Secondly, it reassures you that the incision is not right in the anus (it sometimes *feels* as though it is there) so that the psychological trauma of moving your bowels will be relieved. Some hospitals do "routine" episiotomies for first births. Not all women need these cuts, so ask your doctor to make a note in your record not to do an episiotomy unless really necessary.

94. Sexual activity after delivery

Obviously sexual activity other than intercourse can resume immediately after delivery. Normal intercourse should feel comfortable two to three weeks after: if episiotomy pain interferes, wait for further healing. Birth control should be started as soon as sexual intercourse is—your partner should *use a condom* if you are still bleeding. As long as lochia is present, the cervix is still open, and only a condom or abstinence will protect against infection. WARNING: *Never imagine that you are not fertile after delivery.* Some women (and they can never be sure who they are) start to

152

ovulate again very quickly. Even breast-feeding is not a reliable protection for everyone. *Don't take any chances: use birth control.*

95. Postnatal "blues"

A lot of women feel depressed after delivery, probably aggravated by hormonal changes. It may seem odd that a blessed event should make you miserable, but if it is any comfort, you should remember that writers often feel that way after they finish their great novels and swimmers often feel that way after they have won their great races. You will probably snap out of it in two to three days. If the depression lasts for weeks, or interferes with sleep, then something else may be wrong; seek help.

96. Postnatal exercises

Many exercises taught at childbirth classes before delivery can help retone your abdominal muscles after delivery.

a. If you have had an episiotomy, put off strenuous exercising until three to four weeks after delivery.

b. *Exercises for the abdominal muscles:* Sometimes after delivery the abdominal muscles will separate, leaving a woman with what seems like a hernia at the midline of her stomach. The following exercises, done daily, will pull the muscles back together again. Lie on your back, lift your legs and lower them slowly to a count of ten or fifteen, one leg at a time with the other knee bent. Do sit-ups—lie on your back, lift head and shoulders off the floor.

c. *Exercises for the muscles of the perineum* (the area between the anus and the vulva): These can begin almost immediately after delivery and include stopping and starting the urinary stream each time you urinate, and tightening the muscles 'underneath' (pelvic floor) and pulling them up instead towards the navel.

97. Breast-feeding

The very best food for most newborns is mother's milk, and it is a pity that so few women are breast-feeding today. Breast-feeding is also convenient; no bottles, no mixing, no boiling, no cost (other than the cost of a good diet). Although some babies are allergic to cow's milk, virtually none are allergic to mother's milk. Breast milk is better absorbed than other milk, and some studies show that breast-fed babies are less obese throughout life since they control their own food intake. Important antibodies to fight infections are passed from mother to baby in the milk. Breast-feeding provides contraception (not 100 per cent safe) for as long as it is continued as the only form of feeding for the baby (an advantage for women whose religious beliefs prohibit contraceptives). Finally, psychological studies have shown positive effects from early and prolonged contact between mother and baby. If you can't breast-feed, hold and play with the baby at feeding times. Don't just prop her in a pram with a bottle. It is not only unrewarding; it is dangerous because she may choke.

Any woman who is interested in breast-feeding should do it; and if she isn't interested, she should try to be. True, other children, even a husband, may feel jealous; mothers from the generation that gave up breast-feeding entirely may object; a certain amount of outdated social convention may suggest that breast-feeding is somehow "primitive". However, it is possible to breast-feed, even in public places, without exposing the breast and offending anybody.

If you work outside the home you may be unable to get home, and feed: but even in this case breasts may be pumped and expressed milk stored to be administered by bottle. If you decide that breast-feeding is not for you, don't feel bad; there are several very good premixed formulas on the market.

RECOMMENDATION: There are scattered reports of environmental pollutants appearing in breast milk. *Don't let that deter you from breast-feeding.* Prepared milk undoubtedly has its own pollutants.

RECOMMENDATION: If you are not breast-feeding, keep your breasts tightly bound in a bra or breast binder to prevent the collection of milk in the breasts. Cut down slightly on your fluid intake. Lying in a hot bath allows the milk pressure to be relieved.

98. How breast milk is produced: prolactin, oxytocin, and colostrum

Prolactin is a hormone produced by the pituitary which triggers production of milk in the breasts. Normally, it is inhibited by substances secreted by the hypothalamus. But after delivery, there is an effect on the hypothalamus which stops the prolactin-inhibiting process and allows prolactin to be released, producing milk.

As the baby sucks, more prolactin is released—and more milk produced.

The milk is formed in the glands of the breasts; it is transported to the nipples through many ducts. This process is called the "let-down" of milk to the nipples. The hormone that triggers let-down is *oxytocin,* also produced by the pituitary gland. Suckling causes further release of oxytocin, and increased let-down of

154

milk. (Oxytocin also causes the contractions of the uterus felt during breast-feeding.)

Colostrum, a very nutritious, watery substance, is the advance signal of milk production. During the last few weeks of pregnancy, it usually leaks from the nipples. It is important that the infant nurses early, when colostrum is still present, because it contains antibodies from the mother that protect the infant against infectious illness.

99. Problems with "let-down" of milk

The most common problems with breast-feeding are with "let-down". If a baby doesn't suck hard enough, there may be insufficient oxytocin to stimulate adequate milk flow to the nipples. A woman who is very nervous or anxious may secrete other hormones which inhibit oxytocin production. Mild sedatives, or an alcoholic or milky drink before feeding have been known to help in this case. In addition, nasal sprays of oxytocin may give the needed extra push. Once the baby is breast-feeding regularly, and suckling energetically, then "let-down" is continuous and sure. The first day or two of nursing are usually the toughest, if there is any problem at all.

100. Do not smoke or take drugs while breast-feeding, and watch what you eat

a. The nicotine in cigarettes passes through the milk. Don't pass these poisons to your baby or assail her sensibilities with this relatively strong substance. (See p. 253)

b. Do not take drugs while breast-feeding. If you must, check with your doctor to make sure it will not have an adverse effect on your baby. Do not take oral contraceptives while breast-feeding.

c. Diet during lactation should be similar to that in pregnancy:

1. high in all the nutritious foods,

2. especially high in calcium and the B vitamins (except vitamin B-6 which, in high doses, may inhibit lactation). Drink lots of fluid because you are losing so much in the milk.

d. If your baby is suffering from wind or colic, suspect your diet. Some foods, eaten by the mother, can aggravate the child's stomach or cause wind—chocolate, cabbage, Brussels sprouts, broccoli and garlic are frequently distressing to nursing infants. Some doctors and health visitors suspect that products made from cows' milk cause wind in some babies. They suggest goats' milk products.

155

101. Breast-feeding as contraception

Breast-feeding provides a certain level of contraception, but not enough to rely on—so use a *mechanical* back-up method, a condom or diaphragm. Although women in many parts of the world breast-feed their babies for a year or several years, without supplementary food, women in the western world often start their babies on solid food earlier. As soon as you start adding other items to the baby's diet, the contraceptive effect of breast-feeding begins to diminish.

102. How to prepare breasts and nipples during pregnancy

During the last few months of pregnancy, a woman can prepare her nipples for the challenge of a nursing baby by rubbing them firmly with a towel, rolling the nipples between her fingers, then applying lanolin. These mild abrasions toughen the nipples so they will not be susceptible to fissures and cracks later on. This preparation is not necessary for all women, but helpful for many.

103. How to start breast-feeding

Start immediately after delivery or in the recovery room.

Breasts should not be tender unless they are engorged. It may hurt if the baby grabs only the nipple and not the whole areolar area (the dark area around the nipple). Break the suction with your finger and get her to start again with more of the areola in her mouth.

In the beginning, feed the baby frequently, every one and a half to three hours, as she demands. This stimulates milk production and let-down. Feed from both breasts each time, a short time on each side.

Plan ahead: Rooming in is best when breast-feeding. If you don't have the baby by you in hospital, the baby will be brought to you every four hours, just like children who are being bottle-fed. This means that milk comes into the breast less easily and not co-ordinated with the baby's needs. Women who breast-feed in this situation therefore tend to have more problems than those who have the baby by them and can feed their babies any time it is necessary. Keep the baby with you at night, certainly after the second day when the milk has come in. Sometimes the night staff feed all the babies in the nursery rather than wake the sleeping breast-feeding mothers.

Try not to feed the baby supplementary bottles during the first few weeks. Until her sucking is strong, she will find the bottle easier to get milk from and thus may learn immediately to prefer it.

156

104. Premature infants can be fed with breast milk

A premature baby is usually small and relatively weak and needs the best nutrition possible. *Breast milk is preferable to anything else.* The milk can be expressed out of the breasts by hand or with a pump and fed to the baby through a bottle or stomach tube. If you have your child prematurely, be sure to discuss this method of feeding with the doctor.

105. Breast-feeding has little effect on cancer

Some researchers claim that the virus which causes breast cancer and which is dormant in women is passed on to a baby through breast milk. Other researchers say that the incidence of all types of cancer is lower in people who were breast-fed as babies. Recent large studies have shown no significant difference between the two groups. It is currently believed that the effect of breast-feeding on breast cancer is probably not significant. (Ref. 3) (See p. 333)

106. Weaning from breast to bottle

Start with one feed a day from the bottle; continue this way for a week or more. Then gradually add more bottle feedings. The slow method is easier on the baby, and it helps avoid the problem of breast engorgement as less breast milk is used.

107. There are groups of nursing mothers in most areas of the country

If a woman plans to breast-feed she should find out about organizations of nursing mothers. The National Childbirth Trust and La Leche Leagues throughout the country are available to assist women during breast-feeding. Keep close contact with your doctor, midwife or health visitor or obstetrician if any problems arise. (See References)

Health visitors, who visit every baby when it is ten days old, give advice and support on feeding and all aspects of baby care.

ABNORMAL PREGNANCY AND CHILDBIRTH

108. Problems and abnormalities of pregnancy and birth

A number of things can go wrong for mother and child during pregnancy and delivery. Fortunately, they happen in a small minority of cases. Most can be anticipated with good antenatal care and handled successfully in a well-equipped hospital. But the possibility of complications should motivate any woman to have her children in or very near to a good hospital, with the direct or indirect supervision of a consultant.

109. Breech birth

In 4 per cent of all pregnancies, a baby moves into the birth canal feet first or behind first, instead of head first. This is called a *breech birth*. Its major problem is that the largest part of the baby—the head—comes *last*. When the head comes first, during labour, the baby's bones can mould themselves to fit the pelvis. When the head comes last, the thin parts of the baby's body come out easily, and then it is critical that the head comes out quickly, lest the baby be hurt. (In a breech birth only about three minutes remain for the baby's head to come out before the child is in real danger of brain damage from decreased oxygen flow.)

Even if the pelvis is wide enough for the baby to pass through in breech position, there is still danger to the child in this type of delivery. Damage to the nerves of the neck and arms is common, and so is *cerebral palsy*—various defects (ranging from small speech defects to total crippling) in motor power and coordination caused by damage to the brain during delivery. Many premature babies present by the breech and problems may be more related to this than to the delivery.

To avoid these dangers in a breech birth, doctors will often decide to turn the baby to the normal position around the 35th week of pregnancy. (See *external version,* No. 112) In other cases, a Caesarean operation is necessary. (See Caesarean section No. 135 below) Some breech babies can be delivered safely in carefully selected cases. (Ref. 4) Discuss this with your doctor.

110. Breech birth and other abnormal presentations can usually be detected at regular antenatal examinations or in early labour

Before twenty-eight weeks of pregnancy, the fetus is frequently in the breech position but usually will rotate around before delivery. If it does not, a woman can discuss the possible difficulties with her doctor beforehand. Sometimes ultrasound will be used to determine the size of the baby's head, and X-rays will be taken to determine the size of the bones of the pelvis to see if the baby will have trouble fitting through. Some doctors will advise an elective Caesarean if your first baby is a breech. Unless your pelvis is small or a bad shape, or the baby is very large, you can ask for a "trial of labour". This means that you will be allowed to go into labour and have contractions and dilatation of the cervix observed. If labour progresses well, you will be able to have a vaginal delivery. If the labour does not progress normally, an emergency Caesarean will be performed. Usually the woman fasts and blood is kept ready in case a Caesarean is necessary.

111. Other malpresentations

A "presentation" in obstetrical language is the way in which the baby presents itself over the cervix as it opens during labour. A "malpresentation" is any way that the baby has of entering the birth canal which is not the simple, head-first way. Many of the malpresentations require help during delivery or Caesarean section because it would be impossible to deliver a live, normal baby in that position. For example a transverse (shoulder) presentation means that the baby is lying horizontally across the mouth of the cervix. A compound presentation means that two parts are presenting together, for instance a hand and a foot.

112. External version

External version is the gentle manipulation of the fetus through the abdomen in order to turn an abnormal position such as breech into a head-first position. It is normally done around the 35th week of pregnancy in the antenatal clinic. There are dangers involved, such as the separation of the placenta, and it is important that it is done by a skilled doctor. It is less often done today, as many doctors think that they only succeed in turning those babies which were going to turn themselves anyway.

113. Twins

Twins occur in one in 80 British births. The rate is slightly higher for black families.

a. *Identical twins:* One egg is fertilized by one sperm and early in its development splits into two identical halves and becomes two identical people. In the uterus, the placenta are usually joined.

b. *Non-identical twins:* Two eggs are produced during ovulation and fertilized by two different sperm, producing two people who may look alike to any or no degree. In the uterus, the placentas are sometimes joined, sometimes not.

c. *"Siamese twins"* originally referred to twins from Thailand (then Siam) who were both joined at the rib cage. Today, the term refers to any twins who are joined at any point. This is a rare phenomenon and occurs because the split of the egg for identical twins has been incomplete.

Non-identical twinning is by far the most common type and is hereditary. Usually the parents have family histories of twins on either or both sides. In addition, it is more common in older women.

About 25 per cent of all twins are identical twins. This type of twinning is not hereditary and is not influenced by fertility drugs (see No. 114 below).

Most twins are non-identical and born healthy and normally through the vagina if both are presenting head first. A doctor hearing two heart-beats, feeling two heads, may be able to anticipate twins antenatally. Sometimes, one baby is concealed by the other and comes as a surprise at delivery. The uterus of a woman carrying twins will generally be bigger than that of a woman carrying one child. Breast milk should be sufficient to feed both babies.

114. Fertility drugs increase the chance of multiple births

Clomiphene citrate (a synthetic anti-oestrogenic compound) and gonadotropic hormones (see p. 106) increase the incidence of twins and multiple births by causing greater egg production and therefore multiple ovulation. This does not always happen, but if you are taking these drugs for fertility, be on the look-out for a multiple pregnancy.

115. Problems with twins and multiple births

a. *Prematurity* is the biggest problem with twins. Perhaps because the sheer size of the babies distends the uterus and creates excess pressure that triggers labour, most twins do *not* go to full term.

b. *Smallness*: Even if a woman carries twins to full term, they are likely to be smaller than other babies, simply because they have had to share the same uterus space and the same inflow of nutrition.

c. *Toxaemia* (see No. 149 below) is a greater danger to women carrying twins because of the greater metabolic demands on their bodies, as is

d *Anaemia* (see No. 144 below), red blood cell deficiency, caused by the increased nutritional drain on the mother.

e. *Complications in delivery* occur sometimes with the second-born of the twins, which usually comes within 15 minutes of the first. Most twins enter the world head first; the one lying farthest down in the womb exits, and the second follows. The second most common presentation among twins is that the first baby comes out head first, and the second baby is a breech birth. The diagnosis of twins can be made by ultrasound and usually the presentation of the two babies can be determined too. However, in some cases, an X-ray of the abdomen is needed to see which way the second baby is coming.

f. *Postnatal haemorrhage* is a greater danger in having multiple births because the uterus stretches and may have more difficulty shrinking.

g. *Emotional problems* seem to trouble identical twins as they grow older because it is hard, in a world where everyone else is at the very least unique, to be the same as someone. If a woman has had identical twins, she should be on the look-out for emotional crises and have the advice of people familiar with this syndrome when her children are still very young. The family should stress the individuality of the twins—dress them differently and refer to them singly.

116. A woman who knows she is having twins should be sure to have them in a hospital

Because the risks in multiple births are greater in general, home delivery will only compound an already risky situation.

117. Pseudocyesis: false or phantom pregnancy

This is one of those physiological phenomena whose roots seem to be totally psychological—at least, at our current stage of medical diagnosis. A woman is convinced that she is pregnant. Her periods cease. Her belly grows large. She has many of the discomforts of pregnancy. But she is not pregnant. Every other cause of the signs and symptoms of pregnancy must be ruled out, but then the woman and her doctor must consider the psychological factors. Usually, women who experience false pregnancy have conflicts about child-bearing; they want to be pregnant but they are afraid of pregnancy. Or they don't want to be pregnant but they wish they could satisfy the desire of husband or lover for a child. Infertile women who deeply want a child may also have a false pregnancy. Many cases occur among teenagers who for some deep-rooted reason wish to punish or frighten their parents or please their boy friends. Whatever the reasons, pseudocyesis is a serious emotional disorder and even if it ends of its own accord, it should be treated with psychological counselling. (For a good description of a pseudo-cyetic woman, read Edward Albee's play *Who's Afraid of Virginia Woolf?)*

118. Miscarriage—spontaneous abortion

Miscarriage is the death of the fetus and the passage of tissue and blood from the uterus before the 28th week of gestation. It is estimated to occur in 10–20 per cent of known pregnancies. At least 60 per cent of fertilized eggs are thought to be lost if one considers early abortions before the first period would have been missed. The signs of miscarriage are bad cramps and bleeding; if the miscarriage is occurring early, there may be very little bleeding—a woman may go to the bathroom and pass what seems to be a clot; this is the miscarriage. If you want to be sure that you have been pregnant, save the "clot" in a clean glass jar in the refrigerator, and take it to your doctor for examination. Sometimes, early abortions are caused by genetic abnormalities in the embryo.

For many women who are having problems with fertility, the conceptus simply isn't strong enough to hold on to the uterus, and miscarriages will occur repeatedly. (See p. 114) Heavy smokers have a higher incidence of miscarriage.

Sometimes what looks like the beginning of a miscarriage is just a little cramping and bleeding during the first few months, and the baby grows to term and is delivered safely. WARNING: *Do not take drugs to prevent miscarriage unless you have a specific infertility problem.* (See p. 105) *Most have not been proven effective and may be dangerous to the fetus.*

If you are bleeding significantly, more than during menstruation, get to a hospital immediately. If it is a smaller amount, ask your doctor for advice. Most miscarriages occur without complication, but a woman should be examined to make sure no fetal tissue remains inside the uterus thereby increasing the risk of bleeding and infection.

a. *Incomplete abortion* occurs when a woman is passing clots of tissue and her uterus is open, but the total conceptus does not pass out. She will probably need a D & C (see p. 317) to remove all fragments of tissue so that the womb will close and the bleeding will stop.

b. *Complete abortion* occurs when the whole conceptus is passed and the bleeding stops on its own. If an examining doctor finds no damage, then the woman can go home—no D & C is needed. Very early abortions are usually complete and those after four months can be checked accurately.

c. *Missed abortion* occurs when the fetus dies but does not pass out of the uterus. The uterus does not grow any more; the pregnancy test becomes negative, but the periods do not return as they would in a complete abortion. A D & C must be done to remove the conceptus.

STOP PRESS: Even moderate amounts of alcohol have recently been shown to increase the rate of spontaneous abortion.

119. Immature delivery: loss of the baby during the middle three months of pregnancy

Once a baby is past three months in the womb, its loss becomes more complicated. There are three major reasons why women lose babies up to six and a half months of pregnancy:

a. Maternal illness

b. Incompetent cervix, a condition whereby the cervix opens prematurely.

c. Severe genetic disorders in the fetus.

However, in many cases no clear reason is discovered.

120. Maternal illness (See High-Risk pregnancies No. 156 below)

If a woman becomes very sick during her pregnancy, this can upset the flow of nutrients to the fetus, causing it to die. Severe heart, kidney or liver disease can cause fetal death. However, other serious diseases may not affect the child. Sometimes, if the baby has been in the womb long enough, it can be delivered surgically or by induction, and kept well in an incubator until it is big enough to go home with its mother. This may be necessary (for example with certain diseases) to protect both mother and child. Congenital anomalies of the uterus, or large fibroid tumours, may prevent the uterus from stretching enough to house the baby. In these cases, a woman will usually go into labour and deliver a child prematurely. Paediatric intensive care units can do much to save and restore to health a baby born alive under these circumstances. If you have an illness that may complicate pregnancy, you must deliver in a hospital equipped with intensive care units for you and your child.

121. Incompetent cervix

The cause is unclear, but in some women the cervix loses its strength and begins to open up in the middle of the pregnancy—typically, at four to six months. There is no labour. Suddenly, a woman has the feeling that everything is "dropping out"—and it is. Sometimes the membranes break early and then labour begins.

The cervix should not open before twenty-eight to thirty weeks, even in women who have had many children. A woman who has a history of second-trimester losses should be examined *weekly* starting at twelve weeks, to see if the cervix is opening prematurely. If it does begin to open, she can go to the hospital and under anaesthesia the doctor can put a stitch in the cervix, to hold it closed so that the baby can grow to term. This is called *cerclage*. It is not foolproof, but it has allowed many women who would otherwise lose all their children to bear several normally. Two weeks before birth, or when labour begins, the stitch is cut, allowing the woman to deliver the baby. Rarely the stitch pulls out and has to be replaced later in the pregnancy. It is known as the Shirodkar stitch, after the Indian gynaecologist who invented it.

Once an incompetent cervix has been diagnosed, a woman should have the stitch placed at about fourteen weeks of each pregnancy. She should not wait to see if the cervix will open again—the likelihood is that it will. Early antenatal care is therefore, essential. Some doctors place the stitch while the woman is not pregnant, but this procedure is still being debated.

122. Genetic disorders (See Chapter Seven for complete discussion)

Fetuses with severe chromosomal or developmental disorders have a higher frequency of aborting in the first half of pregnancy. (See p. 131) Any fetus thus aborted should be studied in the lab to determine whether there was any gross disorder, for this will be pertinent to the way the mother and her doctor treat future pregnancies.

123. Ectopic pregnancy

Ectopic (eck-TOP-ic) pregnancy occurs when the fertilized egg implants elsewhere than in the uterus and begins to grow there. It is almost impossible for such a pregnancy to succeed. Ectopic pregnancies usually occur in the Fallopian tube (tubal preg-nancy)—98 per cent—but they can also occur in the ovary, cervix, and in very rare instances, in the abdominal cavity itself.

Tubal pregnancy is more common among women with damaged Fallopian tubes, either because of infection, venereal disease, endometriosis, corrective or exploratory tubal surgery, or an IUD. The incidence of ectopic pregnancy is between 1 in 150 and 1 in 300 pregnancies and may be as high as 1 in 90 live births in urban areas. Some doctors think the incidence is increasing, but others feel that the diagnosis is made more often in early cases because of the use of the laparoscope. The percentage of maternal deaths due to ectopic pregnancy has also risen to 9 per cent. Of the pregnancies that occur in women who have an IUD in place, about 10 per cent are ectopic. (See p. 62) Pregnancies after tubal ligation are more likely to be ectopic (see page 164) as are those which occur as failures of the mini-pill.

124. Symptoms and treatment of ectopic pregnancy

Frequently, the first sign of tubal pregnancy occurs when the fetus grows so large that it splits the tube and blood escapes into the abdominal cavity. This generally happens about six to eight weeks from the time of the last period and causes abdominal pain. Usually some slight vaginal bleeding has occurred. *Seek immediate attention for severe abdominal pain at any stage of pregnancy.*

Sometimes the ectopic pregnancy can be detected before it bursts. In these cases the woman may be having lower abdominal pains, and the doctor detects a mass on one side of the pelvis. An ectopic pregnancy must be differentiated from a corpus luteum which may also be swollen in early pregnancy, so a laparoscopic examination may be performed to look directly at the tube. (See p. 102)

If the laparoscope is unavailable, posterior colpotomy may be carried out to prevent an unnecessary abdominal operation. This is a process in which a needle is put through the vaginal wall into the abdominal cavity to see if there is blood there, indicating a pregnancy.

The surgical procedure usually is the removal of the Fallopian tube on the affected side. This may be achieved through an abdominal incision.

Some surgeons prefer to operate through the top of the vagina in specially selected cases, although this is rarely done in Britain.

Sometimes the conceptus (early pregnancy) can be squeezed out of the end of the tube and the tube repaired. This is the treatment of choice for unruptured tubal pregnancies, especially if one tube has been removed.

WARNING: *The ovary does not usually have to be removed in cases of tubal pregnancy. Many gynaecologists do this routinely. Make sure yours does not, unless the ovary has been damaged.* The loss of the Fallopian tube may be necessary, but the removal of the ovary with its supply of eggs and hormones is not.

Immunoglobulin should be given to all Rh negative women after ectopic pregnancies, as the woman may have been sensitized.

125. Emotional aspects of losing a baby

The loss of a baby through miscarriage or fetal death almost has to affect a woman emotionally; the psychological results may range from simple regret to morbid depression. Very often, the effect is delayed. In the rush and emergency of miscarriage, a woman has no time to think about what might have been. Weeks or months later, she may find herself terribly depressed and anxious. This is a kind of grieving; it may stem from the natural fear that, since one pregnancy aborted, others may not be successful. It is normal to feel very bad after losing a baby. Try and take other emotional pressures off yourself at this time. And if you cannot shake off the depression, seek professional help.

126. Pre-term delivery and low birth weight (LBW)—the greatest single danger to newborn babies

In the last decade it has been recognized that the old definition of prematurity, i.e. a baby weighing 2500g (5lb 8oz) or less at birth, included two different groups of babies. The first pre-term babies are those delivered too early—i.e. before the 37th week. The second group was of babies who were smaller than expected, called small or light for date babies (SFD). Some LBW babies are pre-term but normally grown and the problems they have are related to immaturity of the lungs, liver and nervous systems. The SFD babies which might have grown poorly are more likely to have congenital anomalies or mothers with high blood pressure and need early and frequent feedings, as they suffer from low blood sugar that can cause secondary brain damage. They are less likely to have jaundice and respiratory distress syndrome (RDS) if they are pre-term as well.

In England and Wales in 1979, the perinatal death rate—the number of stillbirths and deaths before one week—was 143 per 1000 births for premature babies who weigh less than 2500 g (5 lb 8 oz). This was nearly ten times the overall perinatal mortality rate of 14.7 per 1000 births. For even tinier babies—those weighing 1000 g (2 lb 3¼ oz) or less—the perinatal mortality rate was 558 per 1000 births.

127. Causes of pre-term delivery

The reason for the majority of these is unknown. The rate is highest in teenage mothers who are unsupported, smoke and are poor. Maternal disease may start a labour early or the doctor may advise induction or Caesarean section to save a baby if the mother's blood pressure is uncontrolled or severe bleeding has occurred. Nearly seven per cent of British women have their babies early.

128. Causes of small-for-date (SFD) babies

About 5 per cent of babies will be defined as SFD, but not all of these will have grown poorly. Some are naturally small because their parents are small. About a third are small because of a congenital defect, such as rubella damage and another third because the mother has hypertension or other chronic disease. The remainder have not grown well for unknown reasons. These babies may be identified antenatally and in suspected intra-uterine growth retardation, doctors may order serial ultrasound tests, urine oestrol examinations or other blood tests.

Doctors tend to err on the side of caution and subject many women to these tests. Don't panic if you have failed to gain weight or a new doctor says the baby is small. The chances are that no problems will be found after the tests.

A sudden drop in the daily number of movements of the baby may be serious so go to the hospital for a heart-beat test (CTG).

One thing you can do is stop smoking if you haven't already, eat well and rest a lot, lying on your side.

129. Problems encountered by LBW infants

a. *Heat loss.* Immature babies cannot control the mechanisms used by adults to maintain body temperature and, in addition, have a bigger surface area in relation to body weight. These babies are therefore nursed in an incubator kept at or near normal body temperatures.

b. *Lack of sucking, coughing and breathing reflexes.* Very immature infants may "forget" to breathe and are nursed with pressure sensitive receptors on the chest wall which lead to an alarm sounding if the baby fails to take a breath in a certain time. Babies born before the 28th week usually require a mechanical respirator to make sure the lungs fill. Lack of a cough reflex means that nose secretions must be sucked out regularly. Because the swallowing reflex may not be adequate until 32 weeks or even later, these babies may be fed milk by a tube inserted into the stomach via the nose. Very small babies may need intravenous feeding and a thin plastic tube is passed through the umbilical cord for this to be done.

c. *Immaturity of organ systems.* The lungs may not be prepared sufficiently for oxygen to pass through and the respiratory distress syndrome (RDS) is the biggest single problem for babies born before 32 weeks. Babies of diabetic mothers may have RDS even later than this. Controlled respiration, extra oxygen and keeping the baby warm at birth have improved these babies' chances of survival and lessen the rate of handicap due to lack of oxygen.

The liver enzyme systems may not be well developed and the baby may become jaundiced. Jaundice is caused by a pigment called bilirubin. Mild degrees of this are treated with ultra-violet light (the baby's eyes are bandaged to prevent damage), but severe jaundice requires exchange transfusion to prevent kernicterus. This is a condition in which the pigment (bilirubin) binds to the brain cells, and may be followed by cerebral palsy.

Infection is more common as the infant's resistance is not

developed. Most pre-term units give antibiotics to all babies.

Babies who have had severe neonatal jaundice should not be given whooping cough vaccine. Their hearing should be checked at 7–8 months.

130. Treatment for premature labour

If there is a reason for the onset of premature labour, such as bleeding or high blood pressure or if the baby seems small, it is better to let the labour progress.

If everything is straight forward and the waters are intact, it is reasonable to try and stop the labour so that the baby can grow more.

a. *Bed rest* with a sedative of a narcotic or tranquillizer may be used and stops labour in about half of all women. Few doctors use these drugs now because they may delay breathing in the newborn baby.

b. *Alcohol* given intravenously was used briefly in this country and about 60 per cent of women went out of labour. Severe headaches like a hangover were a problem and the practice has ceased.

c. *Prostaglandin antagonists* such as indomethacin have given slightly better results but some doubts have been expressed about the effect on the baby if the treatment fails (prostaglandins are important in the change from fetal to neonatal circulation once the umbilical cord is cut). Few units use this method.

d. *β-sympathomimetic agents* such as salbutamol and ritodrine are given intravenously. They block the nerve supply to the uterus and will stop labour for at least 24 hours in up to 80 per cent of women. The side effects, rapid heart beat and flushing, are unpleasant and in women with heart disease, the treatment can be dangerous. Oral treatment may be continued once the pains have ceased in women with a bad record of pre-term labour.

CAUTION: Despite the widespread use of these drugs in the UK and West Germany during the late seventies, the rate of pre-term delivery does not seem to have fallen. If the woman has bled, these drugs may be dangerous.

131. Steroid therapy and pre-term delivery

One study has shown that the babies of women treated for 24 hours with corticosteroids had a lower rate of RDS between 28 and 32 weeks gestation. Many hospitals in Britain try to stop labour for 24 hours to give these drugs. Long term and large scale studies have not been carried out, and some doctors think that the results may be a chance finding or because there were more SFD babies in the treated group.

WARNING: Discuss this with your doctor and do not accept the treatment if your blood pressure is high or the membranes are ruptured.

132. Premature rupture of amniotic membrane

If the bag of waters ruptures *before* the onset of labour, a woman who is near term will probably go into labour very shortly. If she does not, labour should be induced.

If the fetus is very small, however, when the membranes rupture, some doctors will try to forestall further leakage of amniotic fluid by instructing the woman to stay in bed, hoping that the pregnancy will continue for a few more weeks. The risk of this method of treatment is that once the membranes have broken the amniotic sac and the fetus may become infected. This risk must be weighed against the risk of prematurity in each individual case.

Premature rupture of membranes is usually without specific cause; sometimes it is associated with cervical infection, vaginitis, poor nutrition, or due to an incompetent cervix.

133. Steps to take if amniotic membranes rupture

If a woman finds herself leaking fluid without control (enough leakage so that it runs down her leg), she should call her doctor or get to a hospital immediately. WARNING: Some doctors will react by telling a woman to get into bed and stay there. Do not accept this advice. *Insist on being examined immediately,* to make sure that it is amniotic fluid which is leaking, and to make appropriate plans for managing the delivery of your child.

134 Artificial rupture of the membranes to induce labour

Artificial rupture of the membranes (ARM) is a common method of inducing labour when this is necessary. Some obstetricians wait 12–18 hours before setting up an oxytocin drip to make the uterus contract, as 75 per cent of women near term will go into labour naturally. Others set up the drip at the same time. Ask your doctor why he plans to do this, as the oxytocin-induced contractions are often more painful. Infection becomes more likely if the membranes have been ruptured for more than 24 hours before delivery and if labour lasts longer than this. Check if the hospital has a high induction rate. If it does, consider going to another one.

135. Caesarean section

Named after the delivery of Julius Caesar, who was reportedly cut from his mother's womb, a Caesarean (se-ZAIR-ian) section is the major surgical alternative to normal vaginal birth. If you or your baby get into trouble during delivery, it can be done as an emergency operation. If you have had a previous Caesarean section, the delivery can be planned. The delivery of one baby by Caesarean section does not mean that subsequent pregnancies must be by Caesarean, unless the pelvis is very small.

136. Incisions of the Caesarean section

An incision is made in the abdominal wall, either

a. horizontally, at the uppermost edge of the pubic hair, or

b. vertically at the stomach midline, (only done when speed is essential).

RECOMMENDATION: *If there is time to plan the Caesarean, ask for the horizontal incision.* It is usually stronger while healing, and later on will be almost invisible, camouflaged by the pubic hair. (It is known as a "bikini scar".) Ask for it if you are having any abdominal surgery, e.g. a hysterectomy or surgical removal of ovarian cysts.

137. Caesarean section procedure

The uterus is right in the middle of the abdomen, and easy to see after the incision. The intestines are *behind* the uterus, so they do not obscure the surgeon's view. The bladder must be pushed downwards, away from the uterus, so the incision can be made. (A catheter must be placed in the bladder before the operation to drain all the urine.) The incision is usually made horizontally, low in the uterus, in the area of the baby's head; the head is then pulled out and the rest of the body follows as in a vaginal delivery. The placenta is removed. The uterus is sewn back *in two layers.* The bladder is then placed back over the uterus and pinned there; then the abdomen is closed. The whole operation takes about an hour. The reason that the incision in the uterus is made as low as possible is that the uterine wall there is thinner and contains fewer of the major contracting muscles, making the scar stronger and healing easier. In addition, the lower scar makes it easier for a woman to have another pregnancy without the scar breaking. A vertical scar in the upper muscular part of the uterus may be necessary with *placenta praevia* (see No. 151b) or shoulder presentation. *Make sure to ask your doctor what type of scar is left in your uterus.*

Postnatally there is more pain, because there has been an abdominal incision, and postnatal contractions feel worse in an already sore belly. Because of the movement of the bladder during the operation it may be necessary to catheterize the bladder. Even after the catheter is removed, the woman may feel cramping when her bladder is full. Naturally, because of the healing of the abdominal incision, it takes longer to regain full strength.

Unless there is a real emergency, the operation can be done under an epidural anaesthetic. This means you can see and hold the baby immediately. By the first day a woman who has had a Caesarean section will be able to breast-feed if she desires.

138. When is Caesarean section necessary?

a.*Cephalopelvic (KEFF-al-lo-pelvic) disproportion* is a common cause for Caesarean section. This means that the baby's head is too big for the pelvis. Usually a woman will start off making good progress in labour and then the head fails to come down into the pelvis. A doctor who suspects this disproportion may order X-rays (pelvimetry) before making a decision to operate but these are frequently not required. In this case the operation saves the life of the child and the mother who might have died of this complication otherwise. (In underdeveloped countries, cephalopelvic disproportion is a common cause of infant and maternal mortality. The mother labours and labours; the baby, squeezed between the pelvic bones, dies; the uterus ruptures, the mother dies.)

Breech babies and other malpresentations are sometimes delivered by Caesarean section because of the fear that either the head or any other presenting part will not fit through the pelvis. (See No. 110-112 above)

b. *Fetal distress:* If fetal monitoring (see No. 78 above) shows that the baby's heart rate is severely depressed or irregular or if oestriol (See No. 173 below) values are very low and a woman's labour for some reason cannot be induced, then Caesarean section is indicated.

c. *Maternal illness:* Diabetes may be an indication for an elective Caesarean, as it is known that those babies cannot withstand shock. However, with better control of diabetes the woman is usually induced at 38 weeks. A Caesarean section is only then done if the baby is larger, has a malpresentation, or if there is another complication. Similarly, cardiac or other disease alone is not a reason for Caesarean section, but combined with an obstetrical problem it may be the best solution.

d. *Previous surgery on the uterus:* Women who have had fibrous tumours removed from the uterus (myomectomy) (see p. 327) and women who have had a hysterotomy incision for abortion (see

p. 320) are monitored carefully. They have a higher chance of Caesarean section, but the majority deliver normally.

139. Anaesthesia for Caesarean section

In an emergency, when the woman does not already have an epidural anaesthetic in place, general anaesthetic will be used. An epidural or spinal anaesthetic can be used if there is no rush about the surgery. (See No. 74 above)

140. Caesarean section can be performed repeatedly on the same woman

Until only a few years ago, doctors believed a woman could only have three Caesarean section deliveries. Today, advances in surgical technique permit a woman to have several more babies in this manner. Usually, if there was a good reason for the first Caesarean section, the same reason will motivate the next one: for example, cephalopelvic disproportion. However, in some cases—for example, if a section has been done because of fetal distress—a woman may be able to deliver her next child normally, with careful monitoring. Discuss this with your doctor. Make sure you know what type of incision is in your uterus. The low incision makes labouring safer. *Never consider labour and delivery outside hospital if you have had a previous Caesarean section.*

141. Delivery by Caesarean section is increasing

The percentage of babies delivered by Caesarean section has been increasing and is now nearly 7 per cent of all deliveries. A major reason for this increase is the widespread use of fetal monitoring and the detection of abnormalities in the fetal heart rate. It is very difficult to say whether all of these procedures are necessary. One must approach the subject with an open mind at this time. Caesarean sections are done in an effort to prevent a decrease in blood flow and oxygen to the brain (as suggested by abnormal heart rates on the monitor). The major problem is that no one really knows how severe damage will be if an abnormal pattern lasts for a prolonged period of time. Most doctors and their patients are not content to wait and see, once an abnormal pattern is detected.

The other major factor in the increase is that, today, many abnormally presenting infants (e.g. breech) are delivered by Caesarean section. This has substantially reduced the neonatal death rate and brain damage among such babies. (See No. 109 above)

172

142. Postmaturity

There is nothing to the old wives' tale that no pregnancy lasts longer than 40 weeks. About 1 in 11 does. This is nerve-racking for the mother, whose perceptions of the day she conceived are now being challenged by everybody. In most cases, she will go into normal labour and have a normal child without problems. The only time that postmaturity is a danger is when the function of the placenta begins to decline. The baby actually begins to lose weight in the womb and may die. If a pregnancy lasts two weeks past its expected termination, a doctor will check the oestriol (an oestrogen) in the woman's urine and will do some stress testing to make sure the placenta is still functioning normally. (See No. 174 below) If placental function is declining and the woman is still not having her baby, labour will be induced.

Women who conceive immediately after stopping oral contraceptives often ovulate late and go past term. These are not postmature.

143. Hyperemesis gravidarum—pernicious vomiting of pregnancy

A great many women experience nausea and vomiting routinely during pregnancy. (See No. 28 above) However, in a few cases, vomiting is continual; the woman begins to lose weight steadily; she becomes dehydrated. Food and sometimes the mere mention of food make her sick. If the continual retching tears the lower part of the oesophagus (the lower throat) she may vomit blood. Sometimes, the woman becomes jaundiced. Any or all or these symptoms distinguish normal vomiting from pernicious vomiting. An additional sign is that the drugs usually given to control vomiting do not work at all.

Hyperemesis (hy-per-EM-eh-sis) gravidarum (gra-vi-DAR-um) usually starts in the second month—at the same time that normal nausea and vomiting start. The treatment is hospitalization, intravenous fluids to build up her strength again and sedation so that her stomach muscles relax out of the spasms that accompany vomiting. She gets no food by mouth for several days, then gradually is started on fluids, then solids.

As with many diseases, hyperemesis gravidarum may have both psychological and physiological causes, and the relative importance of the two causes is not known. The condition can be successfully treated medically, however, and a few days in hospital are needed.

144. Anaemia—iron deficiency

Anaemia—deficiency in red blood cells—is more common in pregnant women, because greater demands are being made on the blood supply for the nutrition of the fetus.

Most anaemias of pregnancy are related to deficiency in iron. If, as is often the case, a woman has low iron stores to begin with, the extra strain of pregnancy may cause her to become anaemic. (See p. 356) To avoid anaemia before it begins, some doctors think that pregnant women should take an iron supplement. (See No. 19 above) Some women cannot take pills, or liquid supplemental iron, or their bodies cannot absorb iron in this form. In these cases, the iron can be given by injection, but this has side effects. Iron deficiency in pregnancy is a possibility in all women. Particularly affected are those women who have had a child during the previous two years, or women who just don't eat well. Women with a good diet and light periods may not need iron tablets.

145. Folic-acid deficiency anaemia in pregnancy

A simple blood test will frequently tell which kind of anaemia you have. In iron deficiency, the red cells are very small; in folic-acid deficiency, they are usually large. Of course, the two causes may exist together and the distinction would be impossible. An additional blood test for folic acid can be done.

Folic acid is found in leafy green vegetables and liver. Most pregnant women show a marked decrease in folic acid by the last trimester, no matter how well they have been eating. Some specialists believe that folic-acid deficiency may cause premature detachment of the placenta (see No. 151c below, Abruptio placenta), pre-eclampsia (see No. 149 below), and infant anomalies. Folic-acid deficiency severe enough to cause these problems is very rare, and affects only the very undernourished women. REMEMBER: Even if you do not need iron tablets, you may need extra folic acid unless your diet is very good.

146. Effects of anaemia in pregnancy

It is rare in this country (but common in poorer nations) for anaemia to be so pronounced in a pregnant woman that her baby is affected. Mostly the effect is on the mother. She may suffer from fatigue, get headaches, or palpitations of the heart, for it pumps harder when there is less haemoglobin available to carry oxygen to the baby. If a woman is suffering normal shortness of breath and dizziness, these may be aggravated by anaemia.

147. How to prevent anaemia in pregnancy: eat well!

To prevent anaemia eat plenty of liver and green leafy vegetables and take supplements of iron and folic acid. If you become anaemic anyway, you may have a different form of anaemia and this should be tested. (See p. 356) *Adolescent mothers* (see p. 28) are prime targets for severe anaemia because teenagers as a group eat rather poorly to begin with. If you know any teenage girl who is pregnant and have any influence on her at all, make sure she gets excellent antenatal care and eats wisely.

148. Urinary-tract infections

Between 5 and 10 per cent of pregnant women show bacteria in their urine, and 25 per cent of these women will develop symptoms of kidney or bladder infection. (See p. 307) There is a higher incidence in pregnancy because as the uterus grows, it presses on the ureters (the tubes that carry urine from the kidney to the bladder) which are already sluggish and dilated because of the rise in hormone levels during pregnancy. Infection is more likely in the stagnated urine. The symptoms of these urinary tract complications are burning and pain on urination, and urinary frequency. The additional symptoms of kidney infection are often high fever and pain in the back, under the ribs. Treatment is by antibiotics—and if there are any such symptoms, treatment should be sought immediately.

149. Pre-eclamptic toxaemia (PET)

Literally, toxaemia (tox-EE-me-a) means blood poisoning. In pregnancy, this is characterized by hypertension (high blood pressure) and some kidney changes, with or without oedema or swelling.

150. Treatment of toxaemia in pregnancy

The best treatment for toxaemia is good antenatal care, so that it can be detected quickly and treated before it becomes severe. For this reason , blood pressure is checked at every visit; urine checked for protein build-up, legs and feet checked for swelling. If toxaemia is detected in its early stages, observation in hospital is the best course. In the past, mild sedatives were prescribed but this is rarely done today. When a woman has severe toxaemia, and is a likely candidate for seizures, she may be given injections of hydrallazine and Valium or other hyposensitive and antiseizure drugs.

Because of widespread good antenatal care, toxaemia rarely reaches an aggravated stage. Why some women get it and most women don't is still unknown; statistically, it is more frequent in women having their first child; in younger and adolescent mothers generally; and in women who are predisposed to hypertension—for example women who are extremely fat or have a family history of high blood pressure. It may be related to an immunological reaction of the mother to the fetus. Toxaemia usually abates very quickly after delivery.

151. Bleeding in the third trimester is not normal

The only normal vaginal bleeding at this time is the scanty blood show that precedes labour—anything else is a sign of trouble and always should be reported to a doctor.

a. *Cervicitis:* severe inflammation of the cervix can cause bleeding, especially after intercourse. It can be treated by vaginal suppositories or creams, but get your partner checked, as it may be due to non-specific genital infection (see p. 219) which requires erythromycin therapy.

b. *Placenta praevia:* rarely, the placenta attaches to the uterus at an abnormally low point, covering the cervix completely or part-ly. The first symptom is painless bleeding, usually in the seventh or eighth month. A doctor may perform an ultrasound test (see No. 174 d) to check where the placenta has attached. Placenta praevia often requires a Caesarean section delivery. If the baby is still very small, a doctor will admit the mother to hospital and try to get the bleeding under control so the pregnancy can continue for a few weeks. If the bleeding is severe, the operation may have to be done immediately, and the prematurely delivered baby kept in an incubator until it is big and strong enough for the outside world.

Placenta praevia is more common in women who have had many children or who have had a Caesarean section or other uterine surgery.

c. *Abruptio placenta:* Sometimes the placenta separates partly or completely from the wall of the uterus. This can occur before or during labour. The symptoms are severe pain in the uterus and bleeding, although sometimes there is no external bleeding because the blood is accumulating in the uterus.

Abruptio placenta may be associated with hypertension, pre-eclampsia or folic-acid deficiency, and heavy smoking, but the exact cause is unknown.

Treatment is emergency Caesarean section unless the woman is well along in labour and the baby's heart rate is stable.

152. Rh disease in pregnancy

The Rh factor (so named for the Rhesus monkeys in which it was first discovered) is found on the outside of the blood cells of 85 per cent of the population. From the other 15 per cent it is missing. Women with Rh-negative blood in the past could expect problems if they were giving birth to a second or later child with Rh-positive blood. The mother's blood can react against the baby's blood (an immune reaction—the normal way the body has for fighting a foreign element). When, during her first pregnancy, a number of fetal cells enter the circulation of the mother by the breakdown in the placental barrier, the mother can develop antibodies—the body's defence against foreign elements—against the baby's cells. The first baby is usually born unscathed. But the second Rh-positive baby can be developing in a maternal body with predeveloped antibodies against its blood. The antibodies from the mother's blood can pass across the placenta, attack the blood cells of the fetus, making it severely anaemic and in the worst cases, causing such severe loss of blood cells that the baby has heart failure and dies.

153. Detection and treatment of Rh disease

First, the Rh negative mother's blood can be analysed for the presence of the antibody. If it is there, then the chance of Rh disease exists and the pregnancy can be managed accordingly.

If the antibody levels in the mother's blood rise during pregnancy, then the threat to the baby is yet more serious. All mothers who harbour the antibody should have amniocentesis (See No. 174e) at around twenty-eight weeks of pregnancy. A little amniotic fluid can be drawn off. If it contains high levels of bilirubin, the substance that the baby's red-blood cells produce when they are breaking down, then the doctor knows that the baby is being affected.

If the amniotic fluid test shows that the fetus is severely affected, a blood transfusion may be given to the fetus in the uterus. Universal donor (O-negative) blood is injected into the abdomen of the fetus, using special X-ray monitors. Depending on how far along the pregnancy is, this procedure may have to be repeated two or three times, up until the thirty-second week of pregnancy. The baby will probably need another transfusion immediately after birth. It is difficult and nerve-racking, but the baby is frequently saved.

In less severely affected babies, a total blood transfusion may be performed after delivery if the level of bilirubin in the infant's blood stream is dangerously high.

A woman with severe Rh disease can consider artificial insemination with an Rh-negative donor to avoid future problems. (See p. 110)

154. Prevention of Rh disease

Thankfully, today, most Rh disease can be prevented. A shot of immunoglobulin, rich in antibodies, can be given to the woman after any incident in which fetal Rh-positive cells may have entered her blood stream. If the woman's partner is Rh-negative, she need not worry: the fetus will be Rh-negative. These incidents include

a. delivery of an Rh-positive child,
b. abortion or miscarriage,
c. an ectopic pregnancy,
d. amniocentesis for genetic testing. (See p. 214)

The globulin antibodies attack any Rh-positive cells which may have entered the mother's blood stream and destroy them *before* she develops her own antibodies against them. This means that the next pregnancy has the same chance of success as the first. *The injection must be given in each case listed above.* Essentially, it keeps the woman's immune system from going to work against her Rh-positive child, by doing the job the antibodies would have done before they can even get started.

The shot should be given within 72 hours after the incident. Blood is taken before this to measure the number of cells and the dose of anti-D needed. In some areas a test is done six months later to check on the effectiveness of the injections.

All pregnant women should have routine blood-typing. Even if therapeutic abortions are performed, Rh-negative women should always receive the shot of immunoglobulin, unless their partner is also Rh-negative.

155. Too much or too little amniotic fluid can be a danger

a. Sometimes, a woman develops extraordinary amounts of amniotic fluid. Her uterus swells much more than normal. This is called *polyhydramnios* (polly-high-DRAM-nee-ohs). It frequently accompanies twins and diabetes and fetal abnormalities, but may occur in otherwise normal pregnancies.

b. Too little fluid is found when placental function is poor and earlier if there is Potter's syndrome (no kidneys).

156. Medically high-risk pregnancies

Pregnancy carries its own risks even in the healthiest of women, delivering under the best conditions. Some women, however, are in such bad health that they risk doing great damage to themselves and their children just by becoming pregnant. The maternal mortality rate in England and Wales is about 10 deaths per 100,000 births. Many of these women died because of severe additional illness preceding the pregnancy. For babies, the risk of death or injury is much greater with a very sick mother.

Despite the dangers, some high-risk women will decide to have children. This should be a well-thought-out decision, not an accident. *Be aware of the risks if you are considering running them.* Place yourself within reach of a hospital that specializes in obstetrics (usually a medical school hospital); these facilities will have the doctors you need and the intensive care units your baby may need.

Yours is a high-risk pregnancy if you suffer from

a. Diabetes
b. Hypertension
c. Renal (kidney) disease
d. Heart disease
e. Sickle-cell anaemia or thalassaemia
f. Cancer
g. Alcoholism
h. Drug addiction

157. The risk of diabetes

It may be easy to control diabetes in a young woman with insulin and diet; it is much harder to control it during pregnancy. Higher doses of insulin are needed as the fetus grows. Frequently, a diabetic woman will have to be hospitalized for periods during pregnancy for regulation of her disease. Her baby will tend to be heavier than other babies unless the disease is well controlled; or, if the placenta is affected, the baby may be smaller than expected.

Gestational diabetes develops only during pregnancy, usually in women who have a family history of diabetes. Other likely candidates are women who have had overweight (more than 10 lb) babies previously and women with sugar in their urine. These women should have a glucose tolerance test (GTT) at 28 weeks and if this is abnormal, have their blood sugar tested repeatedly during pregnancy. Screening for blood should be done two hours after a large meal. Diabetes is not present at birth but the tendency towards it later in life is inherited. Infants of diabetics have higher risks of congenital abnormalities. Pregnancy should be discussed beforehand with a doctor. Insulin is preferable to oral drugs in pregnancy because of the risk of congenital abnormalities.

158. The risk of hypertension

This is a common disease, especially among older women, obese women, and black women. During pregnancy, high blood pressure can complicate the flow of blood to the placenta, resulting in smaller babies. A woman can have both pre-eclampsia and hypertension in pregnancy. (See No. 149 above) Any severe elevation of blood pressure requires aggressive treatment and close monitoring of the baby. Another possible effect of hypertension is kidney damage during pregnancy, which in turn carries a high risk to mother and child.

159. The risk of renal (kidney) disease
Women with pre-existing kidney disease have many problems with pregnancy. If kidney function deteriorates greatly during pregnancy, abortion or early delivery may be the only ways to prevent maternal death. *Remember: pregnancy is a nutritional interchange.* The waste-elimination function of the kidney is overloaded during pregnancy and therefore it must be in good working order.

160. The risk of heart disease
The work of the normal heart must increase 50 per cent during pregnancy. For the damaged heart this strain may be too great. No matter what the origin of the heart damage—congenital, rheumatic, or hypertensive—the risk to the mother increases during pregnancy. If heart surgery has been performed, discuss anticoagulant drugs with your doctor before getting pregnant.

161. The risk of sickle-cell anaemia and other related diseases
Women with sickle-cell anaemia have great difficulties with pregnancy. Some studies show as high as 50 per cent infant mortality and 25 per cent maternal mortality. The great danger is from blood clots which frequently occur in the lungs and are sometimes fatal. In specialised hospitals such women are able to receive effective therapy in the form of transfusions during the pregnancy, and the risks are lessening. Women with sickle-cell trait may run increased risk of urinary infection in pregnancy. (See pp. 214-19)

162. The risk of cancer
Cancer anywhere in the abdomen rules out pregnancy. If not the cancer itself, then the radiation and drug therapy required to treat it will almost certainly damage the child. Carcinoma in situ (see page 351) of the cervix may be treated conservatively during pregnancy, then more aggressively after delivery. (See p. 352) Breast cancer may be treated during pregnancy, but radiation and mammography constitutes some danger to the fetus, if not shielded.

163. The risk of alcohol excess

Children born to alcoholic women are reported to have many congenital defects. And some reports suggest that children of mothers who drink just moderately may be smaller and more jittery than the average. Pregnant women should try not to drink and should never take more than two drinks per day. (Ref. 5, 6) Binges that go beyond that amount are particularly dangerous to the fetus in early pregnancy.

164. The risks of smoking during pregnancy

Recent studies have shown that babies born to women who are heavy smokers are smaller in size, and more likely to be premature. The incidence of early abortion (see No. 118), bleeding during pregnancy, abruptio placenta (see No. 151c), placenta praevia (see No. 151b) and premature rupture of the membranes (see No. 132) is higher in heavy smokers. (Ref. 7, 8) Women must cut back to less than 5 cigarettes per day during pregnancy; and preferably stop the habit altogether, both for their own and their baby's health. If this is impossible, make yourself eat more than you want and ask for serial ultrasound and oestrio tests.

165. Recommendation: Avoid radiation and X-rays during pregnancy

Any woman who is sexually active and requires abdominal X-rays should only have them during bleeding or the first ten days of her menstrual cycle (counting the first day of bleeding as Day One) when she is sure she cannot possibly be pregnant. If X-rays are absolutely needed in pregnancy, make sure the abdomen is shielded. The risk to the fetus of a diagnostic X-ray series study is very low. The risk of X-ray therapy is very high.

166. Severe environmental pollution is dangerous during pregnancy

There are not yet enough laws or knowledge to control environmental dangers to a pregnant woman and her baby. *A woman has to control her own environment as much as she possibly can.* In July 1976, for example, an industrial accident at the Ismesa Chemical plant in Meda, Italy, created a poisonous cloud, containing the toxic chemical dioxin, that spread over several communities. Doctors warned women in their first three months of pregnancy that they might bear deformed children as a result of the exposure to the poison. Although abortion was at that time against the law in Italy, the government consented to it for these women;

the Roman Catholic Church did not. Each woman had to make up her own mind about what to do.

There is no way to avoid this sort of calamity except by much stricter government regulation of (particularly industrial) pollution. However, an individual woman who ordinarily works with toxic substances must inform herself of the dangers to her baby and should transfer to another job or leave the job as soon as she decides to become pregnant. This is not easy, but it may save your baby's life.

WARNING: *Get out before you become pregnant* if you work with paint, lead, mercury compounds; if you work under the shadow of a big industrial complex; in a plant that produces chemical waste; around an operating room or any hospital or industrial area where anaesthetics are used or produced. (Women working with anaesthetics experience an increase in spontaneous abortion.) Science cannot yet give definitive answers on industrial pollution; sometimes the poisonous effects are not felt for years. So don't wait around for scientists to tell you yes or no; they may not be able to until it is too late.

167. The risk of drug addiction

If a woman with a drug habit continues to take hard drugs while she is pregnant, the baby will be born addicted—and will suffer the horror of withdrawal symptoms after delivery. There is also a higher rate of complications in the pregnancies of addicted women—mainly prematurity. If a woman is a heroin addict, she should try to get into a methadone or withdrawal programme during her pregnancy.

Early but as yet unproven reports indicate that women who take LSD or smoke a lot of marijuana during pregnancy may cause chromosomal damage leading to genetic damage in their babies. *Stay off these drugs if you are pregnant or contemplating pregnancy.*

Other medications are dangerous as well. (See p. 210 and Table 6, Chapter Seven)

168. Infectious diseases contracted by the mother may affect the fetus

Particularly in early pregnancy, some infectious diseases of the mother can cross the placenta and damage the child, or infect the child at the time of delivery. These diseases include rubella (German measles), herpes genitalis, and syphilis and gonorrhoea.

182

169. The risk of rubella

If a woman has been exposed to rubella in early pregnancy, she should have blood tests to determine whether she has become infected with the disease (see p. 219) for it will almost invariably damage the fetus. Check your rubella status before pregnancy. Make sure your daughter has injections at 13 to protect her against rubella.

170. The risk of herpes genitalis

Women who have genital herpes (see p. 295) in the last five to six months of pregnancy may pass this to the infant during delivery and, some doctors believe, while the infant is still in the uterus. If the baby is infected, it develops a disease which looks like smallpox and is frequently fatal. Most consultants advise delivery by Caesarean section if there are any lesions in the vaginal area in the last few months of pregnancy, but even this doesn't completely protect the baby.

171. The risk of syphilis

Syphilis may infect the fetus in the uterus during the last six months of pregnancy and cause severe damage to several organs (brain, bones) if not treated. This is why all women have blood tests for syphilis during the first trimester of pregnancy. If detected early and adequately treated, the baby *may* come through it all right. (See p. 302) If you have had casual sex, have a VD check before trying to become pregnant.

172. The risk of gonorrhoea

Gonorrhoeal infection may cause blindness in the baby if the disease is present in the birth canal during delivery. Testing for this infection should be routine in all pregnant women. To prevent gonorrhoeal eye infections, drops of antibiotics may be placed in the baby's eyes at time of delivery. (See p. 299) If you have taken a chance, have a check before starting your pregnancy.

173. The risks of other infectious diseases

Several other infectious diseases are known or strongly suspected to cause fetal defects. (See Table 5, Chapter Seven)

174. Tests widely used to monitor high-risk pregnancies in late pregnancy

a. *Oestriol detection.* During the last eight to ten weeks of pregnancy, large amounts of *oestriol,* an oestrogen, are excreted in the urine. Oestriol excretion should remain at a constant level up to thirty-four weeks, then increase dramatically. This shows whether the baby's adrenal glands are working well (the adrenal glands of the foetus produce the original substances of oestriol), whether the placenta is normal (for the placenta metabolizes the fetal adrenal substance and changes it to oestriol), and whether the mother's kidneys are normal (the kidneys control the amount excreted in the urine). Oestriol is usually measured in a 24 hour or early morning urine sample or in a blood sample. If the oestriol excretion is abnormally low, further tests will generally be used to evaluate the fetus. WARNING: *Oestrogen cannot be given by injection to correct the oestriol levels!* This in fact may be dangerous. (See p. 334)

b. *Stress testing.* In women with low oestriol levels or who are overdue, a stress test may be given to determine the condition of the fetus or placenta. In the "non-stress" test, the baby's heart rate is monitored as during labour—cardiotacograph (CTG). If the condition of the pregnancy is good, the heart rate of the infant should go up about fifteen or more beats per minute after the infant moves. If this does not occur an exercise stress test can be done. The woman runs up several flights of stairs and the CTG is then done and signs of strain looked for.

c. *Amnioscopy.* This is a test whereby a small cone is placed through the already open cervix; through this cone, the doctor can see the amniotic fluid. If there are greenish-brown stains (known as meconium) on the fluid, that means the fetus is under some strain and has been defaecating into the amniotic fluid. This is not necessarily an indication that the fetus is in trouble; but it does suggest that the baby should be monitored carefully, and that other tests (the oestriol test; the CTG stress test) should be made to check out the situation. Amnioscopy is not widely performed.

d. *Ultrasound:* This is a method of bouncing sound waves off various structures in the pelvis to determine their size. Early in pregnancy, an ultrasound scan can determine the size of the sac in which the conceptus is housed. This is useful if a woman has bled and wants to know if the pregnancy is continuing normally. The fetal heart movement can be seen at five to six weeks. It is usually done before amniocentesis for genetic testing to localize the placenta. (See p. 214) Later in pregnancy, ultrasound can be used to measure fetal growth—the waves bouncing off the head of the baby indicate whether this is occurring at the correct rate. Newer machines measure the circumference of the head and chest or abdomen and can estimate fetal size. They can also determine the location of the placenta. Ultrasound can identify multiple pregnancies. At present it is assumed to be a much safer alternative to X-ray in many instances. The long-term safety of this diagnostic method, and its use in fetal monitoring as well, remains to be confirmed. OPINION: There is *no excuse* for its routine use at every visit, in all pregnancies as is the practice in some places.

e. *Amniocentesis.* This is a test done at various stages of pregnancy, in which a needle is inserted through the abdomen into the uterus to remove a little amniotic fluid for testing. It can tell several things:

—If the baby's kidneys are working. Creatinine can be measured in the amniotic fluid. This substance, produced by the fetal kidneys, begins to rise after thirty-four weeks of gestation.

—If the baby's lungs are working. By measuring the lecithin-sphingomyelin (L-S) ration in the amniotic fluid, the maturity of the fetal lung can be determined. Lecithin and sphingomyelin are lipids, fatty substances, found in the fetal lungs; they increase normally after thirty-five weeks of gestation. If the ratio is high, then the risk of respiratory distress syndrome is less.

—If there are significant numbers of fetal skin cells containing fat in the fluid. This suggests that the fetus is mature.

—How mature the baby is: in late pregnancy it is especially important information when early delivery may be necessary.

—If there are genetic problems. (See Chapter Seven)

—If there is serious Rh disease; bilirubin in the fluid is analyzed.

6

ABORTION

Abortion is the termination of pregnancy by removing the fetus and other contents of the uterus before the fetus is viable—i.e. capable of independent existence. Such a termination of pregnancy involves slight health risks of blood loss and infection. Like other surgical procedures it should be avoided if possible by careful attention to birth control.

The basis of abortion law in Britain is still the Abortion Act 1967, but for most women (and men) abortion involves ethical issues which must be resolved by the individual conscience, not by the law. It should be used as the method of last resort—by women who are absolutely convinced that it is the proper course for them. It must always be a personal decision, not the decision of friends, parents or boyfriends and husbands. In Britain, the law requires that the woman obtains the signatures of two doctors. Counselling is not a legal requirement but is sometimes available. The aim of good counselling is to help the woman make her own decision and be sure that that is what she wants. It should not try to persuade either way.

Legalization has vastly improved the safety of abortion. While abortion was illegal, healthy women were regularly crippled and killed. Good doctors were ruined. Others made illicit fortunes. Wealthy women could afford to travel abroad. Poorer women had to seek back street abortions. It is estimated that at least 70 per cent of women who have had legal abortions would have had illegal ones if the law provided them with no other recourse. (Ref. 1) Some of the methods used were reminiscent of medieval torture: rubber tubing, knitting needles, coat hangers and corrosive douches. They often caused massive infection, perforation and haemorrhage, ultimate sterility, terrible pain and death.

A low estimate of the death rate for criminal abortion is 40 per 100,000, compared with one per 100,000 for legal abortion. Before abortion was legalized, deaths were disguised under various other causes, such as sepsis or haemorrhage, without further explanation. Even so, 463 deaths in England and Wales were officially recorded as being from abortion in 1933. Even in 1969, the first year when the Abortion Act came into force, there were 34 deaths from abortion. But by 1978 there were only five. The complication rate, for example from infections that lead to infertility, are likewise much lower now that abortions are legal.

1. Medical reasons for abortion

Although the vast majority of abortions are requested by the woman with no overriding medical problem, some medical reasons may compel a woman to abort when she would have preferred to deliver the child.

These include:

a. Risks to the woman's own health, from diseases such as:
 1. Severe heart disease
 2. Severe kidney disease
 3. Severe hypertension
 4. Severe diabetes with kidney disease
 5. Sickle-cell anaemia or other related disease
 6. Cancer of the genital tract
 7. Some cases of myasthenia gravis, a neurological disease, that does not respond to drugs

b. Risks of severe genetic defects or illness in the child:
 1. Development of rubella (German measles) or other viral illnesses in early pregnancy (see p. 219)
 2. Exposure (during early pregnancy) to drugs known to cause deformities or disease (see p. 221)
 3. Excessive X-ray exposure
 4. Serious or fatal genetic disorders in the child which can be detected by amniocentesis (see p. 214) (Ref. 11)

Seek another opinion if abortion is recommended for any other "medical reasons" and you do not want it.

2. The risks of abortion increase as the pregnancy progresses, so move fast

Do not allow your GP to delay you by waiting for the results of an NHS pregnancy test (which ian take two weeks) or by suggesting that you return after the next missed period (by which time you are likely to be nine weeks pregnant). It is now possible to get a pregnancy test done on a blood sample which will show a positive result within 14 days of conception. It is sometimes helpful to offer to pay for the test. Family planning clinics will often do the tests free and if your own doctor is unsympathetic will refer you to hospital.

Reputable chemists can do a pregnancy urine test for you which is positive in 90 per cent of women six weeks after the last missed period. The abortion charities (see References) and other agencies registered by the DHSS will carry out these tests for a fee of under £5 in 1980.

3. Routine pre-abortion procedures

a. The doctor who performs the abortion must know the woman's medical history in detail. This includes history of previous pregnancies as well as all past and present medical problems and allergies. Be honest. Conceal nothing. If you do, you are preventing yourself from receiving the best possible care.

b. Certain laboratory tests are essential before an abortion: *a good clinic will do them all.*

1. *A pelvic examination* and *sometimes a pregnancy test* must be done to verify that you are pregnant, and how far along you are.

2. *A blood count* must be done to rule out anaemia.

3. *Blood type* and *Rh type* must be determined. (See p. 177)

4. *Blood pressure* must be taken.

5. *Urine* must be checked for sugar and protein.

6. *A smear* for cervical cancer should be taken if a woman has not had one in the last year or two. (This is an optional test but performed by most good clinics.)

7. *Tests for VD*, especially gonorrhoea, should be taken. If a woman has undetected gonorrhoea in her cervix, she risks infection of the uterus, tubes, and ovaries after the procedure. (See p. 298) The abortion procedure should be postponed until the disease is treated—usually only a matter of a few days.

c. Be prepared to make two visits to the hospital or clinic—one for tests, one for the abortion.

METHODS OF ABORTION

4. Recommended techniques of abortion

The risks of abortion rise as the pregnancy increases, so you must move fast. Only these techniques should be considered.

a. *Menstrual aspiration or extraction* can be used in very early pregnancy or suspected pregnancy up to the second week past the missed menstrual period.

b. *Vacuum aspiration* is the preferred method of abortion for pregnancies in the first trimester—between six and 13 weeks after the last menstrual period.

c. *Dilatation* of the cervix and *evacuation* (D & E) of the uterine contents with sponge forceps (D and E), sometimes supplemented by suction aspiration, is the safest method early in the second trimester (between 13 and 16 weeks). The doctor should not need to dilate the cervix beyond 10 mm in a first pregnancy or 12 mm in a later one.

CAUTION: If the gynaecologist says you are too late for suction and must wait two or three weeks for an injection method, return to your GP for referral to a unit which will do the vaginal method quickly.

d. *Intra-amniotic injection of prostaglandins* with or without urea, or of saline are considered the safest methods over 16 weeks in Britain. *Extra*-amniotic prostaglandin with or without syntocinon is used in some units.

In the United States the latest figures show that D & E is the safest method up to 20 weeks and probably later than that. In the hands of an experienced doctor this is probably true in this country as well.

CAUTION: Some gynaecologists will suggest hysterotomy (a mini-Caesarean section which leaves the uterus scarred) or even hysterectomy (where the womb is removed). Do not accept these more dangerous methods without a second opinion, even if you have to pay for this.

5. Menstrual aspiration or extraction

For women who recognize that they are pregnant within two weeks after their first missed period, menstrual aspiration is the ideal method of abortion. It can be done with anaesthetic and involves only minor discomfort.

Firsl, a speculum (SPECK-you-lum) is inserted into the vagina as in an ordinary pelvic examination. The vagina and the cervix are grasped with a tenaculum (ten-ACK-you-lum), a small surgical clasp. If local anaesthesia is used, it is injected at this point into the cervix—causing a little pain. A flexible plastic cannula (CAN-you-la) attached to a syringe is then inserted into the cervix. (*Cannula* comes from the Latin word for cane or reed, and that's what a cannula looks like—a reed, thin as a drinking straw.) Suction is applied with the syringe and the lining of the uterus, including the pregnancy, is removed.

6. Routine procedures after menstrual aspiration

After menstrual aspiration, the woman should wait at least thirty minutes for a blood-pressure test. Bleeding should be checked. A follow-up examination should be scheduled for no more than three weeks later, to make sure that there are no complications or side effects, including the possibility that the procedure has failed and the pregnancy has not been ended. (See No. 31 below)

7. When should menstrual aspiration be performed?

Menstrual aspiration should be performed no later than two weeks after a missed menstrual period, and no earlier than the date the period was expected, unless a serum test for HCG (human chorionic gonadotrophin) has confirmed pregnancy earlier than this.

8. Who should perform menstrual aspiration?

Only a doctor trained in sterile technique and with experience in doing pelvic examinations and abortions should perform menstrual aspiration. The procedure should not be done by an untrained person because of the greater risk of infection. Even when doctors perform menstrual aspiration, the complication rate is higher for the first 20 operations they perform.

9. Where should menstrual aspiration be performed?

Menstrual aspiration may be performed in an out-patient clinic; hospitalization is not usually necessary. In Britain, the hospital or clinic must be licensed for abortions under the 1967 Act. There is pressure to remove this legal requirement.

10. Advantages of menstrual aspiration

a. Menstrual aspiration has a lower incidence of complication. The biggest advantage is that the cervix does not need to be dilated. This is important because any damage caused to the cervix while dilating it can lead to second trimester abortion or premature delivery in subsequent pregnancies. The immediate complications of the procedure appear to be very few—a 1 per cent incidence of infection, excess bleeding, cramps and spotting. In about three per cent of cases the procedure does not work. This is why the examination two or three weeks afterwards is very important.

b. Now that the serum HCG test for pregnancy is available, it is possible to terminate the pregnancy by menstrual aspiration very early. This is obviously preferable psychologically and emotionally as well as medically and is especially useful after cases of rape.

190

c. In countries where the termination of a proven pregnancy is not legal or acceptable, menstrual aspiration can be used prior to a positive pregnancy test and provides a safe and legal solution to the problem of an "overdue" period.

11. Menstrual "regulation" by non-surgical means

WATCH FOR NEWS of prostaglandin pessaries. Work in Oxford using synthetic analogues of prostaglandins and research in Sweden is promising. The pessary is inserted into the vagina when the period has been missed and it stimulates the uterus to expel its contents. At present, the dose needed for a complete abortion tends to make the woman sick or have diarrhoea, but this problem should be overcome in the next few years.

The advantage of this method is that no instruments invade the uterus, so that, as long as the abortion is complete, the risk of infection is minimal and uterine trauma is nil. Secondly, a method like this which could be used by the woman herself would make abortion freely available to all women.

12. Vacuum aspiration

Vacuum or suction termination of pregnancy (VTOP or STOP) is the preferable procedure for terminating pregnancies of six to 13 weeks duration.

Anaesthesia is always used—either general or local (paracervical block, an injection of local anaesthetic into the cervix). If local anaesthesia is used, a woman will sometimes receive a sedative before the procedure begins.

A speculum is placed in the vagina. The cervix is grasped with a tenaculum and the anaesthesia is injected into the cervix. Both of these steps may involve a short-lived pain until the anaesthetic takes hold. There should be very little pain during the procedure after that.

The cervix is gradually widened with a set of successively larger dilators until it is just wide enough to receive the plastic curette connected by tubing that is connected to a suction pump. The pump sucks the tissue of pregnancy into the tubing and thence into a container in which it is collected and sent for pathological examination. After the suction, some physicians scrape the inside of the uterus with a metal curette, to make sure all the tissue is removed from the uterine wall. ("Curette" comes from the French word *curer,* which means "to clean.")

13. Routine procedures after vacuum aspiration

The woman should rest several hours in a recovery room after the operation, where her blood pressure and pulse will be monitored frequently, and she will be observed for amount of bleeding. She should be prepared to stay until the sedative wears off and she feels well enough to go home. Some centres routinely give prescriptions for medications to take to contract the uterus, and for infection if it develops later. While the woman is still in the recovery room she will usually receive the first dose of ergometrine, the drug to contract the uterus and to lessen the bleeding. Do not expect to take any other drug at this time.

Arrange a follow-up appointment with the hospital, your own GP or family planning clinic for four weeks later.

14. When should vacuum aspiration be performed?

Vacuum aspiration may be performed up to 13 weeks of pregnancy—*but it is much preferable to do the procedure before twelve weeks,* for the complication rates rise sharply after that.

15. Who should perform vacuum aspiration?

It is important that the doctor is well practised in the procedure and does not overstretch the cervix. The more procedures any doctor performs, the lower the rate of complications. If you have the choice, a hospital or clinic which does a large number of abortions is usually better than one that does a few.

16. Where should vacuum aspiration be performed?

Vacuum aspiration can be done safely as an outpatient procedure up to 12 weeks of pregnancy. Some hospitals have day-care units and the charities (see References) and some private clinics are now licensed to do abortions on a day care basis. Women whose pregnancies are further advanced or those with any medical problem are not suitable for day care. There must be a person available to stay overnight with the woman at home in case she has an adverse delayed reaction to the anaesthetic.

17. Dilatation and evacuation (D & E): a supplementary procedure for abortions between 13 and 16 weeks

In this procedure vacuum aspiration is used after the uterus has been partially emptied using sponge forceps.

Discuss with your gynaecologist whether he or she feels competent or prepared to do D & E after 16 weeks. We have limited information about the incidence of cervical damage from this procedure, but some doctors are very skilled and do not dilate the cervix more than 12 mm, even if doing an abortion at 20 weeks. (Refs. 3, 4)

18. Intra-amniotic methods

This method is used to terminate the majority of pregnancies between 16 and 26 weeks. A concentrated solution of salt or of prostaglandin with or without urea is introduced into the uterus in exchange for the amniotic fluid around the fetus. Saline solution and urea both kill the fetus. Prostaglandin, a hormone, produces uterine contractions which expel it.

The woman empties her bladder, lies on her back, and the lower part of her abdomen is washed with antiseptic solution. A small amount of local anaesthetic is injected into the skin over the uterus. Then a long needle is inserted through the abdomen into the sac around the fetus. The fluid is removed through the needle and replaced by the saline solution or by prostaglandin with or without urea. Some physicians thread a small plastic catheter through the needle before it is withdrawn in case a second dose is needed.

A general anaesthetic is not needed, and it helps for the woman to be awake during this procedure. The reason for this is that occasionally the saline solution is injected into a blood vessel, causing dizziness and headaches which the woman must be able to report immediately to her physician.

The prostaglandin solution may be injected intravenously, and the woman then feels sick and may get diarrhoea and flushes. Her blood pressure drops. This is treated by setting up an intravenous infusion and giving anti-nausea drugs. The addition of urea speeds the procedure and ensures that the fetus is not delivered alive.

Within two to twenty-four hours, the uterus begins cramping. This will last for several hours until the fetus is delivered. Frequently, as the cramps begin, some fluid will leak from the vagina. The placenta will be delivered after or with the fetus. The whole procedure takes between twelve and thirty-six hours. Sometimes the placenta does not deliver itself, and a curettage (a scraping of the uterine lining) must be performed. The cervix is already open, so dilatation is not needed. During the contractions with a saline abortion, a woman will need analgesic drugs.

In theory the urea and prostaglandin method is safer than saline, but in Britain, where saline has been used in the non-NHS sector and prostaglandins in the NHS, the statistics do not show a difference. (Refs. 5, 6, 7)

RECOMMENDATION: At present, the combination of D & E with vacuum aspiration is safer for 13 to 16 week pregnancies. (See above)

19. Routine procedures after intra-amniotic methods

Remain in the hospital until the abortion is complete. Blood pressure, bleeding, pulse should be monitored for at least six to twelve hours afterwards. Allot several days for recuperation at home and schedule a follow-up appointment for no longer than four weeks later.

20. When should intra-amniotic methods be used?

Intra-amniotic abortion should be performed preferably after the sixteenth week of pregnancy—the complication rate is lower then. It should, of course, only be performed by a qualified gynaecologist in a fully-equipped hospital.

21. Extra-amniotic prostaglandin

In this method a speculum is introduced into the vagina and a rubber tube is inserted through the cervix. The tube is kept in place by a balloon which can be blown up after insertion. A solution of prostaglandin specially prepared for this use is then slowly run into the tubing. It runs between the membranes and the uterus.

The main disadvantage of this method is a higher risk of infection, since it is difficult to sterilize the vagina. Secondly, it is more likely to fail, in which case syntocinon is given intravenously to stimulate contractions. The cervix is sometimes torn severely during this procedure and water intoxication leading to brain damage has occurred with this combination of drugs.

CAUTION: If your hospital rarely does late abortions, this method is probably the most dangerous. You should ask for referral to another hospital or clinic, or accept hysterotomy.

22. Utus paste should not be used

This old-fashioned method which involves inserting medicated soap through the cervix should not be used. The risk of infection is high and it often fails. In 1978, 14 women, all in NHS hospitals, were subjected to this method despite the reiterated condemnation of the method in the Department of Health's enquiries into maternal deaths. (Ref. 7)

23. Hysterotomy is not a good method

Hysterotomy, a kind of mini-Caesarean section, was used widely for abortion between 16 and 26 weeks before intra-amniotic methods became available. It is a major operation with a high mortality rate as well as other complications. Hysterotomy should only be used as an abortion technique in the rare eventuality that intra-amniotic drugs fail several times, if infection or haemorrhage occur, or to spare the women's feelings where there are psychiatric complications. Even in cases where the woman herself wants to be sterilized, hysterotomy is not a good choice of method. It is safer to do the abortion and sterilization separately.

24. Hysterectomy is not a proper method of abortion

WARNING: Hysterectomy, the removal of the uterus, is sometimes recommended to women who want an abortion and no further pregnancies. The only good medical reason for doing a hysterectomy is if there are large fibroids preventing vacuum aspiration or hysterotomy. There are safer forms of abortion and tubal ligation is a vastly safer form of sterilization. In the latest figures available from the Office of Population Censuses and Surveys (OPCS) (Ref. 8) there are marked regional variations in the use of hysterotomy and hysterectomy for pregnancy termination. In London and Oxford fewer than four hysterotomies are performed per 1000 abortions. In the North-west the figure is 27; in Yorkshire and Merseyside 19; in East Anglia 18 and in northern region 17. Similar variations apply to hysterectomies, which range from 4 per 1000 abortions in the South-East Thames region to 5 per 1000 in Yorkshire. (Ref. 9)

Get your partner or a friend to support you whilst discussing the reasons for the decision with the gynaecologist. If you are not satisfied, get a second opinion, most easily from the abortion charities.

25. Abortion and sterilization

Although the shock of an unwanted pregnancy may make coincident sterilization seem a rational choice, studies have shown that up to 25 per cent of women regret the decision later. Secondly, when Peter Huntingford compared large groups of women who have had abortions alone with those who have had abortion and sterilization together, he found a risk six times as great when the operations were done together. Most of this extra risk is because of thrombosis which is more likely during pregnancy and in overweight women. Allow yourself to recover from the abortion before making the final decision of sterilization.

Again, OPCS figures show a marked difference between the NHS and non-NHS practice and between regions. In 1977, over 15 per cent of women in the NHS were sterilised with their abortions, compared with under two per cent in the non-NHS sector. Regional variations ranged from only 4.8 per cent of abortion patients in North-West Thames region being sterilized with their abortions, to over 11 per cent in Northern, Trent and South-west regions, over 12

195

per cent in North-West and Wessex regions, and 15.6 per cent in East Anglia. (Ref. 9)

RECOMMENDATION: If you cannot get an assurance from your GP that your local gynaecologist will do your abortion quickly, vaginally, and without pressure for sterilization, go to one of the charities where you will have competent treatment and humane advice. (See References)

NORMAL POST-ABORTION COURSE
26. Routine care and normal after effects of abortion

a. Do not leave the clinic or hospital without a twenty-four-hour-a-day phone number to call in case of emergencies.

b. Even if you feel fine, have an examination three or four weeks after the abortion, which you should schedule before you go home from the abortion procedure.

c. Bleeding from an abortion usually lasts one to two weeks—it may last only a few days or up to four weeks. The bleeding is usually very light (less than a menstrual period) after the first two days. A series of a few small clots in the days immediately following the procedure is normal. Large clots and constant heavy bleeding are not normal. If the amount seems too great, contact your physician or clinic *immediately*.

d. Mild cramps are normal for the first few days after the abor-tion. Frequently medications are prescribed to help the uterus contract back to normal size and these may cause more severe cramping in the first two to three days. Also, the later the abortion, the more frequent and severe the cramping, for the uterus has to shrink back to normal from a much larger size. After early abortions it is also normal to experience no cramping at all. If constant, severe pain is experienced, especially if accompanied by heavy bleeding or fever, a woman should contact her doctor or clinic *immediately*.

e. Infection sometimes occurs after abortion, so a woman should check her temperature several times daily for the first few days after the procedure and tell her doctor if it is over 100°F (37.8°C). A foul-smelling vaginal discharge is another sign of possible infection.

f. The first period after an abortion should occur within fifty days. If it does not, see a doctor.

g. Breast tenderness may occur, especially after late abortions. Oestrogens are no longer given to counteract this as they increase the risk of thrombosis. *A tight bra or binder is the best and safest treatment.* (See p. 154)

h. Resume showering, bathing, washing hair, and eating immediately after abortion.

j. Intercourse should be avoided for the first few days. If resumed within the first two weeks, the man should use a condom to safeguard against infection through the still open cervix.

k. Fatigue is normal after an abortion, even an early one—because of blood loss and the release of tension. Plan for at least two days' recuperation to get your strength back completely.

27. Resume contraception immediately after abortion

Many women ovulate very shortly after abortion, so plans should be made before the procedure for the use of contraception. Birth-control pills may be started immediately after the procedure. They may also be started after the first period; ask your partner to use condoms until that time.

The IUD is usually inserted during the first menstrual period but not before four weeks after the procedure (to decrease the chance of perforation, see p. 60). Use condoms until this time. Some physicians insert IUDs immediately after an *early* abortion procedure and this is safe. Other doctors prefer to wait four to six weeks, because of the difficulties in diagnosis if pain or bleeding occur. However, IUDs should not be inserted immediately after a *late* procedure because the uterus is still too large and expulsion rate very high.

If a woman uses a diaphragm, this should be fitted at least three to four weeks *after* an abortion so that all the relaxation effects of the pregnancy on the vagina will be gone.

28. Anti-D administration is routine post-abortion treatment for women with Rh-negative blood

Even in the termination of early pregnancies, a woman may become sensitized to Rh-positive red cells and therefore have problems with future pregnancies. (See pp. 176-8) For this reason, all women having abortions should be tested for blood type and, if Rh negative, should receive anti-D after the procedure. Check with the clinic or doctor ahead of time about this if you know you are Rh negative. If you know that the man who fathered the pregnancy is Rh negative, you do not need anti-D.

29. Warning: Do not accept hormone treatment to bring on your period until you are sure you are not pregnant

Sometimes women who are late with their periods are given hormone tablets to bring it on. *Recent warnings suggest that synthetic progestogens given during pregnancy may cause fetal malformations.* So don't accept this medication until you have had a pregnancy test and are absolutely sure you are not pregnant. These medications do not induce abortion; they only bring on a period if you are *not* pregnant. Primodos and Amenorone forte are the trade names of these preparations.

30. The earliest abortion is the safest abortion

The later in pregnancy the abortion is performed, the greater the risk of complications. On the other hand, when performed before the eighth week of pregnancy, abortion is one of the safest of all surgical procedures. It only becomes dangerous when indecision, fear, or misinformation delay it. *So don't wait.* If your doctor tells you to wait, or suggests a pregnancy test which has to be sent away, ask for a referral then and there. If he refuses, visit your local family planning clinic or Brook Advisory Centre for a second opinion. Chemists or licensed pregnancy advisory services do tests on the spot, and the latter will also provide counselling. Studies have shown that many women who come early are delayed by doctors or by the system.

ABORTION COMPLICATIONS

31. Major complications of abortion

Most serious complications occur in later abortions. These include:

a. *Haemorrhage.* There can be several causes of post-abortion haemorrhage:

1. The tissues of conception have not been completely evacuated, and the remainder is delivered with a lot of bleeding afterwards.

2. The uterus has not completely contracted after the abortion, causing sudden severe bleeding.

3. Lacerations or perforations of the uterus have occurred without anyone noticing.

The symptom of haemorrhage is heavy bleeding that persists; *if it occurs, don't wait to reach a doctor by phone; go to the doctor or to the nearest casualty department immediately.*

In an early abortion, excess bleeding will be detected more frequently while the woman is still in the clinic: in later abortions, haemorrhage generally occurs after the woman has gone home. Haemorrhage is much more likely after a late abortion than after an early one.

b. *Infection* of the uterine lining, or endometritis, (en-doh-mee-TRY-tis) occurs in about 2–3 per cent of all abortions, but is more frequent in procedures after twelve weeks. The symptoms are:

    1. A vaginal discharge which may be foul-smelling
    2. Persistent lower abdominal pain or cramping
    3. Fever

See a doctor immediately if you suspect infection. Antibiotics will be prescribed which should arrest the infection within 24 hours; generally they should be taken for seven to ten days. In severe cases, hospitalization may be in order.

Extension of the infection to the Fallopian tubes and general abdo-men is rare after legal abortions—although it was fearfully frequent with illegal abortions.

c. *Perforation of the uterus* is a complication of suction abortions which again increases in incidence as the pregnancy increases in duration. It occurs in about one in 500 abortions. It is usually caused when an instrument used in the procedure (either a dilator or suction curette) accidentally pierces the upper part of the uterus. With a perforation in the uterus the woman will be observed for signs of bleeding into the abdomen and excess vaginal bleeding. Many physicians will recommend laparoscopy (la-par-OS-co-py) for women in whom uterine perforation is suspected. (See p.60) In this operation, the doctor inserts a type of periscope through the navel to view the uterus directly and see whether there is a hole, or significant bleeding, in which case there would have to be further repair. If perforations are not detected at the time of the procedure, later signs could be severe abdominal pain and bleeding into the abdomen. Before nine weeks of pregnancy, this complication is very rare.

d. *Cervical lacerations* can occur in both early and late abortions. In the suction procedures, these are usually caused by the tenaculum tearing through the soft cervix, or by dilators, and can almost always be repaired easily, with little long-term problem. In the later procedures (especially when prostaglandin abortions are augmented with syntocinon) severe cervical lacerations can occur with very forceful contractions working against a cervix that is very tightly closed. If the lacerations are severe, a complicated repair may be needed. In the United States, laminaria (a form of seaweed which dilates the cervix) has been inserted into the cervix before the abortion procedure and may reduce this complication. Cervical lacerations occur in one of every 1000 procedures. (Ref. 10)

e. *Injection of solution into a vein during intra-amniotic methods.* This can sometimes occur *during* the saline or urea procedure or, when blood absorbs the solution, in the hours immediately afterwards. It will be detected by blood tests showing increased salt or urea in the blood. Early symptoms will be severe headache, thirst, dizziness, nausea and abdominal pain. The nurse or doctor should be notified if you have these symptoms so that a doctor can treat it immediately. Prostaglandin injection causes a fall in blood pressure, flushing, vomiting and diarrhoea and must be treated quickly with intravenous fluids and anti-emetics

f *Blood-clotting disorders* are rare complications of abortion, reported in association with saline procedures. Some women, during the process of the abortion or shortly after, develop a disorder called *disseminated intravascular coagulation* (DIC) in which small clots occur in the blood vessels, and all the substances important for blood clotting are used up. The symptoms are uncontrollable bleeding from the uterus as well as the gums and nose in some cases. The treatment is the administration of plasma or fresh blood and the rapid delivery of the fetus.

g. *Allergic reaction to local anaesthesia.* This can often be avoided by careful attention to pre-existing allergies and medical history before the procedure begins.

h. *Failure to discontinue the pregnancy.* In 0.5–1.0 per cent of menstrual and vacuum aspirations, the pregnancy is not ended and a very disappointed woman will have to return for another procedure. In saline procedures, between three and five per cent of women will have to receive a repeat injection of saline because they do not go into labour within 24 to 48 hours.

i. *Water-rentention from syntocinon.* Contractions tend to be unpredictable when extra-amniotic prostaglandin is used, and some doctors augment the contractions by administering syntocinon. This synthetic hormone has mild water-retaining properties and some women have been overloaded with fluid. A few have sustained brain damage or died as a result. If this method is suggested to you, find out whether the unit has done these regularly and knows the dangers. If not, ask if you can have an alternative method (intra-amniotic urea or prostaglandin) or could be referred elsewhere. It cost over £200 to have a late abortion done by one of the charities in 1980.

32. Can a woman die from an abortion?

You are in less mortal danger with a legal abortion than with a normal term delivery. Data from a very large sample of abortions performed in 1972–76 before eight weeks of pregnancy, show a death rate of 1 in 100,000. Between nine and 10 weeks, the risk is 2.8 per 100,000 and between 11 and 12 weeks, 4.7 per 100,000. After 12 weeks, the mortality rate becomes much higher: 13 deaths per 100,000 women having abortions between 13 and 15 weeks; 26.8 deaths per 100,000 women having abortions between 16 and 20 weeks. At 21 weeks or more the death rate was 44.7 per 100,000. (Ref. 11)

It is only when the abortions of over 12 weeks are encountered that the death rate exceeds the death rate for childbirth. At present about ten women die every 100,000 pregnancies. This figure refers to *all* deaths due to *all* complications in pregnant or recently pregnant women. *So in the first three months of pregnancy, abortion is ten times safer than giving birth.* Thereafter, it becomes an increasingly dangerous procedure which should be avoided if at all possible by early action. Each year that abortion has been legal, the death rate has gone down. This is partly because women are obtaining earlier abortions, and doctors have learned the techniques of abortion.

33. Long-term effects of abortion

a. Uncomplicated early abortions probably have no effect on a woman's ability to conceive or bear children in the future. However, if the procedure is complicated by uterine and tubal infection, infertility may result as from other pelvic infections. (See p. 199)

b. There is conflicting evidence about the effect of second trimester abortions, but it seems likely that the risk of miscarriage is increased slightly (from one per cent to two per cent) by abortions in the second trimester. If the cervix has been over-stretched, premature delivery or too-rapid labours may also occur.

When studies have matched women very carefully for all the variables—age, parity, social class, height, smoking etc.—no significant difference has been found in complication rates after one first trimester abortion, and no statistically significant difference after one second trimester abortion. (Refs. 12, 13, 14)

c. There is some evidence that *repeated abortions* can cause a higher incidence of premature deliveries in future pregnancies. Some Eastern European countries where abortion is widely used as a method of birth control show much higher prematurity rates than the rest of Europe. (Ref. 15) This is thought to be related to the termination method of dilatation and curettage which may damage the endometrium.

34. Emotional effects of abortion

The major emotional effect of abortion is relief at the safe end of an unwanted pregnancy.

Those women who go into the abortion with severe, unresolved doubts may come out of it with feelings of guilt and depression that can last for weeks. Sometimes women who thought they were sure about the abortion are plagued by depression afterwards. This may be more likely to occur after late abortions, when a woman has had time to feel and look pregnant, and the abortion itself has been so similar to delivery. (Ref. 16) These feelings of depression generally pass quickly. They have to do as much with the emotional shock of discovering you are pregnant when you don't want to be as with the abortion itself.

Post-abortion depression is not punishment for a crime! It is just a depression, the after-effect of a harrowing experience, supported by endocrine changes that affect your mood. Treat it the way you would treat a depression for any other reason—with a change of scene or a change of pace, lots of company or pleasant solitude, a little self-indulgence, the distractions of work and entertainment.

It is important to remember that the loss of a pregnancy, whether by therapeutic abortion or spontaneous abortion, may produce a reaction similar to mourning. For this reason it is important to be able to remind yourself that you did not want the pregnancy, could not have continued it—and abortion was the only way to end it.

In the event that depression continues and becomes more severe, seek help from your GP or family planning doctor who may refer you to a qualified psychiatrist, psychologist or counsellor.

35. How to get a safe abortion

Surveys have shown that 25 per cent of general practitioners believe abortion should be more difficult to obtain. Most of these doctors will make their position clear, but if you find that you are being delayed unnecessarily or that the hospital gynaecologist is unsympathetic, go to an abortion charity (see References) without further delay. Commercial private abortions often cost more, and the charities have a wealth of experience.

Still only 50 per cent of abortions are done on the NHS. The percentage varies from six per cent in Dudley to 96 per cent in Newcastle. Also, the rate varies, so that women in East Anglia are less likely to have an abortion than those in London.

36. Travelling away for an abortion

If you have to leave your home area to have the abortion:

a. Try not to go alone or return alone—company is comforting when you're in a strange town.

b. Tell someone in your home town where you are going and how they can reach you.

c. Do not make a long return trip the same day as the abortion; try to arrange to stay at least one night.

d. Make sure you return home with all the prescriptions you may need, including written advice on over-the-counter drugs and post-abortion care.

e. See your doctor four to six weeks after returning home. A discharge summary should be sent to him.

37. Never have an abortion in secret

Even though abortion is a woman's legal right, many women—especially young girls—do not want to tell anyone they are pregnant and go into the abortion procedure in secret. This is foolish and unnecessary and immeasurably increases the emotional wear and tear on the woman. If you cannot tell your parents, tell a trusted friend.

If you cannot tell anyone you know, go to an abortion-counselling agency and tell someone there. Your confidence will be respected. Frequently you can walk into the local hospital and ask to see a social worker—you should be able to get good advice and strictest confidence here.

It is vital not to have any operation in secret, because complications may arise which must be taken care of immediately, and which you cannot treat yourself.

Also, there is no comfort to match the comfort of a friend when you are in a tight spot, when you are worried and tense, facing a new experience and wrestling with unfamiliar fears.

38. Counselling comes with abortion

Any accredited clinic or hospital which provides abortion services provides counselling of some sort. At worst, you will be asked some questions about why you want the abortion, how many other children you have, etc., which waste your time and seem more like the collection of material for a school essay than a real effort at guidance. At best, you can find yourself provided with a wise and sympathetic counsellor at a time when many women really need one.

Counselling in NHS hospitals is often rushed and minimal. Ask whatever questions you want answered. Ask to see the medical social worker if you have any doubts or further questions.

Counsellors at the abortion charities are well trained to find out what it is you really want. Other agencies may assume that you have already decided. In exactly the same way, a visit to an anti-abortion counselling agency, or some clergy, may get you the same sort of one-sided advice. If a woman is married and able to provide a family home for her child, many counsellors who would otherwise recommend abortion will try to dissuade her. This variety of bias will be apparent if you look hard at the prospective counsellor. Try to see people who are not likely to impose external social criteria on your personal situation. Because of the newness of the legality of abortion, many women do not know what they think about it—and counselling can help a woman think through her ideas on abortion and come to a conclusion that is right for her. (Ref. 17)

39. The law in Britain

As the law stands in Britain, the woman has to convince two doctors of her reasons for wanting an abortion. The abortion can be done:

1. If your life is at greater risk by continuing the pregnancy than by terminating it.

2. If your physical or mental health is more likely to be injured by continuing with the pregnancy than by terminating it. This is the reason most often used.

3. If the physical or mental health of any existing children you have is more likely to be injured by your continuing with the pregnancy than by terminating it.

4. If there is a reasonable chance that the baby may be abnormal or deformed.

If you are under the age of sixteen, one of your parents must sign a form consenting to the operation. If you are sixteen or over, you can sign the consent form yourself.

A few doctors justify abortion on demand early in pregnancy with the argument that an early abortion is safer than pregnancy and childbirth.

ACTION: If you feel these grounds are too restrictive, join your local branch of the National Abortion Campaign, so that women have a right to choose whether to have an abortion. NAC is at 374 Gray's Inn Road, London WC1 (01-278-0153). Doctors should join Doctors for a Woman's Choice on Abortion (DWCA), c/o Judy Bury, 8 Magdala Crescent, Edinburgh 12 (031-337-8999).

40. The law in Australia

The law on abortion differs very much from state to state. While every attempt has been made to be as up-to-date as possible, a woman seeking an abortion in Australia should make sure that no changes in the law have been made since the time of writing.

The grounds on which abortion can be legally performed and the restrictions on its implementation (if any) are:

1. *South Australia:* abortions may be performed only if there is a risk to the life or physical or mental health of the woman, or if there is a danger that the fetus is abnormal or deformed. The abortion must be performed by a medical practitioner in a prescribed hospital within twenty-eight weeks. The woman must obtain a second opinion except in emergencies, and she must have been resident in South Australia for at least two months.

2. *Victoria, New South Wales* and *Australian Capital Territory:* abortions may only be performed if there is a risk to the life or physical or mental health of the woman; they can also be performed in the case of fetal abnormality, rape, incest or for a socio-economic reason if any of these can be interpreted as a risk to health. In all three states, abortions can only be performed by medical practitioners, and in Victoria they must be performed within twenty-seven weeks.

3. *Northern Territory:* abortions can only be performed if there is a risk to the life or physical or mental health of the woman, or if there is a danger of fetal abnormality. The abortion must be performed by a gynaecologist in hospital within fourteen weeks for 'broad indications' and within twenty-three weeks for 'grave' physical and mental indications. The woman must obtain opinions from two medical practitioners and, if under sixteen, must obtain consent from a parent or guardian.

4. *Western Australia, Queensland* and *Tasmania:* abortions can only be performed if there is a risk to the life of the woman or, in Tasmania, if it is considered to be a 'reasonable' performance of a surgical operation. In Queensland it must be performed by a doctor. In Western Australia and Tasmania, it can only be performed at a stage of pregnancy which would be considered 'viable'.

41. The law in New Zealand

Abortions can only be performed if there is a risk to the life or physical or mental health of the woman, and only if the danger cannot be averted by any other means. The abortion must be done by a registered medical practitioner at a licensed institution, and the practice is to perform abortions only up to twelve weeks. The woman must obtain medical opinions from two certifying consultants, one of whom must be a practising obstetrician or gynaecologist.

7

GENETICS and ANTENATAL DIAGNOSIS

Genetics—the science of heredity—will provide us with some of our most brilliant medical advances and some of our most excruciating moral dilemmas in the coming decades. New discoveries in genetics and related fields such as eugenics (you-GEN-ics), molecular biology (mo-LEK-u-lar), environmental medicine, and biophysics are coming thick and fast. Eugenics is the science of making improvements in genetic inheritance; molecular biology, the study of the microscopic particles that make up the cells of life, may be used to affect the cells that control inheritance; environmental medicine is the study of how factors like housing and pollution affect our health, including the health of our unborn children and grandchildren; biophysics applies what physicists know about matter and energy to the human body; the ultrasound (see p. 184), which uses sound waves to assess the health of a fetus, is a technique of biophysics. All these fields, now in their flowering, feed the study of heredity. Their technology is often baffling to the non-scientist; however, we must understand something about that technology if we are to keep control of our own lives.

The questions asked of genetic research often sound like science fiction (remember, visiting the moon sounded like science fiction a few years ago?). Ask yourself this: What will happen to society if children can be created *routinely* by the union of sperm and egg in a laboratory? What will happen to the human species if human beings can be created *without* sexual union—by making an egg reproduce itself without a sperm, so that it becomes an exact duplicate of its parent? (This is called *cloning*; it has already been accomplished with bacteria.) (See p. 111)

If genetically inherited disease can be wiped out by genetic medicine, can *any* inherited quality be bred in or out? For example, can we breed for blue eyes or musical talent? When technology makes the production of "perfect" people possible, what will happen to those of us who are "imperfect"? And who will control the definition of perfection?

If molecular biologists create new forms of life by recombining the genetic material of different organisms, will these new forms be good for humanity or will they destroy us all? (Ref. 1) How is it possible even to *experiment* with these new forms of knowledge and keep the world safe from biological disaster either through accident or through design?

In days gone by, poor women were wet nurses for rich women who didn't wish to be bothered with suckling a child. Genetic engineering allows us to envisage the day when a woman who doesn't want to be bothered with *carrying* a child can allow her egg to be fertilized in a laboratory and implanted in another woman, whom she has hired to carry the baby for her.

And what will happen, in a world where most people still prefer sons, when genetic technology allows us to predict *and control* the sex of our unborn children?

It is not possible to consider these questions in this chapter, which confines itself to genetic technology that specifically affects the health of women and their unborn children.

But it would be wise for women to read further in this field, which promises so much and threatens so much and about which we must all be educated enough to make *personal* decisions, so that the final decisions will not be entirely out of our hands.

NORMAL DEVELOPMENT— THE ROLE OF CHROMOSOMES

1. Chromosomes and their component genes contain the genetic material that determines individual characteristics

A chromosome (CROW-ma-soame) is a human cell part made up of long strands of DNA (deoxyribonucleic acid), and protein. DNA is the material of inheritance. Each person has twenty-three pairs of chromosomes: twenty-two pairs control all physical and mental characteristics; the twenty-third pair determines which sex a person will be.

Genes are the tiny components of the chromosomes that control each individual characteristic that is inherited. There are one or more genes for virtually everything in the human body—blood, bones, hair, skin colouring—everything.

Chromosomes have two major functions.

207

a. They control individual heredity.

b. They regulate *differentiation* (see Nos. 6, 7 below), the process by which the fertilized egg grows and develops into different kinds of cells forming the different parts of the body.

2. Mutation: a change in chromosomal pattern

A mutation is a change in the pattern of heredity, leading to the development of a new characteristic—or the absence of an old characteristic—in a new generation. For millions of years, mutations could only be caused gradually by such things as environmental pressures and natural accident; the patterns of dappling, for example, that occur in nature evolved over time—in zebras, in poppies, in the infinite colouring of fish.

In recent years, especially since the industrial revolution and its pollutants and the great breakthroughs in physics that led to the harnessing of atomic energy, mutations—usually rare in the physical world—have probably become more frequent. It is now quite likely that man will injure nature through environmental pollution so that the injury is passed on to future generations, if not in humans, then in the other plants and animals with which we share this planet.

For example, radiation and food additives are known to cause genetic mutations and cancer in laboratory bacteria and small animals, and potentially have the same effects on humans.

3. How the pattern of chromosomes is studied

a. A sample of tissue scraped from the inside of the mouth will give a guide to the number of sex chromosomes in an adult. This is a rapid test (though not entirely accurate), sometimes used to determine the sex of athletes or infertile women.

b. Lymphocytes (LIM-foh-sites)—white blood cells—taken from a blood sample are grown in cell culture and then analyzed for their total chromosomal pattern. This is the test commonly used to test the parents of an abnormal child to determine whether one or both of them is a carrier of the abnormal genes, and is more accurate than the smear test. This test can also be used to determine the true sex of a child who has abnormal genitals. (See p. 265)

c. Cells from the fetus, obtained in a sample of amniotic fluid, can also be grown in cell culture and analyzed. The cells can be studied for chromosome patterns as well as for enzymes and chemicals which indicate certain diseases.

4. How sex is determined

The sex chromosomes for men and women show a differing pattern. Most females have two X chromosomes and most males one X and a smaller Y chromosome.

Each sperm and each egg have twenty-three chromosomes. When they combine at fertilization, they become a union with forty-six chromosomes—twenty-three from the mother and twenty-three from the father. Since a woman has two X chromosomes, she can only produce eggs with X chromosomes. Since a man has one X and one Y chromosome, he can produce either kind of cell as his sperm. *Thus, the father determines the sex of the baby.* If he sends along an X sperm that fertilizes the egg, that will create an XX fetus—a girl. If he sends along a Y sperm, that will create an XY fetus—a boy.

5. Cell division immediately after fertilization

After the sperm fertilizes the egg in the Fallopian tube, the cells rapidly divide and multiply. By the time the conceptus (con-SEP-tus) reaches the uterus, there are about eight cells in it, all born of the original two cells (sperm and egg) that created the original fifty-fifty chromosomal split between mother and father. Implantation in the uterus begins about five days after fertilization.

6. How cells differentiate after conception (embryogenesis)

From the time of implantation (Day six or seven) to the fifty-fifth day after conception, the cells are differentiating. Initially all the cells are the same, but soon they change (differentiation), some of them becoming the heart, some becoming the fingernails, etc. Some people believe that the process of differentiation begins as early as the stage when the conceptus consists of only four cells. (Ref. 2) The chromosomes have a major role in controlling differentiation, but how they do this is not completely understood. Genetic clocks which switch on the growth enzymes have been suggested.

7. Induction: the geography of differentiation

Very little is known about how differentiation starts. However, it *is* known that once this process begins, an orderly arrangement of cells is necessary for differentiation to continue normally. Certain kinds of cells must be arranged next to certain other kinds of cells; their effect on each other allows them to develop properly. This is called induction.

8. Birth defects: congenital or inherited

a. *Defects caused by outside influences in early pregnancy.* Up to fifty-five days after conception, a number of factors may interfere with the chemical messages among the dividing cells of the fetus and affect differentiation and induction, leading to birth defects.

Thalidomide was a *drug* which was found to interfere with the induction of the cells that form the arms and legs.

Rubella (German measles) is a *virus* that interferes with differentiation of cells that form many body parts including brain, eyes and heart.

High-dose radiation is an *environmental factor* which can interfere with any groups of cells in the body, causing defects that are obvious when the baby is born or which show up later in life (for example, a late-developing cancer).

Such birth defects are *congenital*. The child is *born* with them but has *not inherited* them from previous generations.

b. *Defects caused by outside influences later in pregnancy.* After fifty-five days of gestation, the fetus is less vulnerable to substances affecting differentiation and induction. The kinds of birth defects that can be caused at this time are often more insidious in that they affect the *rate of growth* of certain body parts or the body as a whole. Malnutrition of the mother, for example, may lead to an underweight baby with higher risk of infant death or small brain size. Maternal diseases that interfere with the blood supply to the fetus (such as high blood pressure, or kidney disease) may cause brain damage by impairing oxygen flow to the brain. Damage to the fetus during labour and delivery would be included in this group of defects.

Again, birth defects of this kind are *congenital*. The child is *born* with them but has *not inherited* them from previous generations.

c. *Birth defects caused by abnormal genes or chromosomes.* Some birth defects are caused by disordered messages from abnormal genes or chromosomes. Many of these disorders can be passed on from generation to generation.

Tay-Sachs disease, sickle-cell anaemia, and cystic fibrosis are passed on this way, along with other relatively rare conditions (see below). Sometimes, the defect is unimportant—for example, colour blindness, or oddly shaped fingers. Sometimes it is very severe—for example, haemophilia (bleeder's disease), caused by the inherited malfunction of one of the 12 clotting factors in the blood.

These birth defects are *congenital*, in that the child is born with them. *They are also inherited,* in that the child has *inherited* them from previous generations.

Antenatal testing and amniocentesis have been most useful for detecting some inherited disorders; much less so for other congenital defects.

9. Recessive genes: the source of most inherited diseases

All chromosomes are present in pairs, so all genes are paired as well. This means that two genes, one from the father and one from the mother, determine each characteristic. Some genes are *dominant,* and the traits which derive from them are *dominant traits.*

For example, the gene for brown eyes is stronger than that for blue eyes. Thus, if a child has a blue-eyed parent and a brown-eyed parent, the child will most likely express the dominant trait—and have brown eyes.

Most abnormal genes exist in "carrier state". This means that some people carry an abnormal gene which is masked by the normal gene of the pair. The abnormal gene is called *recessive*; the trait which derives from it is called a *recessive trait.* The abnormality can only express itself in a child who has two carrier parents.

If both parents carry the recessive gene for the abnormality, 25 per cent of their children will express the abnormality.

Many recessive genes are associated with particular ethnic or family groups. Between 5 and 10 per cent of black people of West African parentage carry the recessive gene for sickle-cell anaemia. If two people who carry the gene have a child, there is a 25 per cent chance that the child will be stricken with sickle-cell disease; that is, one out of four children born to such a couple will have the disease. (See p. 214)

Similarly, cystic fibrosis, a genetically determined disorder of glandular secretions which leads to respiratory ailments affects children of families in northern Europe, but does not turn up in Italian families, for example. Eastern European Jews (Ashkenazim) must watch out for Tay-Sachs disease, a neurological degeneration of young children leading to loss of brain function and death. Jewish people from the Middle East (Sephardim) are generally not affected.

10. How recessive-gene diseases originate

Most recessive-gene diseases are clouded in history; they probably originated through a mutation in a particular family in a particular locality. In fact, the mutation may have occurred originally because it was *needed*; it was *selected* in the evolutionary process. For instance, part of the persistence of the gene for sickle-cell anaemia is attributed to the fact that people who were carriers of this disease were more resistant to malaria, which is endemic in West Africa.

11. Sex-linked genetic disorders

Sometimes, a recessive gene for a disease is present on the X chromosome. In girls, if one X chromosome carries the defective gene and the other X chromosome is normal, the disease will not show up. However, the woman who carries the disease recessively on one of her X chromosomes will pass the disease on to *half* of her sons. This is because half of her eggs will contain the abnormal gene, and the genes on the Y chromosome are not strong enough to counteract the effect. Haemophilia and muscular dystrophy are the major sex-linked recessive-gene diseases.

12. Dominant gene diseases

Diseases arising from dominant genes are the least common type of disease. They usually arise by spontaneous mutation and the child may die in the uterus or in infancy, and so never reaches an age where reproduction is possible. One exception is Huntington's chorea, characterized by spasmodic movements of the face and hands gradually leading to loss of mental ability and then death.

The first generation may suffer and die after having had children. This second generation will then have to decide whether to accept the 50:50 chance of having the disease and have children knowing that they will not know until their children reach adolescence whether or not they have passed the disease on.

Certain kinds of skin disorders or extra fingers or toes may be passed down from one generation to another via harmless dominant genes.

13. Diseases associated with abnormal numbers of chromosomes

In recessive and other gene diseases, the chromosomes remain normal in number and appearance. However, there are some birth defects which are caused by chromosomal disorders. Usually these can be detected antenatally by checking the chromosomes in a sample of amniotic fluid cells (amniocentesis).

Chromosomal anomalies in a fetus are usually accidental; they do not pass from generation to generation. Most are caused by an accident during division of the germ cells (the cells which produce the egg and sperm). If an egg or sperm has too many or too few chromosomes, a severe chromosomal disorder may be passed on to the fetus.

If the chromosomal number is too great, the fetus usually dies before birth, as in the case of *triploidy,* in which the fetus has chromosomes in triplicate, not duplicate (sixty-nine instead of forty-six).

If the chromosomal count is not too severe (for example, one extra chromosome or one too few), then the resulting child may live to be born, with a gross abnormality.

14. Non-disjunction: the cause of most chromosomal abnormalities which the fetus can survive

Non-disjunction describes the situation in which, when germ cells divide, one set of chromosomes sticks together. Therefore, after union with the egg, the two-by-two division does not apply for all twenty-three sets of chromosomes. One set of chromosomes may be a triplet; or one set may be a single.

15. Diseases caused by non-disjunction

The most frequent variety of non-disjunction is *Down's Syndrome* (*mongolism*) in which three chromosomes are present on the twenty-first set.

Trisomy 18 (multiple congenital defects) is another variety; it occurs when three chromosomes are present on the eighteenth set.

Klinefelter's Syndrome is a case of non-disjunction in which a male child has an extra X chromosome in the twenty-third set determining sex. Instead of being XY, he is XXY. Such a boy will have underdeveloped testicles and may have other developmental problems.

16. Down's Syndrome: a form of retardation that can be lessened with antenatal testing

a. Down's Syndrome is a kind of mental retardation that is responsible for almost 30 per cent of all the severely retarded children in the western world. (Ref. 3)

Down's Syndrome (and all other disorders caused by non-disjunction) occurs in greater frequency among the pregnancies of older women. The approximate risk of mongolism is as follows:

age 30–35:	1 in 900 births
age 35–40:	1 in 300 ”
age 41–45:	1 in 100 ”
age 45 + :	1 in 40 ”

In short, a woman under age thirty-five has a slight risk of having a child with Down's Syndrome; over age thirty-five, the risk is significant. Because the risks of amniocentesis are about equal to having a child with Down's Syndrome at age 35, many hospitals use this as the age at which amniocentesis is offered.

b. Another less frequent type of Down's Syndrome occurs in children of younger women; in these cases, some genetic material from one of the twenty-first set of chromosomes (either the one from the father or the one from the mother) is displaced on to another chromosome. When the cells divide, one of them has more genetic material than the rest, and the result is a mongoloid child. This type of disorder can also be detected antenatally. There is a 5–10 per cent chance that if it happens once, it will be repeated. This is higher than the chance of repetition with the mongolism that occurs with older women (see above).

In these younger women a chromosomal test on her blood and that of her partner will enable them to know whether they run this increased risk or not. Sisters or brothers of these carriers can also ask for a test if they want this information before embarking on a pregnancy.

GENETIC TESTING AND AMNIOCENTESIS

17. Genetic testing and amniocentesis: ways to test for and prevent birth defects

a. Genetic testing is the testing of mother and father for genetic traits which might, in combination, damage the child. Some recessive-gene diseases like sickle-cell anaemia, thalassaemia and Tay-Sachs, affecting particular ethnic groups can now be tested for and discovered, so that men and women who find that they are carrying the disease traits can rethink whether they wish to have children together or plan for further testing after conception.

b. The chromosomes of the fetus can be checked by testing some amniotic fluid cells, obtained by amniocentesis. This antenatal test will discover most major chromosomal abnormalities early enough in pregnancy for the mother of an afflicted child to have an abortion, if she chooses.

c. Amniotic fluid cells can be tested for substances that indicate recessive diseases which involve abnormal metabolism such as Tay-Sachs disease. Over 3000 rare metabolic diseases (where an enzyme is missing) have been detected. These tests are only offered to couples with one affected child. The test can also detect some physical abnormalities such as spinal-column defects.

d. Other procedures such as fetoscopy and ultrasound (see Nos. 28 and 29 below) may detect structural defects in later pregnancy.

18. Amniocentesis

Amniocentesis is a simple test by which some of the amniotic fluid around a fetus is drawn off between 14 and 16 weeks of gestation, and the cells tested for chromosomal patterns and other substances. Generally, an ultrasound scan (see No. 29 below) is performed first to locate the placenta so that the practitioner who inserts the needle to withdraw the fluid may avoid it. Thereafter, 10–20 ml of amniotic fluid is withdrawn and placed in a culture medium in the laboratory, where the cells grow. Within two to four weeks, the chromosomal pattern (and any abnormalities in it) can be detected and various specific chemicals can be identified in metabolic disorders. The test must be performed under sterile conditions in hospital. In over 95 per cent of cases, an adequate number of cells for testing can be grown. In the remainder the test may not work and may have to be repeated.

19. The risks of amniocentesis

As with other specialized procedures, it is best to go to a centre where amniocentesis is performed frequently and where the practitioners and the labs are experienced. There is conflicting evidence about the risks. There is very little risk in this test for the mother (very rare cases of infection, bleeding, fainting, and amniotic-fluid leak). The risks for the fetus are more severe, but still *rare:* for example, the needle might go through a part of the fetus. Another risk is that the test may cause early labour, but, when done by experienced people, this risk is probably only a little greater than for pregnancies without amniocentesis. (Refs. 4, 5, 6, 7) A woman may become sensitized to the Rh antigen during amniocentesis or fetoscopy, so all Rh negative women should receive the shot after these procedures. (See p. 176)

20. The limits of amniocentesis

At present amniocentesis can only discover chromosomal abnormalities and some inherited metabolic diseases and structural defects of the spine. *It cannot discover damage to the fetus that is caused by virus, X-ray, drugs, and thousands of other factors that could conceivably cause a birth defect.*

21. Who should consider having amniocentesis?

a. Women over thirty-five.

Many women are putting off having children until later in life in order to establish careers. Since chromosomal abnormalities increase considerably after age thirty-five, women over this age may want to avail themselves of the test. (Younger women may consider amniocentesis, but the risk of Down's Syndrome for them is less than the risk of the procedure causing a miscarriage, at present.)

b. Younger women who have previously borne a child with Down's Syndrome or a child with some other chromosomal abnormality.

c. Women with a high possibility of a specific inherited metabolic disease.

This includes, for example, the woman who along with her husband, carries the trait for Tay-Sachs, or a woman who has previously borne a child with some other inherited metabolic dis-order. If a couple has a family history of any rare disease, they should check with a genetic counsellor to determine their risk of having a child with a similar problem.

d. Women who are carriers of sex-linked disorders (like haemophilia).

e. Women who have had children with neural tube defects. (See No. 24)

22. Tay-Sachs disease can be controlled by genetic testing and amniocentesis

The gene for Tay-Sachs disease occurs in one in thirty Ashkenazi Jews (Jews from families that originated in Central and Eastern Europe). Carriers can be detected by a simple blood test which will discover the level of the enzyme hexosaminidase A in the blood. If two carriers have children there is a 25 per cent chance of each child born having and dying of Tay-Sachs. If parents know themselves to be carriers, they can conceive a child and then resort to amniocentesis, to check for a deficiency of the enzyme in the amniotic fluid or in the cells derived from it. High-risk couples whose religious observance normally prohibits abortion should seek counselling with rabbinic authorities before proceeding with the amniocentesis. An alternative way to prevent the disease is to use artificial insemination. (See p. 110)

Do not wait until you are pregnant to find out if you and your partner are carriers. Have yourself tested before you decide to have children. Know what risks you are—and are not—running when you conceive a child.

23. Amniocentesis as a test for sex-linked genetic disorders

Amniocentesis can determine the sex of the child: if this is the only information being sought, the test is certainly not worth the trouble, with one medical exception: women who carry the trait for sex-linked genetic disorders, such as muscular dystrophy or haemophilia, may expect 50 per cent of their sons to be affected. In this case, a woman might not wish to carry a male fetus to term and amniocentesis is probably in order. Women who are carriers usually know who they are because the disease is in the immediate family. Watch for news of antenatal diagnosis of haemophilia and muscular dystrophy.

24. Amniocentesis for alpha-fetoprotein and antenatal diagnosis of neural tube defects

Alpha-fetoprotein is a substance present in the amniotic fluid. Its concentration rises until the twenty-eighth week and then remains static or becomes lower. Between 16 and 18 weeks, the range of values is narrow for normal fetuses. A high level is usually found when the fetus has a neural tube defect.

Defects which can be detected in this manner are anencephaly (in which the infant has no head), spina bifida with meningomyelocele (me-NING-go-my-ell-o-seel) (a structural defect in the spinal column in which some vertebral arches may be missing and some of the spinal cord tissue and nerves may protrude).

Women who have previously had children with these disorders run a risk of recurrence and should be tested. *The test for alpha-fetoprotein is performed routinely in most centres, even when the amniocentesis is done for another reason.*

WATCH FOR NEWS: Ninety per cent of the cases of spinal and brain defects occur in the children of couples with no family history of these problems. Until now, they usually had to wait until they had an affected child to know whether further pregnancies should be tested. A screening test on the mother's blood during pregnancy may soon be widely available to detect which women might be at higher risk for carrying an abnormal fetus, and thus amniocentesis would be strongly suggested in these women, to detect the spinal and brain defects.

25. Diagnosis of sickle-cell anaemia

People who think that their ancestors may have originated in West Africa should have themselves tested for sickle-cell trait (a simple blood test) before they have children. If both parents have the trait each pregnancy carries a 25 per cent risk of producing a child with sickle-cell anaemia.

Once a child is conceived, antenatal diagnosis of whether that child will suffer from sickle-cell anaemia is available on a limited basis.

26. Amniocentesis for thalassaemia

Thalassaemia is a severe condition, mainly affecting people from Cyprus and Turkey. The children affected receive frequent transfusions and often die in their teens. Amniocentesis for thalassaemia is available at a few centres.

27. Amniocentesis for cystic fibrosis: not yet available

Cystic fibrosis is a severe, chronic respiratory disease caused by recessive genes. If a couple has had a previously affected child, they should be referred to a genetic counselling centre. Amniocentesis may soon be able to detect whether a fetus is affected by this disease, and a simple blood test may soon be available to identify carriers.

28. Fetoscopy: a form of antenatal testing

Fetoscopy requires the insertion of a needle carrying lenses into the uterus to look directly at the fetus and at times to obtain a small amount of fetal blood for laboratory evaluation. This is difficult for several reasons:

a. A rather large hole has to be made in the uterus and amniotic sac to extract the blood, with a danger of complications for mother and child.

b. When the blood is extracted, the mother's blood may also be present, confusing the sample and preventing an accurate lab reading.

Fetoscopy can also be an important detector of structural defects in the infant, such as spina bifida (see No. 24 above)—an outpouching of the lower spinal cord—because these can be directly visualized. However, these defects can usually be detected more safely by ultrasound and amniocentesis. Fetoscopy may be useful if these methods give different results.

29. Ultrasound can be used to detect some structural defects in the fetus.

An ultrasound (see p. 184) is a test by which sound waves are bounced off the fetal sac to indicate the shape of the baby. An abnormal pattern of waves will indicate a structural defect.

30. Counselling is important

Couples who participate in genetic testing for potential defects in their children can anticipate severe emotional strain. If an abnormal fetus is detected, this may have a devastating effect on the individuals or their relationship. Marriage or psychological counselling is a must at this time. Expert advice and support may be provided for the rarer types of defect. Otherwise it might be carried out by the obstetrician. Make sure your G.P. is involved also.

INFECTIONS AND BIRTH DEFECTS

31. Rubella and antenatal testing

Rubella—German measles—is a virus which, if contracted by the mother early in her pregnancy, causes severe or minor malformations, including mental retardation, in 10–90 per cent of affected pregnancies.

Thus it is absolutely essential for every woman to be vaccinated against rubella if she has not had the disease in childhood and developed a natural immunity to it.

Whether you have had rubella or not, get a blood test for it. If the results show a high level of antibody, then you can be assured that you have had the disease and are immune. If there are no antibodies get vaccinated.

If you are pregnant and think that you may have had contact with rubella, and are unsure whether you had the disease or vaccination before, get a blood test immediately. Generally if the antibody count is high, you're safe; there is no need for worry or for further testing. If the antibody count is low, a second test should be taken about three weeks later. If the levels are higher in this second test then this is proof that a woman has recently had the disease.

If the blood test shows that you have contracted rubella, you may wish to consider abortion. *If you are less than fifty-five days from conception when the infection occurred, the chances are very high (about 30–50 per cent) that the infant is damaged.*

Antenatal diagnosis is not able to determine fetal damage by viruses.

Other viruses which may damage the fetus if infection is in the early stages are listed in Table 5. These viruses usually do not affect the fetus as virulently as rubella, but help should be sought if you are infected during pregnancy.

32. The symptoms of rubella

These include a fine rash over the chest and back and swollen glands in the back of the neck. Even if a woman does not develop these symptoms, she should be tested if she has been in contact with any other person with the symptoms.

33. When to be vaccinated against rubella

The best time to be vaccinated is before pregnancy is even a remote possibility, because the vaccine uses a weak form of the virus, which could affect a developing embryo. Since you must wait three months after the vaccination to become pregnant, consider being vaccinated immediately *after* giving birth. In fact, hospitals tend to test for rubella routinely after women have given birth.

Most reports now say that it is safe to be vaccinated during breast-feeding: the vaccine does not appear to cause any problems for the newborn.

34. Warning: Avoid vaccinations with live virus during pregnancy

Some immunizations involve the injection of a very low dose of live virus to allow the person to build up immunity to the virus as protection. The live vaccines include rubella, smallpox, oral polio, measles, mumps and yellow fever. Routine vaccinations should be avoided during pregnancy because the live virus can infect the fetus. However, if there is an epidemic of a disease, the vaccination may be safer than risking the infection. Consult community health officials in these cases or your G.P.

OTHER CAUSES OF BIRTH DEFECTS

35. Radiation exposure and antenatal testing

No one really knows what dosage of radiation can cause fetal damage during pregnancy. In general, the risk of single films or diagnostic X-rays is very low. If X-ray treatment for diseases such as cancer is given to the pelvic area in early pregnancy, the risk is very high.

Fetal damage by X-rays cannot be determined by antenatal testing.

36. Warning: Avoid radiation if you are pregnant

Even though the *exact* risk is unknown, the *potential* for radiation damage should lead pregnant women to avoid any unnecessary X-rays. If chest X-rays or dental X-rays, for instance, are absolutely necessary, the abdomen should be shielded with a lead apron.

37. Warning: Any drug given in pregnancy may potentially damage the fetus

Table 6 lists the drugs that are known or suspected to cause damage, but the sensible woman will avoid any medication not absolutely essential, especially during the first three months. This includes over-the-counter drugs. *Damage by drugs cannot routinely be detected by genetic testing.*

38. Choosing the sex of your baby: the Shettles hypothesis

Dr. L. B. Shettles has propounded an hypothesis, for which he claims 80 per cent success, to help parents get the baby of the sex they want. There is no guarantee of success in this procedure, but it is probably harmless enough, and those who wish to try it need fear nothing more than the arrival of a bouncing baby of the sex they didn't want.

Shettles claims that, by altering the times of coitus and using acid or alkaline douches or gels his patients have much success in getting children of the sex they prefer. (Ref. 8) Other physicians report success by spinning down the semen and thus separating the X- from the Y-bearing sperm.

TABLE 5
INFECTIONS WHICH MAY AFFECT YOUR BABY

Chicken Pox	Mycoplasma
Chlamydia	Rubella (German Measles)
Coxsackie B	Streptococcus (B-haemolytic)
Cytomegalovirus	Syphilis
Hepatitis	Toxoplasmosis
Herpes Simplex	Vaccinia (from Smallpox
Influenza	immunization)
Listeria	

TABLE 6
SOME DRUGS KNOWN TO AFFECT YOUR BABY

Alcohol
Antibiotics, (tetracycline, chloramphenicol, streptomycin)
Androgens (male hormones)
Anti-cancer drugs
Anti-convulsants (phenytoin, trimethadione, phenobarbitone)
Anti-coagulents (phenindione [Dindevan], warfarin)
Diethylstilboestrol (DES), a synthetic oestrogen
Nicotine
Sulphonamides
Thalidomide

SUSPECT, BUT NOT PROVED

Amphetamines
Anti-emetic drugs
Aspirin
Barbiturates
Caffeine
Diuretics
Hexachlorophane
Iodine in high doses
Lithium
LSD
Marijuana
Oral drugs for diabetes
Phenylmercuric acetate (PMA)
Progestogens (synthetic progesterones)
Thiouracil
Tranquillizers (diazepam [Valium], meprobamate [Equanil or
  Miltown], chlordiazepoxide [Librium]

8

EVERYDAY GOOD HEALTH

The best way to stay healthy is to make a personal judgement regarding the healthiness of everything you do and everything you put into or on your body. This is very difficult. But there is no other way.

From childhood someone has to decide which foods are good, which cosmetics are good, which social habits are healthy, which hygiene regimes are worthwhile. A parent cannot just trundle down the aisles of the supermarket throwing everything the children want into the trolley; many of the things they want are at best nonnutritious and at worst harmful to the body, even though they may be delicious and brilliantly advertised and packaged. A woman cannot accept the notion that if a product is in her chemists, it is *ipso facto* safe. It may not be safe for her. It may be safe for her—but it may be ineffective and a waste of her money.

Everyday good health is created by the individual woman, rendering judgements on every single aspect of her daily life and that of her family. Though everyone else may be smoking, drinking, wearing six-inch heels, the individual woman must stand aside, make her own decisions and join the crowd *only* when it suits her personally.

As a general rule, the movement towards a more natural, untreated, undrugged existence is a good one. It can be a grave mistake to underestimate how healthy you are normally; to weaken your legs by driving when you are strong enough to walk; to weaken your intestines by taking laxatives when your body is strong enough to eliminate on its own; to take medications for colds that your system could fight off independently. A healthy body stays healthier if it is used; underuse may be tantamount to misuse.

The environment both inside and outside the body is up for grabs today, by every economic and political interest in the country. The consumer, who is also the patient, who is also the voter, who is also the parent must try with all the self-knowledge and power at her command to control her own environment, and decide what sort of life is healthy for *herself*.

RECOMMENDED HYGIENE

1. Recommendation: Preferred hygiene is plain soap and water

Hygiene is understood in the traditional sense as cleanliness, which is said to be next to godliness. Today, cleanliness sometimes goes beyond what is actually healthy; we are encouraged to eradicate every smell from our bodies, and in so doing we sometimes eradicate the odour-causing bacteria which are natural to our bodies and protect our general health. We wash our hair so much that we dry it out beyond repair. We wipe the hair off our bodies with products that sometimes irritate the skin. We use easy-drying fabrics because we are always washing our clothing; yet for many women, these fabrics are not as healthy as natural fibres which may take longer to dry and sometimes don't look as clean.

A woman who is simply trying to keep clean and fresh can do so with plain soap and water. She must make a critical judgement about every additional product she uses to keep herself, her house and her clothes clean. In general, it can be said that not much besides soap and water is actually needed.

2. Natural bacteria are essential to good health

A healthy body is covered with friendly bacteria. Bacteria which endanger are usually picked up by the hands, transported to the mouth and into the stomach or picked up from the air and absorbed into the respiratory system. The purpose of bathing is to protect the body from unfriendly bacteria without killing off the natural bacteria that live on the body and in many cases protect its normal functioning.

3. Sensible bathing

A daily bath or shower will control body smells and make a woman feel good—but she does not have to bathe her entire body *every day* to maintain good health.

Hands and lower arms, the areas most exposed to outside dirt and bacteria, should be washed frequently during the day; before every meal; and after every trip to the bathroom.

It is important to wash out the mouth frequently, if only with

224

plain water, and, ideally, to brush teeth after every meal to prevent accumulations of food that cause odour and decay.

Wash under arms and the pubic and vaginal area daily to prevent odour. The face is washed mainly to remove dirt and excess oily secretions. It is quite normal for a woman to find that soap dries her skin more than she likes and to choose instead plain water and/or cleansing cream.

4. Vaginal hygiene

The vagina is a clean place; normal urine does not enter and, anyway, urine is sterile; normal semen does not make it dirty, for it also is sterile. The national advertising campaigns on vaginal hygiene products might make a woman think that her vagina is a hotbed of soil to be washed and perfumed away incessantly. A mature woman should know better. The natural secretions of the vagina are there to protect a woman's health, and too much washing (see No. 7 below) may actually wash away her defence against outside infection.

The bowel contents are not sterile—and it is very important to wipe the anus from behind, so as not to draw bowel contents towards the vagina, inviting cystitis and vaginitis. (See p. 287) This habit should be taught to young girls when they are toilet-trained. It will protect them for a lifetime. In addition, the urethra and vagina should be wiped after urination from front to back.

5. Vaginal odour is usually held not by the vagina but by the pubic hair; wash it away

If you are bothered by vaginal odour, wash the outer pubic area; in most cases, it is the hair that catches and holds the odour. Wash the hair and labia and you clean the odour away. In addition, try cotton pants which are more absorbent and deodorizing than synthetics. If these methods do not work, check with a doctor, for odour may be an early sign of vaginal infection. (See p. 287)

6. Avoid perfumed products for vaginal hygiene

Perfume may cause irritation; it is not a necessary part of vaginal hygiene and may give some women trouble. *It is nice to smell nice, but it is better for general health not to smell at all.* And, remember, a foul vaginal odour may be a sign of infection. By perfuming the vagina regularly with sweet-smelling soaps, douches, or vaginal sprays, you may be concealing an odour which is a vital early warning signal of a problem.

OPINION: Do not use "feminine hygiene sprays". They contain

perfuming agents which frequently cause allergic reactions. In the past, some contained hexachlorophane, causing both allergic reactions and potential fetal damage in pregnancy, so they are now banned. *If you find a vaginal spray with hexachlorophane on the shelves where you shop, tell the store manager to get rid of it.*

7. Routine douching is not necessary for good health

Douching (doosh-ing) is the flushing of water up the vagina with a thin hose or syringe to clean the vaginal canal, and is a popular practice in America. This job can also be done by the upward spurting water of a bidet (bee-day), a special tub for cleaning the vaginal and rectal areas often found in bathrooms abroad.

8. Body odour

Most body odour comes from perspiration and the growth of bacteria in the armpits and pubic area. Soap and water will help in eliminating the bacteria and excess perspiration. Shaving the hair will also help. Deodorants for the armpits are safe, *but don't use them in the pubic area.*

Tight-fitting clothing, clinging, synthetic undergarments and slacks aggravate body odour, especially in hot weather. Try not to wrap up so tightly in the summertime and choose clothes of natural fibres.

9. Bad breath

Bad breath usually comes from food left over in the mouth, deteriorating under the impact of natural salivary juices, or from the left-over smell of strong foods, drink or tobacco. Brushing teeth and rinsing the mouth will usually wash it away. Mouthwashes are fine but not necessary. Many people find that plain water is just as good.

Persistent bad breath may be a sign of serious dental decay. Some times generalized disease will cause it as well; a woman may notice that when she has a bad cold or sinus infection, her breath will smell bad. If this persists suspect a chronic tonsillar infection. If your breath smells foul, and repeated rinsing and brushing cannot control it, see a dentist or doctor.

10. Hair removal is a cosmetic decision, not a health matter

Hair does not make a woman's body dirty. Whether she removes it, from her legs or armpits, for example, is entirely a *cosmetic* decision, unrelated to good health.

a. *Hair may trap perspiration and its odour.* The areas of the body most thickly covered with sweat glands also tend to be covered with hair. So in hot weather particularly, hair may trap perspiration and the natural odour it causes. Many women remove underarm and pubic hair in the summer to avoid this. However, hair removal does not solve an odour problem completely; *you still have to wash.*

b. OPINION: *Shaving is the safest method of hair removal.* A light lathering with soap before shaving will make the blade run more smoothly. An electric razor is fine as well. *Make sure you're dry when you use it.* When hair is shaved, its early regrowth looks dark and stubby; it only looks that way; in fact the old wives' tales that shaved hair grows darker or more thickly are quite wrong. Bleaching, tweezing or electrolysis (see No. 10f below) for unwanted hair on your face tends to be more effective.

c. OPINION: *Depilatories (chemical hair-removers) should only be used on the legs.* Most depilatories (de-PILL-a-tories) can irritate skin, eyes and/or nostrils. Therefore, use them only on your legs and test a small area first for allergic reaction. If the skin puffs up, or a rash develops, go back to shaving.

d. *Waxing is a more permanent way to remove hair from legs.* A woman can do it at home or have it done professionally. Wax is melted, cooled a little so that it does not burn, then smeared on the legs. Pieces of cloth are placed on it. The wax dries. Then cloths and wax are ripped off, pulling the hair out with them. The hair does not grow back for quite some time and women who use wax for years may find eventually that it does not grow back at all. Waxing is uncomfortable; imagine an adhesive bandage being pulled off the hairy side of your arm.

e. *Facial hair should only be removed by bleaching, tweezing or electrolysis.* The first order of treatment is bleaching with plain hydrogen peroxide. Plucking the darkest hair with a tweezer is also effective and harmless (after years of tweezing, these hairs may not come back). Shaving is safe but not permanent. WARNING: *Do not use depilatories or hot wax around your eyes.*

f. *Electrolysis is the most permanent type of hair removal.* A needle is touched to the hair follicle, a tiny electrical current is applied, destroying the hair base, then the hair itself is tweezed out. Electrolysis hurts. Most women cannot take too much of it at one time and must go back for repeated short appointments. This can become enormously expensive: about £250 for 20 minutes.

OPINION: Generally, permanent hair removal is so protracted, expensive, and uncomfortable that only women who feel severely disfigured by excess hair should consider it.

g. *Sudden new growth of hair in unexpected areas should take a woman to her doctor.* This may be caused by a hormone imbalance or other illness. It should be checked. Don't try to remove the hair until the reason for the growth has been discovered.

COSMETICS

Cosmetics, as distinct from drugs, are not absorbed by the body. The Department of Trade regulates their safety.

11. Allergic reaction is frequent with cosmetics

Many women react badly to certain ingredients in cosmetics such as perfumes, hair dyes, and mascara, usually by itching and swelling or redness. All cosmetics are now required to list such ingredients on the label. *Read the label.* Read the warnings about possible irritation or allergy; use the product on a small area first to see if it affects you badly.

If it does, look for a product with different ingredients. *Report the reaction to your local trading standards office* and to the manufacturer.

Some face make-up seems to aggravate acne: this is the reason so many actors who wear heavy stage make-up end up with rough skin. If you are having trouble with acne, and wear face make-up routinely, shop around for another product and/or get a medical opinion. (See p. 32)

WARNING: *Never try to cover a skin condition with a cosmetic without asking medical advice first.* You may need medication.

12. Hair care

Many young girls have oily hair that requires frequent washing to keep it looking clean and fresh. The same people may grow up into women who have hopelessly dry hair that splits at the ends, breaks off, even falls out—because by that time they may have bleached it, dyed it repeatedly, used a blower to dry and curl it, a curling iron to iron it—all of which slowly but surely hurt the hair. There are an enormous number of hair products to choose from, and as with other cosmetics, a woman should be wary of advertising. Several things should be kept in mind:

a. No product will increase the actual *volume* of hair. A body wave and some shampoos and rinses may add a *feeling* of thickness.

b. Protein conditioners do help to make damaged hair more manageable.

c. Some conditioning rinses eliminate knots and make it easier to comb through hair when it is wet.

d. Comb—do not brush—your hair when it is wet. Brushing may damage the hair.

e. Baby shampoo lacks the hard washing ingredients that make eyes sting; therefore, it is excellent for little children whose hair tends to be thinner and easier to clean anyway. Older women may find that baby shampoo cannot get their hair as clean as they wish.

f. In general, a detergent shampoo washes the hair cleaner than an acid shampoo.

g. Lemon juice makes oily hair more manageable. Use actual lemon juice, not the reconstituted type.

h. The aniline (ANN-ih-line) based hair dye and rinses may create allergic reactions in some women. Before dyeing either at home or in the salon, do a patch test. Apply a small amount of the eye solution with a cotton swab to a patch of hair behind your ear or on the skin inside the crook of your elbow. In the case of dye, two solutions must be mixed together; use the combined solution, not each of the two separately. Wait twenty-four hours. If any red blotches appear, do not use the product. (Ref. 1)

WARNING: Avoid products containing dye substances, 2,4-diaminoanisole (2,4-DAA), and 4-methoxy-m-phenylenediamine (4-MMPD). These have been shown to cause cancer in lab animals. Concern about these products has increased, with recent studies that suggest beauticians have an increased risk of lung cancer. These conclusions are not definitive, because none of the studies have taken into consideration the smoking habits of the subjects (see pp. 253-5; Refs. 2 and 3) or the possibility that hair sprays may be a factor.

While waiting for further studies women should use dyes containing other compounds—henna is a good alternative.

Never apply dye or tint to your eyebrows, for your eyes may be sensitive to the fumes of the solution (not to speak of accidental direct application) even if your skin is not.

i. Some women find they are much more sensitive to the chemical in hair dye when they are pregnant. In general, it is a good idea to avoid hair colouring at this time.

j. If your hair is falling out more than a few strands at a time, don't just experiment with different products infinitely. Seek professional advice.

k. *Hair sprays:* Concern about the propellants used in aerosols causing damage to the atmosphere has now led to a reduction in the amount of chlorfluorocarbon added. To reduce this risk to a minimum, be sparing in your use of aerosols.

13. Deodorants and antiperspirants

A *deodorant* does not stop wetness. It may mask the smell of perspiration by killing or limiting the natural bacteria that create the smell, or by merely adding a fragrance to conceal the smell.

An antiperspirant contains aluminium salts which temporarily close the openings of the sweat glands and stop wetness. In addition, it may contain an antibacterial agent to fight odour-causing bacteria.

An American study in 1975 showed that of all toiletries on the market, deodorants and antiperspirants produce the most adverse reactions. Some women find they are allergic to the aluminium salts, some to the perfume. If redness or swollen glands develop under the arms, switch to a brand without perfume. If redness continues, stop using the product altogether. Frequent washing and the application of non-irritating powder will do just as well for many people. (Ref. 4)

OPINION: Roll-on and stick deodorants are the best value. Manufacturers may begin to push these now, reacting to the drive to remove propellant sprays from the market.

14. Perfume and contact dermatitis

Contact dermatitis (dur-ma-TYE-tis) is a general term for reactions of the skin to substances applied to it. Perfume is perhaps the most common substance to cause contact dermatitis. Many women develop reactions to perfume in the form of an itch, a rash, stinging or red blotches. If you experience these reactions, switch to non-perfumed products (soaps, toilet paper, tampons, deodorants, etc.). In addition, oil of bergamot—an ingredient of some perfumes—can cause a photosensitive reaction (dark skin blotches) if worn in the bright sun. *Be careful.* Don't wear perfume while sunbathing.

15. Mascara and eye infections

Eyes are very sensitive, easily infected by small numbers of bacteria which would not hurt the body elsewhere. In order to prevent infection with *pseudomonas* (soo-do-MOAN-as), which can grow in eye products, manufacturers include an antibacterial mercury substance, to keep the products (and therefore the eyes) sterile. *Other than this, mercury compounds are not allowed in cosmetics.*

A recent study on five hundred women showed that mascara can also become contaminated with *staphylococcus epidermidis,* which can cause chronic lid infections called *bacterial blepharitis* (bleh-far-EYE-tiss). (Ref. 5) The trouble arises mainly because water-based mascaras do not contain adequate preservatives to keep out bacteria. Bacterial blepharitis symptoms are: redness along the eyelid, eye irritation, loss of lashes. If you experience these symptoms, stop using your mascara and see your doctor. If you scratch your eye with a mascara brush and pain or redness persists for more than twenty-four hours, get to your G.P. If the mascara was infected, fast treatment can save you from severe eye problems.

Any trouble with mascara or any other cosmetic products should prompt you to write to the manufacturer and trading standards officer.

16. Nail polish is fine, but give your nails an occasional rest from it

Polishing nails in and of itself is not dangerous; but some women find that if they leave polish on all the time, the nails get brittle and crack easily.

17. Infections in the finger and toenails

The fingers come in contact with more dirt and more moisture than any other part of the body. It is logical therefore that fungus infections, which thrive in moist places, should easily lodge around and under the fingernails. Treat these with local applications of medicine, prescribed by your doctor.

These infections may rarely be confused with psoriasis (sore-EYE-a-siss), a skin disease often affecting the scalp, elbow, and knee areas. Fungus infections in the fingernails may be the source of recurrent vaginal infections.

Assume that any recurrent or long-term scaling and itching around the nails is worth checking with a doctor.

OVER-THE-COUNTER DRUGS

18. The regulation of over-the-counter drugs

An over-the-counter drug is different from a prescription drug in one regard; it is considered to be a drug, in that it is absorbed by the body, has an effect on the body, *but the government deems that it can be safely taken at the discretion of the consumer.*

There are two types of over-the-counter drugs:

a. *General sale drugs*, e.g. indigestion tablets. These are on sale in many shops other than chemists and are regulated for safety and quality.

b. *Pharmacy medicines.* These are drugs available only in chemists' shops. They can be sold only under the supervision of a trained chemist, e.g. Benylin. These drugs are controlled for safety, quality and effectiveness.

Prior to 1967, a drug manufacturer could, essentially, market any product that he could manufacture. It didn't make much difference whether the over-the-counter product was actually *effective* or not, so long as it was fairly safe.

After 1967, every drug product has had to pass certain more stringent guidelines to obtain a licence. And in the years since then, the Committee on the Safety of Medicines has been slowly examining over-the-counter products for both safety, quality *and* efficacy. As the test results accrue, the regulations become more stringent; the labels on drugs become more complex, more worth reading. But as the CSM has over 30,000 drugs to test, it will clearly take a long time.

Today, several rules should be followed when you buy any over-the-counter drug.

a. *Read the label before buying—the whole label.* Take seriously every direction; it has been placed there for your safety; it is based on thorough evaluation of the method of action of the drug. This evaluation is costing the taxpayer large amounts of money, so use what you have dearly purchased.

b. *Do not take any drug, even an over-the-counter drug, in early pregnancy if not absolutely needed.*

c. Every ingredient in over-the-counter drugs has probably been evaluated or soon will be, so the formulations of some products are changing. If you find that an over-the-counter drug has, in your estimation, seriously misrepresented what it can accomplish in its advertising, call that fact to the attention of the trading standards officer. And if you suffer any adverse effect from the drug, stop taking it; write to the medicines enforcement section of the DHSS. You may be wrong; that is, you may think the drug is doing something to you that is actually caused by something else entirely. *But be suspicious.* In a free market, the testimony of consumers is a vital guide, both to the regulatory agencies and to the manufacturers themselves.

d. When buying over-the-counter drugs, compare the ingredients. When faced with two products which have the same ingredients in the same quantities, *buy the cheaper.* They have all been regulated in exactly the same way, and if they say they are the same, then they are the same. A brand name in this case gives no advantage over the store's own brand, for example.

19. Over-the-counter pain-killers: aspirin, paracetamol, aloxiprin and codeine combinations

a. *Overdoses of these drugs are dangerous, especially for children. Keep these and all other drugs out of reach.*

b. *Aspirin is quite safe if used in moderation.* Soluble aspirin is the best form. It should always be taken with milk, antacids, or food so that it will not irritate the stomach lining. *It should not be taken during pregnancy unless prescribed by your doctor.* (See p. 134)

c. Paracetamol is also effective against pain and does not irritate the stomach lining as aspirin may. However, it doesn't work against arthritic pain as well as aspirin. (See p. 362)

d. Combination pain-killers usually have aspirin as their major ingredient but may have substances like antacids to make them more palatable. Check the labels *and* the prices! OPINION: Aspirin taken with milk is usually a cheaper, equally effective combination.

WARNING: In Australia these compounds in chronic high doses were found to cause kidney damage, *especially when used with laxatives.* Always take them with plenty of fluid. (See No. 23 below)

20. For sleeplessness, exercise is the best medicine

Some people feel refreshed with four hours' sleep; some need a full eight to ten hours; some are satisfied with frequent catnaps. However you get your rest, it is vital to your health that you get it *regularly.*

a. Accumulated tension often causes sleeplessness; a tranquillizer may relax you temporarily, but it won't relieve the underlying tension that made you wakeful in the first place. For tension and resultant sleeplessness, the very best medicine is exercise. *Try exercise first.* USE SLEEPING MEDICATIONS WITH THE UTMOST CAUTION AND GREATEST POSSIBLE INFREQUENCY!

b. Try these time-honoured methods repeatedly before indulging in a sedative:

—Take a hot bath before retiring.

—Drink a glass of warm milk. Avoid coffee or tea in the evening.

—Exercise strenuously, then wait an hour or so before going to sleep.

—Do not eat immediately before retiring. Leave a couple of hours between your last meal and sleep.

—Do not watch visually stimulating or frightening TV programmes immediately before going to bed.

—Keep an unexciting/relaxing book by the bedside to read.

c. The major causes of disturbed sleep are:

—Situational stress (ongoing problems)

—Specific stress (something you're worried about)

—Physical pain (a toothache is worse at night when nothing distracts you from it)

—Circadian rhythm upset (otherwise known as "jet lag")

—Increasing age (older people sleep lightly and fitfully; this is *normal*)

—Medical problems such as angina, asthma, and duodenal ulcers may display their symptoms more boldly at night.

d. *Depression* affects the body's metabolism as well as its sleep patterns. A depressed person may sleep excessively because she feels tired all the time or because she's so low that she would rather not be awake. Another sign of depression is a pattern of waking up at three or four o'clock every morning.

21. Care of the bowels

Early in this century, it became a popularly accepted notion that a daily bowel movement was necessary; children were taught to move their bowels at the same time every day, without fail. Otherwise, it was supposed that the uneliminated waste products in the bowel would poison the body.

Of course, regular elimination is essential to good health. But "regular" does not mean every day, or the same time every day. "Regular" means "at regular intervals": a bowel movement every other day, every two or three days may be perfectly sufficient.

22. Over-the-counter laxatives

Because the rigid definitions of regularity have such a hold on our people, we take too many laxatives. Laxatives are fine occasionally, to relieve the discomforts of constipation. But when taken regularly, they encourage dependence; the bowel loses its natural strength, and the cycle may perpetuate itself.

Keep several things in mind when using a laxative.

a. Know when you are really constipated. If the stool is anything short of rock-hard, then you are probably not constipated.

b. If you are constipated, try a combination of bran cereal, fresh fruit, leafy vegetables, and lots of water to relieve the diet. Exercise will help too—for it improves circulation and food metabolism. If you have got into the habit of taking a laxative try the same treatment. It may take a few days for your body to adjust, you may experience some assorted discomforts with withdrawal, but the changeover is vital to your good health.

Troublesome signs such as narrowing of the stools or of blood in them should prompt a medical examination. Some drugs such as narcotics, codeine, oral contraceptives, iron and some antacids, can cause constipation.

c. If constipation persists, try a *stool softener*. These are usually Dorbanex preparations with cellulose which create a bulkier, softer stool. They draw water into the stool, putting greater pressure on the bowel, encouraging it to move naturally. WARNING: *If you are on any prescription drug, check with your chemist about possible interference from a non-prescription drug such as a laxative or stool softener.*

d. Most laxatives on the market are safe (Ref. 6) but every effort should be made not to rely on them for a bowel movement, for in the long run, laxative dependence weakens the bowel and general health.

23. Laxatives, pain-killers and kidney disease

Recent reports say the incidence of kidney disease may be higher in people who take large amounts of aspirin, paracetamol or phenacetin, especially when the same people are chronic users of laxatives. (Ref. 7) Avoid as many medicines as possible!

24. "Wind" pains, colonic spasm, one of the most common everyday afflictions

Most people occasionally suffer from wind pains and learn from experience that they will eventually pass. The symptoms of indigestion are usually pain in the lower abdomen or under the rib cage. Typically, the pains move around in the abdomen and are accompanied by excessive belching or passing wind from the rectum.

Sometimes a particular food causes wind. If you're suffering, avoid leafy vegetables, beans, onions, spicy foods, carbonated beverages, beer. Some people react to stress or food allergies by spasm of the colon, associated with a retention of wind. Try keeping a diary of when the pain occurs in relation to what you have eaten. You can then pinpoint the trouble.

Another cause is air-swallowing. Many people, when they are nervous, tend to swallow repeatedly and since there is nothing in the mouth, most of what they swallow is air. You may be able to control this if you are *conscious* of the way you react to tension.

Several products on the market containing activated dimethicone or charcoal are good absorbers of wind. Or try lying on a firm surface and rubbing your stomach clockwise to relieve the pain. Stool softeners may help if constipation is also present.

Persistent pain, fever, or bleeding should take you to a doctor.

25. Over-the-counter drugs for allergy

Millions of people suffer from allergies to pollen, animal hair, home dust or to air pollution and occasionally require antihistamines and decongestants to relieve runny noses and itching eyes. These complaints are so frequent that the consumption of this class of drugs is enormous; in fact, many people take them on a continuing basis. RECOMMENDATION: If you plan to take allergy drugs more than once in a while, consult a doctor. You may need stronger medications than those available over the counter; you may require allergy testing and desensitization shots. Changing your bedding to pillows and duvets made with synthetic fillings helps those sensitive to feathers.

WARNING: *Wheezing* is not a normal symptom of everyday allergy; it may indicate asthma, or heart disease and should not be treated without a doctor's supervision.

26. How to use an over-the-counter drug

a. *As infrequently as possible.* A drug is defined as a drug because it is absorbed into the blood stream and affects the body. A healthy person who eats and exercises properly should have need for drugs only occasionally, and should not make a habit of taking any medication. Avoid *all* drugs in pregnancy.

b. Ask your chemist any questions about any drug which you may have forgotten to ask your doctor. A chemist knows about any possible side effects and any possible bad reactions from the interaction of several drugs being taken simultaneously. This is especially true if you are taking drugs prescribed by *several different doctors.*

c. Many over-the-counter drugs have package inserts which are vital reading for the well-informed consumer.

d. *Do not use over-the-counter drugs instead of doctors.* Many people use a variety of different products over prolonged time periods, trying to avoid a medical visit. *If any symptoms occur for which drugs of any kind are needed for more than one week, a doctor should be consulted.* The persistence of a symptom may signify a serious problem that you should check more thoroughly, or a simple one which responds quickly to the correct treatment.

27. Hygiene during menstruation

As well as the traditional belt-with-pad and tampon, there are some newer items on the market:

a. *Beltless sanitary towels* have a strip of adhesive on the underside which sticks to pants or tights and holds the pad in place without a belt. If you wear loose underwear, these won't work.

b. *Very small pads* are advertised as useful for the few days of extremely light flow. However, they were undoubtedly developed because millions of women on the pill normally experience very light flow. They tend to fold in at the sides.

c. *Plastic-encased tampons* work exactly the same as the cardboard-encased variety. *Keep in mind, however, that the plastic is not biodegradable.* It does not break up into natural components and disappear back into the earth when discarded, and so it eventually pollutes the environment. Thus, bathing beaches may become littered with plastic tampon containers, disposed of at sea and washed up intact on the shore. Even the rolling, salty oceans cannot destroy them. OPINION: If tampons are all the same to you—*and they should be*—opt for those which have biodegradable casings, or no casings at all.

d. *Perfumed tampons and artificial fibres in pads* are irritating to some women, and can cause contact dermatitis, redness and itching around the vulva. If this happens, switch to other products. Perfumed pads and tampons are unnecessary to combat odour during menstruation anyway. Washing is preferable.

e. *Do not use tampons in between periods!* Some women use tampons when they are not bleeding to absorb an unusually heavy vaginal discharge. This is potentially dangerous. The tampon acts as an irritant in the vagina and may actually make the situation worse by causing vaginal ulceration and severe infections. The tampon may absorb the normal vaginal mucus that fights infection and thereby rid you of your natural defences.

f. *Toxic Shock Syndrome (TSS)—a new disease that may be associated with tampon use.* In the U.S., about 800–900 cases of a new disease have been reported within the last two years; some cases have been fatal. The disease involves a high fever, vomiting, diarrhoea, headache, sore muscles and later a very red tongue, a peeling red rash on the hands and feet and shock—a sudden drop in blood pressure that may lead to kidney failure. Ninety-six per cent of the cases were in women: of these, 95 per cent were menstruating at the time the disease occurred, and most were using tampons which were superabsorbent, made of man-made fibre. Almost all

237

of the afflicted women were found to have *Staphylococcus aureus* in cultures of their vaginas. A powerful toxin released by these bacteria seems to get into the body and cause the disease. At least, this is the current theory.

Pending settlement of the issue, we recommend the following for safe tampon use. Change tampons frequently; do not use them when flow is very light or in between periods. (See 27e) Avoid super-absorbent tampons. Some are so absorbent that they adhere to the walls of the vagina, and many women notice pain when pulling them out. This is because the superficial layers of the vagina are also being damaged.

28. Over-the-counter drugs for menstrual discomfort

The main compound in these is aspirin or salicylamide (sal-ih-SILL-ah-mide), which is very much like aspirin. More expensive than ordinary aspirin, *they are no more effective* for the average woman.

Some contain *mild* diuretics, such as *parabrom,* caffeine or ammonium chloride, which only help women who have fluid retention contributing to their menstrual discomfort.

COSMETIC SURGERY

29. Voluntary (cosmetic) surgery

Surgery is "voluntary" when it is not needed for reasons of health but is desired nonetheless by the patient. Although unnecessary surgery should be avoided as a rule, some women feel so disfigured by a particular feature that they opt for this alternative; the cosmetic and psychological benefits can be very considerable. However, it is important to remember that a nose job—for example—will not solve all your social problems; it will just straighten your nose. If the psychological problems are severe, treatment on the National Health Service might be available. Otherwise cosmetic surgery must be done privately.

30. Who is a qualified cosmetic surgeon?

Plastic surgeons are expected to obtain the fellowship of the Royal College of Surgeons and then take a training course of several years at specialist plastic surgery units.

Ask your GP to refer you to a plastic surgeon. Do not reply to newspaper advertisements. Recent reports have identified unqualified personnel working in some of these clinics.

31. Rhinoplasty ("nose job")

This is the most common kind of cosmetic surgery. The nose is broken and the cartilage is reshaped under local anaesthesia with a sedative. The patient is usually in the hospital three to five days, and will have severe bruising, black eyes, and swelling around the nose and cheeks for two to three weeks thereafter. When this heals, there will be no visible scar. There are a few complications to this procedure: rarely, an infection or scarring inside the passage. Sometimes, the "new" nose does not come out exactly as expected and this possibility must be anticipated. However, in most cases, the result is very satisfactory.

32. Wrinkles

The skin wrinkles because it has been weathered and stretched and used with time. The only way to get rid of wrinkles is by cosmetic surgery or by covering them up with make-up. Some things do contribute to faster ageing of the skin:

a. Heredity;

b. Too much exposure to sun and wind, particularly ocean wind;

c. Excessive drinking, for alcohol dries the skin;

d. Heavy smoking, which impairs circulation in the skin of the face (as well as the hands and feet);

e. Excess creaming and massaging of the face (this is a relatively new theory; see No. 33 below) and

f. Frequent weight gain and loss (the weight gain stretches the skin; when the weight is lost, the skin sags and wrinkles over the diminished flesh).

It is unfortunate that in our youth-oriented culture, wrinkles, which express the character and personality of a person so well, must be viewed as things to be eliminated. Try to stand by yourself and leave your wrinkles alone.

33. Massage and facial exercise may actually lead to wrinkles

Although facial massage and exercises have been heralded for years as a way to keep the skin looking young, it is now thought to promote wrinkles. (Ref. 8) The theory is that collagen fibres in the skin are responsible for skin tone and that massage and exercise break it down, causing the skin to sag and wrinkle. Collagen is a protein that helps to hold tissue, cartilage and bone in shape (the word itself comes from the Greek root *koila*, meaning glue). Wrinkles appear where the face moves the most, where movement has damaged the collagen so that it cannot replenish itself fast enough and do its work of holding the facial tissues in shape. This theory, if it is true, means that the least wrinkled face is the one that never moves, never laughs or suffers or feels the blast of a fresh wind. Surely, it is better to be wrinkled.

34. Rhytidectomy ("face lift") (rye-tih-DECK-toe-me)

This operation is usually performed because the patient thinks he or she is excessively wrinkled and has too much overfolding tissue under the chin (double chin). An incision is made across the top of the scalp, behind the ears and under the chin. Local anaesthesia is generally used. A rim of tissue is removed all around. The skin is attached again, more tautly than before. There will be no visible scar. This operation keeps a woman in the hospital four to five days; three weeks or more are required before the swelling and the bruising clears up.

35. What can be expected from a face lift?

Anyone who has a face lift looks better for a while. However, natural ageing processes will eventually begin to wrinkle the newly smooth face again and many people who are desperate about their wrinkles will have the face lift more than once. A face lift makes *only* the face look more youthful. The rest of the body is ageing normally.

36. Opinion: Oestrogen creams do little to fade wrinkles, and are to be avoided.

Face creams containing hormones make wrinkles fade a little, temporarily, because they force the skin to hold more moisture, to swell up and press out the wrinkles. They must be used continuously to have any significant effect and may cause oestrogen to build up in the body, creating unpleasant side effects.
They are best avoided. Other moisturizing creams without oestrogen will have essentially the same effect. Mask applications also make the face tissues retain water temporarily. The high-dose oestrogen creams are available only by prescription.

37. Facial discolourations

As a woman gets older, her body has undergone many hormonal changes: years and years of menstruation; pregnancies; climacteric. These hormone cycles sometimes have an effect on the pigment cells in the skin, so that freckles, "liver spots" and other small discolourations may appear. If these grow unsightly, some may be removed by simple surgery. If you have them removed and they grow back, don't have them removed again—use make-up to cover them. Creams that are available over the counter which claim to fade these spots and freckles are generally not effective. The best and cheapest answer is make-up.

38. Blepharoplasty (eyelid repair) (BLEFF-ah-roe-plass-tee)
A small piece of skin is removed from each upper and lower lid so that the remaining skin will stretch more tautly. Vision is not impaired; the eyelid crease hides the scars. Frequently, this procedure is done in conjunction with a face lift.

39. Breast surgery
Women often seek cosmetic surgery to increase or decrease breast size, to even out the size or to replace a breast lost by mastectomy. This highly complicated surgery should not be undertaken lightly either from a medical or psychological point of view. Over-large breasts may severely limit a woman's mobility and these operations may be done on the NHS.

40. Warning: Never accept silicone injections in the breast!
In the 1960s when female nudity became so prominent in magazines and in "topless" nightclubs, women, their managers and doctors began experimenting with injection of silicone into breast tissue to increase the size of the breasts and offset natural sagging. *This was a catastrophe!* Infections, poisoning, necrosis (tissue death) of breast cells and even cancerous growths resulted in many cases. *Never* use this procedure, and if you know anyone who is considering it, *warn her off!*

41. Solid silicone implant to increase breast size
The only relatively safe procedure to increase breast size today is *implantation of a solid chunk of silicone* in the base of the breast; where it will not interfere with breast function, including breast-feeding. The implant can be made with local or general anaesthesia; the incision is relatively simple. In a few cases, there are complications; haematoma (blood clot) or infection, or, at a later date, formation of a capsule around the implant, and there is the possibility that the body might reject the implant. *The procedure should only be contemplated by a woman*
    a. after mastectomy, or
    b. when breasts vary greatly in size one from the other.

42. Breast reduction is more complex than breast enlargement
Breast reduction surgery takes two to three hours in the operating room, sometimes requires blood transfusions, and leaves

rather large scars under the breasts. The *only* women who should consider it are

a. those with grossly large breasts which create serious secondary discomforts—trouble in breathing, chronic backache, irritation from pulling bra straps; or

b. women with one breast which is much larger than the other.

43. A developing procedure: breast augmentation after mastectomy (see page 342)

Artificial prostheses to make breasts look normal under clothing are widely available and very satisfactory for many women who have undergone mastectomy. However, women who are not content with the prosthesis may wish to consider silicone implants. *At present, there is no indication that these implants encourage a recurrence of malignancy.*

The implant can be done at the time of surgery itself (especially if the tumour is very small and a simple mastectomy or subcutaneous mastectomy is possible). Not all surgeons are willing to perform this replacement if a radical mastectomy is needed (see p. 343) and prefer to wait 1-2 years to ensure that the tumour has been completely removed. (Ref. 9)

The implant can also be done in women who had mastectomy in the past.

Remember that the replacement breast will not look just like the other breast. However, techniques are improving and there are now even ways of simulating a nipple by tattooing or by grafting skin from the vulva or from remaining nipple on to the new breast.

DENTAL CARE

44. Tooth decay: a preventable epidemic

Latest figures show that 29 per cent of British adults have no teeth and that on average adults have two teeth which have decayed and need attention. This figure could be improved very simply with fluoridation of the water supply in all areas. Diet is also an important factor.

45. What causes tooth decay?

a. Plaque (pronounced "plack") is a thick gel formed by saliva and bacteria combining in the mouth, which sticks to the teeth. As the bacteria digests sugar, an acid is formed which eats away at the enamel of the tooth. If the plaque stays on the tooth and hardens, it forms calculus (a calcium substance, so hard it has to be chipped and scraped away). Calculus can cause irritation and infection of the gums.

b. Sugar (carbohydrate), especially the "free" sugar in sweets and cakes, causes bacteria in the mouth to thrive, encouraging plaque formation. The more sugar in the diet, the more bacteria to digest it, the more acid forming to destroy tooth enamel. We have one of the highest free sugar consumption rates in the world; one survey estimated that the average Briton eats about *100 pounds (45 kg)* of refined sugar each year! That is dental suicide.

c. Heredity determines the innate strength of tooth enamel to a very great degree. *Know your family's dental history.* If it is bad, take every step to protect yourself and your children.

46. Preferred dental hygiene

a. Virtually all medical and dental authorities now agree that fluoride in a water supply can help prevent cavities—people living in fluoridated communities experience 60 per cent less tooth decay in the first twelve years of their lives. If the water in your area is not fluoridated, get fluoride treatments at your dentist yearly; brush with a fluoridated toothpaste. Children in such areas should take vitamins with fluoride in them daily for the first five years and fluoride alone until 14 years. (Fluoride in water may also help prevent osteoporosis in later life, see p. 282)

b. Avoid the sweet-type vitamins for children. If you cannot find unsugared vitamins because of the current fad to the contrary, give your kids an ordinary combined vitamin *plus* a fluoride pill.

c. Brush after every meal; this helps prevent plaque build-up. A new theory suggests that if you brush before the meal plaque is removed and food does not then stick to the teeth.

d. Don't use a very hard toothbrush; it may hurt your gums.

e. Use non-waxed dental floss daily to prevent food that is caught between the teeth from rotting and causing decay.

f. RECOMMENDATION: Do not use toothpastes with whiteners routinely. The whiteners may be abrasive to tooth enamel. Remember: absolutely white teeth look false, and abnormal. There is nothing unhealthy about slightly yellow teeth; if you want your teeth to look whiter, try a different colour lipstick; white often looks brighter or duller depending on the colour that is around it.

g. RECOMMENDATION: Avoid toothpastes with chloroform and formaldehyde in them. These are dangerous substances, even in low concentrations.

h. See a dentist at least twice a year.

i. There are now tablets which can be taken which discolour the areas of plaque and enable you to brush away plaque more efficiently. If you are bothered by constant decay, try them.

j. Don't smoke. It will turn your teeth yellow or even brown and cause gum infections. Calculus in particular stains easily and looks terrible.

k. If you have teeth removed, see that you have the appropriate bridgework done. The teeth hold each other in place; when one goes, all the rest weaken, may change position and get loose. If your bridge doesn't seem to fit, or is irritating you, have it refitted immediately. Badly-fitting bridges that irritate the gums, can cause much more serious infection and illness. Get a second opinion or a referral to a nearby dental school from your G.P. if you think you are being pressurized into expensive private bridgework.

l. Calculus should be removed regularly by the dentist.

m. If you have bad teeth, with lots of fillings and an obvious tendency towards decay, have your teeth X-rayed yearly.If you have good teeth, avoid the X-rays or have them infrequently; they are an unnecessary risk to you. If you're pregnant, try to avoid dental X-rays. If you must have them, make sure your abdomen is completely screened.

47. Gingivitis and pyorrhoea: common gum ailments

When plaque along the gum line calcifies, it can cause an inflammation called gingivitis. This should be treated immediately by removal of the calculus and medication to relieve the inflammation. Sometimes, the plaque and calculus creep around between the gum and the teeth; the constant irritation can lead to pyorrhoea, a more serious gum inflammation, loosening of the teeth, or sometimes loss of them.

48. Smoking is terrible for your teeth

Smoking discolours your teeth and discolours calculus, which starts off white. It increases the risk of gum disease, especially in young women. *Smokers are twice as likely to lose their teeth as are non-smokers of the same age,* though this may not be entirely due to smoking but to other factors.

49. Dental anaesthetics

Dental surgeons have had some months of training in anaesthetics and are qualified to administer general anaesthesia, for example, for tooth extractions, although it is preferable to have an anaesthetist carry it out. If you have any medical problems of any sort, do not allow yourself to be anaesthetized in the dentist's chair; you can have your tooth extracted in the hospital or under local anaesthesia.

A local anaesthetic is safer; a dentist can numb your mouth totally without the risk and complexity of general anaesthesia. WARNING: *Never have a general anaesthetic for dental work during pregnancy*— because you run the risk of decreasing the oxygen supply to your baby. Never have a general anaesthetic given by your dentist working alone. An anaesthetist should do the anaesthesia and the dentist do the dentistry.

THE IMPORTANCE OF PROPER DIET

50. A nutritious diet is rare

Very few people now follow a basic, nutritious diet without excess calories or junk food. The table of basic food substances found at the end of this chapter (Table 8) shows the average needs of an adult. If you do heavy work, you need more calories and nutrition; if you do sedentary work, you need less.

The way a woman eats as an adult derives partially from patterns set in childhood (e.g., not liking spinach) and partially from adult conditioning patterns (e.g., eating very fast). Individual metabolic rates vary, so that the same diet and same exercise pattern will result in different body weights for different individuals. A woman should embark on a well-balanced diet for herself, and if she has children should discourage non-nutritious foods which add nothing but fat or carbohydrates to the body. *Exercise must go together with diet.* If you don't develop a good exercise pattern, you cannot eat as much as you want; it's as simple as that.

51. Nutritional values

A calorie is a unit of energy supplied to the body by food. The body burns calories in response to its energy requirements. There are three categories of foods:

a. Fats
b. Proteins
c. Carbohydrates

Carbohydrate calories burn off the fastest; fat calories more slowly; protein calories least quickly. Most reducing diets therefore suggest a decrease in fats and carbohydrates and maintenance of proteins. A body which does not receive enough protein will suffer from malnutrition. Thus, some of the fattest people who look quite well nourished are actually malnourished, because their diet is too rich in fat and carbohydrate and deficient in protein, and some people who are slender and appear to be in great shape are actually malnourished because they are not receiving enough calories of all the different food groups. For example, a person who *looks* thin can have an excess of cholesterol in her system from excess saturated fat consumption.

52. Healthy shopping and cooking
Health foods are not processed, preserved or recoloured; they *may* be healthier than processed foods because they are more natural, but one does wonder why they should be so much more expensive.

a. One excellent, and less expensive, way to put "health foods" into your daily diet is to cook. Cook the broccoli fresh instead of buying it frozen. Cook the chicken yourself instead of buying it prefried. Make the biscuits yourself instead of buying them packaged, with all their preservatives, sweetenings and processing. You may not get fewer calories with your own baking—but you'll get fewer chemicals.

b. When you buy fresh produce, wash it very well. There's no sense in eating the spray that kept the aphids away.

c. Powdered non-fat dry milk is just as nutritious as any other milk on the market. In addition, it lacks the butter fat which adds calories and cholesterol to your diet.

d. Fish is high in protein, low in calories, and can be the staple of a well-balanced diet. Try to cultivate a taste for fish and eat it several times a week. Cook it plain; avoid rich sauces and frying in batter. Grill.

e. Trim the fat off beef and lamb before cooking; there's enough fat inlaid in a good piece of meat to keep the flavour.

f. There is worry about the cancer-causing potential of the nitrites used to prevent botulism in processed meats such as hot dogs, corned beef, ham and bacon. Try to limit your intake of these meats. Encourage the development of safe alternatives and of a further reduction in nitrite levels.

g. Most bread is re-enriched with the vitamins and minerals which were otherwise processed out. Thus, white bread is generally just as nutritious as other kinds, although it may lack fibre and whole grains.

h. Among the most dangerous food additives are those we put in ourselves—salt and sugar. Salt promotes retention of water, and this may be particularly dangerous to people with a personal or family history of hypertension. Train yourself—and your children—not to add extra salt to food that has already been prepared with salt.

Refined sugar (that is, not occurring naturally in fruit, for example) has very little nutritional value except for supplying fast-burning calories. It contributes greatly to obesity and to tooth decay. (See No. 45 above)

Avoid sweetened breakfast cereals.

Avoid fruit or tinned fruit juices containing extra sugar.

Drink coffee or tea without sugar.

Eat protein or fresh fruit snacks rather than sugary or salty ones.

53. Sugar substitutes

Sugar is bad for you and saccharin may be bad for you (studies show the potential to cause cancer, at least in animals), so at present, the best policy is to use both as sparingly as possible. The data currently available shows that small amounts of both substances are reasonably safe. Watch for further news. (Ref. 10)

VITAMINS

54. Opinion: Healthy women should avoid large vitamin supplements

Ever since Linus Pauling, who received the Nobel Prize for chemistry and not for nutrition, suggested that large doses of vitamin C could prevent the common cold, people have been infatuated with the notion that vitamins—truly a natural medicine—could be used to create good health. There is no proof that they will—and some evidence that too many vitamins can hamper good health.

Overdoses of vitamin A can cause mental disorientation and skin disorders: also growth retardation in children.

Overdoses of vitamin D can put too much calcium in the blood.

Overdoses of vitamin C are thought to aggravate gout and kidney stones and to lower fertility.

Vitamin E is sold for everything from smooth skin to increased energy and control of hot flushes in menopause. No one has proved that it works for anything except as an anti-oxidant which *may* help to keep the body's oxygen supply steady.

Do not take too many vitamins. A balanced diet will provide all your normal vitamin needs.

(Megavitamin therapy to cure mentally and physically ill people is another, still experimental, matter.) (Refs. 11 and 12)

55. Vitamin deficiency and the oral contraceptives

Some studies have shown that the blood levels of several vitamins go down when a woman is on the pill—vitamins B-6, C, and folic acid in particular. (Ref. 13) A woman should make sure she eats foods high in these vitamins while she is on the pill.

OBESITY

56. How obesity threatens good health

About half the adult population of Britain is overweight. This makes people more susceptible to:

a. Endocrine disorders (including irregular periods and infertility)

b. Elevated blood sugar (diabetes is four times as common in overweight people)

c. Increased incidence of breast and endometrial cancer. (See pp. 333-8, 353)

d. Lung disorders

e. Osteoarthritis (see pp. 365-6)

f. Heart attack; stroke; other cardiovascular illness such as hypertension

g. Gall-bladder disease

h. Complicated pregnancy and delivery

i. Psychological disorders, including depression

j. Venous thrombosis in particular following surgery.

57. Psychological aspects of overeating

Many people overeat because of tension, emotional problems, boredom, or unhappiness (for example, prolonged grief). In fact, some people eat in order to get fat: fatness is psychologically useful to them. It may help them avoid situations which they fear—for example, athletic or social competition.

Never forget that it is unhealthy to be fat. You can adjust psychologically to overweight—but you should still try to lose the excess, because undoubtedly it is shortening your life. (Ref. 14)

58. Diets

Most people get fat from underexercising *and* overeating. Very few people get fat from glandular malfunction or "thyroid trouble": in fact, such people are usually very sick in other ways as well and being overweight is often the least of their problems.

Too many people who seek out special diets harbour some mystical belief in a magic formula or pill that will make them lose weight and still be able to eat whatever they want. *This just isn't possible.* If any advice can be given at all, *it is probable that a book about nutrition—not about dieting—will serve you best.*

Here are some general guidelines about diets:

a. WARNING: *Avoid taking pills for dieting.* Will-power doesn't come in a bottle or syringe. Amphetamines, which take away your appetite, also make you nervous, sleepless, unable to concentrate. People may become addicted to amphetamines. If your doctor prescribes them, get another doctor, for this is now considered bad medicine. The only exception to this rule is a case of massive obesity, a health emergency. (See No. 59 below)

b. WARNING: *Do not accept HCG (Human Chorionic Gonadotrophin) injections for weight loss.* They have not been proved effective, and HCG is too powerful to use in this way.

c. Do not go on a one-food or fad diet. All types of food are needed for good nutrition.

d. Do not go on a crash diet. Rapid weight loss is dangerous to your health. *Three pounds (1.5 kg) a week is the most a healthy woman should lose.* Remember that at this rate you would lose more than 10 stone (63.5 kg) in a year!

e. Never go on a diet without an appropriate companion plan of exercise. As you lose weight, this will keep your skin and muscles in good shape: it will also speed the weight-loss process.

f. OPINION: Use one of the following two methods as an aid in sensible weight reduction:

1. Group plans such as Weight Watchers work for many people. The advantage of these plans is that they advocate good, nutritious diets and slow, steady weight loss, rather than drugs and rapid weight loss. Besides, some women find it easier to diet with the help of others in the same situation. The expense helps others.

2. Behaviour-modification plans work well for some people. Basically, these programmes hope to change eating habits so that food is eaten more slowly and under better conditions (e.g. early in the day, when metabolism is faster).

3. Dietitians in the NHS will see you regularly to advise on your diet and give you the support needed to change your eating habits.

4. A reputable hypnotist may 'suggest' dietary changes which help people to lose weight.

TABLE 7
HEIGHT/WEIGHT CHART FOR WOMEN

HEIGHT	AVERAGE HEALTHY WEIGHT (+/—10%)	DANGEROUS WEIGHT (MORE THAN 25% OVERWEIGHT)
6' (1.83 m)	11 stone 11 (75 kilos)	14 stone 9 (93 kilos)
5' 10" (1.78 m)	11 stone 1 (70 kilos)	13 stone 13 (88.5 kilos)
5' 8" (1.73 m)	10 stone 5 (66 kilos)	13 stone 3 (84 kilos)
5'6" (1.68 m)	10 stone (63.5 kilos)	12 stone 7 (79 kilos)
5'4" (1.63 m)	9 stone 9 (61 kilos)	11 stone 11 (75 kilos)
5'2" (1.58 m)	9 stone 4 (59 kilos)	11 stone 1 (70 kilos)
5' (1.52 m)	8 stone 8 (54.5 kilos)	10 stone 10 (68 kilos)

59. Massive obesity: a health emergency

If you weigh twice as much as you should for your height, you have a problem which should be treated as an emergency. No leisurely experimenting with diets will do in this case. You are in great danger and must act now.

a. Consult your doctor who will refer you to an endocrine specialist.

b. Have all the appropriate blood tests to determine, scientifically, which specific diet plan you require.

c. Lose weight under carefully controlled medical conditions. These should be set only by specialists in conjunction with an extensive weight reduction programme. The doctor may suggest you go into hospital.

d. "Health farms"—special resorts where diet and exercise are carefully controlled—often succeed in getting their guests to lose weight. Check the *bona fides* of the doctors in charge of them. You should leave them with dietary instructions you will stick to. They are expensive.

60. Calculate the risk: the intestinal bypass operation to prevent obesity

If all other methods fail for the massively obese person, a surgical procedure is possible in which a section of the small intestine is eliminated from the normal flow. This should be used only as a last resort, for risk of complications is high. About one person in 20 does not survive the operation. Diarrhoea and frequent bowel movements may persist more than six months afterwards. Liver disease has also been reported. (Ref. 15) An alternative surgical procedure which may be safer is stomach stapling. (Ref. 16) Watch for news.

61. Involuntary weight loss may indicate ill health

Weight gain may or may not mean you are sick—but *involuntary weight loss means that something is wrong*. Get a medical examination, especially if you have any other abnormal symptoms.

62. Coffee, tea, cola, caffeine and tension

Caffeine is a relatively powerful stimulant which occurs naturally in coffee, tea and the cocoa bean from which cola-type drinks (including diet cola) are made. WARNING: Each cup of coffee contains between 100 and 125 mg of caffeine; if you drink coffee after every meal, you are getting a lot of caffeine; if you drink two or three cups after every meal and a couple more during the day, you may be overdosing with caffeine.

Symptoms of excess caffeine may be extreme nervousness, heartburn, heart palpitations, and diarrhoea. It was believed for some time that caffeine caused ulcers, colitis, and heart disease. However, a recent study showed that even *decaffeinated* coffee is associated with ulcers. (Ref. 17) And no good evidence has confirmed an association between caffeine and heart disease. (Ref. 18) There is some suggestion that excess caffeine intake may aggravate cystic disease of the breast, but at present, all we can say is that caffeine is a powerful stimulant which may cause some medical problems in susceptible people. (Ref. 19) It should not be used excessively.

63. Cholesterol is not a great danger to most women before the menopause

Cholesterol is a kind of fat (lipid), present in butter, and other saturated fats and oils, high-fat meats such as pork, untrimmed beef and lamb, whole milk, and eggs. In the body it is manufactured in the liver and is then metabolized into steroids, hormones, and bile acids and is present in cell membranes. If cholesterol and other lipids are present in the blood stream in high levels, they may build up in the interior of the arteries, causing a narrowing of the passage. This process is called artheriosclerosis or hardening of the arteries.

Women seem to have a lower risk of artheriosclerosis before the age of the menopause. It now appears that an important factor in determining whether a person is adversely affected by cholesterol build-up is the type of complex molecule by which the cholesterol is carried in the blood stream. Some of the cholesterol is carried as high-density lipoproteins (HDL) which are large molecules, high in protein and low in cholesterol. The rest is carried in low-density lipoproteins (LDL) which are high in cholesterol and low in protein. The HDLs appear to have a protective effect on cardiovascular disease; the higher the HDL/LDL ratio, the less the risk of cardiovascular disease, such as heart attack and stroke. HDL levels are increased by cutting back on saturated fats and by strenuous exercise. Women, before the menopause, seem to have higher HDL levels and therefore less risk of cardiovascular disease. This protection is decreased by obesity, smoking, use of oestrogens (and perhaps some progestogens) and a diet high in fat. Women should have their cholesterol levels measured periodically—especially over age forty. Values less than 200 mg/ml of blood are normal. Watch for further news in this area. Some doctors are encouraging the routine determination of the HDL/LDL levels, especially in high-risk people. (Refs. 20, 21)

64. High-fibre foods and cancer of the colon

It has not been proved conclusively that high-fibre foods, like vegetables, salads, whole-grain breads, and unprocessed cereal grains, will prevent cancer of the colon—but they will make your intestine work better by helping the waste move faster through it, and may save you from the discomfort of constipation. (Ref. 22)

65. Lactose intolerance

Lactose is a natural sugar occurring in milk and milk products. Many people find that after babyhood (and sometimes during infancy), they are unable to digest milk. A glassful gives them a stomach ache, nausea and diarrhoea. Cheese and yoghurt, which are lower in lactose content, are better tolerated. These people have a deficiency in the intestinal enzyme, *lactase,* which might be added to milk before drinking. Watch for developments in this area. If you suffer from excess wind and colitis, consider that lactose intolerance may be the cause. People with southern European and African ancestry seem to be the most affected.

66. Acidophilus replacement

Lactobacillus acidophilus is a bacteria normally present in the colon, where it assists in digestion of milk products. (This is very similar to the lactobacillus normally present in the vagina.) Under certain circumstances such as prolonged antibiotic usage, the normal bacteria of the colon are killed off and some people believe that for good digestion to continue, the acidophilus must be replaced. Special milk with acidophilus is sold at rather high prices: live yoghurt, which contains another lactobacillus, probably works just as well.

67. Exercise is essential for good health throughout life

It is probably true that people who exercise regularly look better, live longer, and stay healthier.

a. Exercises done regularly every day keep your body in shape, assist body systems in functioning, and clear your head. A woman may select any system, depending on what is best for her. (For example, a pianist or typist will prefer different exercises from those needed by a saleswoman or cook, because the first may suffer from cramped back muscles, the second may suffer from aching legs and feet.) Those who work under tension may prefer a system like yoga, which stretches the muscles while relaxing the mind as well. Many women find that it is helpful to learn the exercises in weekly, or twice-weekly classes and continue practising at home.

b. *Avoid now-and-then strenuous exercise.*

If you have stopped exercising for some time, don't leap into strenuous exercise suddenly. Too many tennis players and joggers have been struck down by heart attacks because they did not build up to strenuous exercise; because they overestimated their strength, or, rather, underestimated their accumulated weakness. See your doctor before undertaking strenuous exercise if you are over forty. Do not do any strenuous exercise in the midday sun if you are out of shape.

c. Swimming is a good all round exercise for everyone. You don't have to swim fast or with perfect form to enjoy the benefits of relaxation and improved muscle tone that comes with swimming.

d. Exercise prevents or alleviates many of the conditions that chronically make women feel ill; for example, it helps to prevent osteoporosis; alleviates dysmenorrhoea and constipation; by strengthening muscles, it makes childbirth easier.

SMOKING AND HOW TO STOP

68. Smoking is terrible for your health

It is almost ludicrous and trite to mention that smoking is bad for you. Everyone over age three knows that! Smoking is just about the worst thing a woman can do to herself. Smoking is a major factor in the development of (among other things) lung cancer, bronchitis, emphysema, heart attack, hypertension, stroke, severe gum disease and loss of teeth, early menopause, bladder cancer and bad facial wrinkles. (Refs. 23–27) Women who smoke and who take oral contraceptives are at much greater risk of heart attacks and strokes than non-smokers. (See p. 45) It seems likely that the smoking is a greater factor than the pill. Women who smoke and who do not take the pill are at greater risk of these problems than are non-smoking pill takers. If smoking among women continues to rise female deaths from lung cancer will soon exceed those from breast cancer.

There is no getting around the fact that smokers are voluntarily doing irreparable harm to their bodies. Pregnant women who smoke are voluntarily exposing their babies to great danger, including fetal death. (See p. 181) A recent article puts forward the *theory* that the children of women smoking during pregnancy may be at increased risk of developing cancer when they grow up. This is only a hypothesis but only time will tell if there is truth in it. Why take the risk? (Ref. 28) It is truly a futile exercise for a woman to follow all of the other advice in this book and then continue to smoke.

69. Some women are smoking more than ever

Since the medical evidence, published in the 60s, showed the dangers of smoking, there has been a decline in smoking. But women have been slower to give up than men and among working class women, smoking is still increasing. Tragically advertisers have succeeded in making women equate smoking with liberation.

70. How to stop smoking

A number of products may help you stop smoking, although there are no magic cures. Some Area Health Authorities, GPs and hospitals have set up group therapy clinics to help kick the habit. Children are very useful in the fight to stop, for they have been convinced by health education in schools that smoking will kill their parents and feel justified in tearing up and throwing away cigarettes. The protesting adult feels foolish struggling with a six-year-old for possession of a tube of tobacco which the adult knows full well is poisonous to the system. Hence, the final reason for a halt to smoking is simple shame.

Taste-distorting lozenges can be helpful, since they ruin the taste of the cigarette. Very strong mints, for example, are quite good. If you are a person who smokes most when you are under a lot of tension, substitute another oral satisfaction. Chew on something. People who think they smoke to *relieve* tension very often find that the smoking itself caused them to be more tense than they had to be. Many people find that after they stop smoking, they gain weight (perhaps because they are compensating their oral needs by eating more).

A new chewing gum containing nicotine, called Nicorette, has been used successfully in small scale trials and has now been marketed for use on prescription only, and is not yet available on the NHS. Ask your doctor about this.

Whichever method you try, what really counts is your genuine desire to stop. Many women succeed after they have tried one or more times already, so it is always worth trying again. It is a good idea to choose a day in advance, preferably one when you will not be under special stress or in the company of smokers. Tell as many people as possible that you are giving up—their support will be very helpful.

ALCOHOL AND ITS DANGERS

71. Alcoholic beverages in moderation are not medically dangerous

At present, well-nourished people who have a drink or two a day seem to show no adverse medical effects. Some studies have actually shown that they live longer than non-drinkers. The key word, of course, is moderation. There is great concern currently over the rising number of female and teenage alcoholics. In a recent survey, six per cent of men and one per cent of women admitted drinking more than the upper limit recommended by the Royal College of Psychiatrists of the equivalent of three pints of beer a day.

72. How to avoid getting drunk or having a hangover

If you want to drink to be social, but don't want to get intoxicated or suffer too much the following day, consider these ideas:

a. Eat while you drink. It makes the drink last longer—and may slow down the amount of alcohol entering your blood stream.

b. Sip your drink slowly; nurse it; make it last; dilute spirits with tonic water, or ginger ale.

c. If you anticipate a hangover, drink several glasses of milk, water or juice before bed to replenish fluids and soothe the stomach. Analgesics may help, but the chances are that nothing will prevent a hangover entirely, if you have drunk too much.

73. Is alcohol becoming a problem for you?

Ask yourself the following questions, and answer them *honestly:*

a. Do you take a drink in the morning?

b. Do you drink at lunch every day without fail?

c. Do you get merry every night, or do you absolutely need to drink to get to sleep?

d. Do you feel you *need* a drink at the end of your working day . . . or before?

If the answer to any one of these questions is "yes", you may be on your way to a drinking problem. *If the answer to two or more is "yes", you probably need help immediately!*

74. The medical risks of alcoholism

The most serious medical problems associated with alcoholism are:

a. Cirrhosis of the liver (destruction of the liver cells—often fatal)

b. Peptic ulcer, alcoholic gastritis, oesophageal varices (with bleeding into the bowel)

c. Malnutrition and vitamin deficiency

d. Severe anaemia

e. Heart disease (damage to the heart muscle)

f. Severe mental disorders (hallucinations, loss of memory, later, actual destruction of brain cells), depression, paranoid delusions

g. Seizures (often associated with withdrawal from alcohol)

h. Fetal alcohol syndrome (see p. 181) in babies born to mothers who are alcoholics.

i. Even moderate amounts of alcohol (up to 3 glasses a day) increase the risk of a mid-term spontaneous abortion. (Ref. 29)

75. Organizations that help alcoholics

a. A general practitioner, social worker or health visitor can start counselling for an alcohol problem but will probably refer the patient to an Alcoholic Treatment Unit or voluntary organization.

b. Alcoholics Anonymous has been most successful in helping alcoholics stay away from drink. They offer clear rules, understanding and a mutual sharing of a terrible problem.

c. Al-Anon provides counselling for the family and friends of alcoholics; Alateen deals with the problems of teenage alcoholics.

d. There are many alcoholic treatment units throughout the country funded by the health authorities for both inpatient and outpatient therapy. Usually the treatment begins with several weeks' hospitalization, followed by outpatient therapy.

e. Local Councils on Alcoholism are voluntary bodies, thoughout Britain, which also help problem drinkers and their families.

TRANQUILLIZERS

76. Warning: Tranquillizers and other drugs affecting the emotions are dangerously overprescribed and overused by women

Tranquillizers (anti-anxiety drugs) are the most commonly prescribed drugs in this country. (See Table 9) These drugs, while very effective in relieving anxiety, are very powerful and potentially addictive. If high doses are taken, withdrawal symptoms may occur when a woman tries to stop the drugs.

Women receive most of the prescriptions for tranquillizers, not only for anxiety, but for a myriad of complaints which may or may not be related to anxiety. There is a prevailing bias among doctors that women's disorders are far more likely to be "psychoneurotic" than men's. Frequently, they are prescribed when the doctor doesn't take the time to discuss the woman's problem fully or to do a complete examination. *Don't let this happen to you.*

When a woman feels nervous, she should attempt to determine why. If she has increasing tension and sleeplessness, then she may need professional counselling with a psychiatrist, psychologist or marriage or young people's counsellor to help determine the cause of the problem. In the long run, counselling is far better for a woman's health than drugs. It is important that a woman learns to deal with her problems rather than become dependent on long-term therapy with potentially addictive drugs. *Don't accept tranquillizers just to mask anxiety without determining the cause.*

If tranquillizers are absolutely necessary for treatment of severe anxiety attacks, they should be taken in low doses only and for short periods of time *unless* they are prescribed in combination with counselling.

77. Avoid drink or marijuana if you are taking tranquillizers or barbiturates

The combination of alcohol or marijuana and tranquillizers is dangerous to your health; excesses of the two can cause blackouts or have other severe potentially lethal effects on your nervous system. For example, your ability to drive a car may be limited–but you may not realize this. NEVER COMBINE THEM!

78. Marijuana

An estimated 5 million people smoke marijuana regularly in Britain. It provides a mild "high" without the hangover and ill health associated with heavy drinking.

Attempts to find some adverse effect of marijuana to discourage pot-smokers have failed generally. There are some reports of acute psychosis; fast heart rate; impaired coordination because of adverse effect on the brain. Some tests show that marijuana smoke can cause malignancies and lung damage just like tobacco smoke. Reports of genetic damage because of marijuana smoking by pregnant women remain unproved. *However, marijuana is a drug and it certainly is a good idea not to use it, or any other drug, during early pregnancy.* (Ref. 30) One new study indicates that prolonged use can lead to a decreased sperm count in men. (Refs. 31, 32)

A new development: Recently, there have been some reports that marijuana has good effects on the disease glaucoma, in which pressure builds up in the eye because of poor drainage of internal optic fluids. If you suffer from glaucoma and other treatments have failed, ask your doctor about marijuana.

Reports that sex is "better" when the partners are under the influence of marijuana are yet to be proved. Individuals can judge for themselves whether they prefer to be more, or less, bereft of their senses when making love.

Other "hard" drugs are disastrous for a woman's health. Avoid them at all cost!

79. Energy, stress, and fatigue

Energy is a natural endowment; good nutrition, adequate exercise, and enough satisfying sleep will maintain it in full measure. Yet few women (or men) receive these simple basic ingredients, and as more women go to work, fatigue—lack of energy—becomes a great problem.

"Quick energy" is that extra little burst of steam you can get from a chocolate bar (fast-burning carbohydrate) or from emotional stimulation which causes the release of adrenaline. This kind of energy is vital—but you can't live on it.

80. Poor nutrition may cause fatigue

A breakfast of coffee alone, which has no nutritional content, will eventually contribute to fatigue. The caffeine, and the sugar, in the coffee may provide quick energy. But the protein in whole wheat bread or whole grain cereal or an egg plus a glass of unsweetened orange juice provides the energy that the body needs *all day*.

81. Lack of exercise may cause fatigue

It is almost axiomatic that the people who feel most tired are those who have worked for years in an office or factory, at a sedentary job. Exercise renews the body's oxygen supply by increasing the flow of oxygen through the circulatory system: thus, if you can't get any exercise at work, run in the morning or play tennis or work in the garden in the evening.

82. Stress may cause fatigue; prolonged stress may cause disease

When you are under a lot of stress, your body reacts to help you cope with it; your muscles tighten; your mind races; your blood pressure and cholesterol levels rise. Over time, stress of this kind can predispose the body to serious disease—heart trouble and ulcers, for example. WARNING: *Fatigue is the first signal that you may be under too much stress for your own health.* If you are exhausted every day after work, curtailing your social life, unable to read or enjoy a film, then maybe the fatigue you are suffering from should be regarded as a warning—and you should take a second look at your work.

Research during International Women's Year (1976) showed that the hardest-working person in the entire world is the woman who works a full day and then comes home to cook, clean and otherwise care for house, children, and husband.

Do not accept crippling fatigue due to stress as the *sine qua non* of your everyday life. Depending on your personality and your individual circumstances, you may be able to organize a less stressful situation and get back your energy, and your good health.

TABLE 8

FOOD SUBSTANCES—RECOMMENDED DAILY REQUIREMENTS

	ADULT WOMEN	PREGNANCY AND LACTATION	BODY FUNCTION	FOOD SOURCES
Carbohydrates	2000–2500 Calories	2400–2750 Calories	Main source of energy – excess stored as fat (cellulose bulk)	breads, sugar, cereals (cellulose – dried fruits, grains, nuts, vegetables)
Fats			energy, fatty insulation of the body	eggs, liver, kidney, butter, milk, oils
Protein	47–62 g	60–69 g	body structure	meat, poultry, fish, milk, cheese, eggs, soya beans
Minerals *Calcium*	500 mg	1200 mg	bones and teeth, regulators of muscle contraction, blood clotting and nerve function	milk and milk products
Phosphorus	800 mg	1200 mg	bones and teeth, co-enzymes in metabolic pathways	meat, poultry, fish and eggs
Magnesium	300 mg	450 mg	co-enzyme in metabolic pathways	leafy green vegetables, nuts, soya-beans (average diet deficient)

	ADULT WOMEN	PREGNANCY AND LACTATION	BODY FUNCTION	FOOD SOURCES
Iron	12 mg	13–15 mg + (may need supplements)	blood cells	liver, meats, egg yolks, leafy vegetables, raisins, prunes, apricots, seafood and seaweed, iodized salt
Iodine	100 mcg	125–150 mcg	part of thyroid hormone	seafood and seaweed, iodized salt
Zinc	15 mg	20–25 mg	co-enzyme, hair, bones and male sex gland function	animal protein

Fat-soluble vitamins – avoid excess intake – these are stored in body if present in excess

	ADULT WOMEN	PREGNANCY AND LACTATION	BODY FUNCTION	FOOD SOURCES
Vitamin A	750 mcg	750–1200 mcg	visual pigments, skin and mucus membranes	whole milk, butter, egg yolks, liver, kidney, yellow fruits and vegetables
Vitamin D	400	10 mcg	calcium absorption and bone metabolism	egg yolk, milk, butter, liver (exposure to sunlight allows body to manufacture its own requirements)
Vitamin E	30 IU	30 IU	inhibits oxidation of unsaturated fatty acids – rest of activity not proved	vegetable oils, leafy vegetables, whole grain cereals

Water-soluble vitamins – excess is excreted

	ADULT WOMEN	PREGNANCY AND LACTATION	BODY FUNCTION	FOOD SOURCES
Vitamin C	70 mg	100–150 mg	formation of connective tissue and adrenal gland function	citrus fruits, berries, melons, leafy green vegetables
Total folate (including folic acid)	300 mcg	500 mcg	co-enzyme in synthesis of nucleic acids – deficiency = anaemia	whole grain cereals, leafy green vegetables, meats, milk (supplements may be needed in pregnancy)
Niacin (nicotinic acid)	15 mg	18–21 mg	co-enzyme in fat metabolism	liver, kidney, brewer's yeast, tuna, muscle meats, poultry, peanuts
Riboflavin	1.3 mg	1.6–1.8 mg	co-enzyme in metabolism of carbohydrates, fats and proteins	brewer's yeast, glandular meats, milk, cheese, eggs, veal, beef, leafy green vegetables
Thiamine	0.9 mg	1.0 mg	co-enzyme and important in nerve function	brewer's yeast, wheat germ, whole grain cereals, pork, nuts
Vitamin B-6	2.0 mg	2.5 mg	co-enzyme especially in protein metabolism. Needed for chemical reactions in brain.	muscle meats, liver, vegetables and whole grain cereals
Vitamin B-12	6.0 mcg	8.0 mcg	red-cell production, co-enzyme in many cell processes	animal foods, especially liver, brewer's yeast (vegetarians may need supplements)

TABLE 9

FREQUENTLY PRESCRIBED TRANQUILLIZERS

GENERIC NAME	MAJOR BRAND NAMES	USUAL DOSE (total/day)
Chlordiazepoxide	Librium	20–40 mg
Clorazepate dipotassium	Tranxene	30 mg
Diazepam	Valium	8–30 mg
Doxepin HCL	Sinequan	up to 150 mg
Hydroxyzine	Atarax	75–300 mg
Meprobamate	Equanil	1200–1600 mg
	Miltown	
Oxazepam	Serenid	40–60 mg
Lorazepam	Ativan	1–4 mg

9

LITTLE GIRLS

Most family doctors like dealing with children and will take the time to be gentle and win their trust. Do press for referral to a paediatrician if you think yours has not got to the root of the problem. For little girls with vaginal or other genital problems, paediatricians may be less frightening to visit than gynaecologists.

NEWBORN CHILDREN

1. Breast enlargement is normal in newborn infants

Up until two to three weeks of age, a newborn female infant may have breast enlargement due to high levels of female hormones present during pregnancy. There may be a small amount of cloudy secretion from the nipples, known as "witch's milk". By three weeks, the maternal hormone levels no longer affect the baby's body. Very frequently, boy babies will show exactly the same breast enlargement, and this is normal.

2. Genital swelling and discharge is normal in newborn girls

When a baby is born, genitals frequently appear swollen; the clitoris may seem to be very large; the labia may appear swollen. Often, a mucus discharge comes from the vagina. Like breast enlargement in infants, this comes from the effect of the maternal hormones. The internal organs, including the uterus, are slightly larger at birth as well. As the hormone levels fall, there may be a few drops of blood from the shrinking uterus and this appears as vaginal bleeding. At three weeks, when maternal hormones no longer achieve high levels in the baby's blood stream, these effects will disappear. They are perfectly normal, indicating a healthy body that is responsive to hormone stimulation.

DEVELOPMENTAL PROBLEMS

3. Imperforate hymen

The hymen is the thin membrane that partly covers the entrance to the vagina. It has a hole in it normally. Shortly after birth, the girl should be examined to make sure that an opening is present—that the hymen is not imperforate (im-PER-for-it). It is not always routine and there have been some cases in which a girl got all the way to puberty before an imperforate hymen was detected. Imperforate hymen will not cause any pain or any difficulty except that as puberty approaches, the normal discharges of the vagina may be caught behind the hymen, creating secondary problems of pain and swelling in the lower abdomen.

If the hymen is imperforate, it must be surgically opened in the hospital. This involves one or two days in hospital and is a simple procedure causing very little discomfort for the child.

4. Confusion as to the sex of a baby

In *extremely rare* cases, the clitoris of a newborn female infant seems almost as large as a penis; or in boys, the scrotum is not completely fused in the midline, creating a vagina-like cavity. In these circumstances there may be real confusion as to the sex of the child.

A scraping of cells from inside the cheek can be checked for chromosome count or a test on white blood cells can be done to prove the sex of the child. Thereafter, appropriate surgery can be done to establish genital sex and create a more normal life for the infant. If any such confusion exists, have it cleared up with a chromosome test immediately, and thereafter with the appropriate surgery. Occasionally, a child has been reared as the wrong sex—and it has been shown that after two to three years of age it is psychologically impossible to successfully reverse the gender identity of the child, i.e., the person thinks of themself as the wrong sex.

5. Premature development of breasts and pubic hair

Very often little girls (three to six years old) will develop small amounts of pubic hair and breast tissue. *This is almost always nothing to worry about.* A fast, simple vaginal smear can be taken to check if female hormones are actually elevated, and premature puberty is taking place. Most often, the hormone levels are normal for the age of the child. If the smear is normal and the general physical examination is normal, forget it. There is nothing to worry about. The breast growth and pubic hair growth will limit itself, and normal puberty will occur later on. If the tests are not normal, you should see an endocrinologist (a doctor specializing in body chemistry and hormones).

The biggest problem with this self-limiting early development is that parents become terribly anxious about it, constantly examining their daughter and making her feel self-conscious and deformed. Try not to let your girl see that you are worried, so the episode can pass—as it probably will—without abiding trauma.

WARNING: *Make sure your daughter has not taken your birth-control pills or other hormonal medication, for these can cause breast changes.*

VAGINAL DISCHARGE AND RELATED PROBLEMS

6. Vulvovaginitis: the most common gynaecological problem of little girls

Irritation of the vulva and vagina is common in little girls aged two to six. Most often it is caused by:

a. Contamination of the vagina by organisms from the bowel. Teach your daughter to wipe from front to back, so that she does not wipe bowel contents towards the vagina. If you find any bowel stains on her underwear, suspect that she is not wiping herself completely and correct the situation. The vagina of a little girl is thinner than that of an adult woman and therefore more susceptible to this kind of infection.

Other causes of vaginitis symptoms—itching, odour, and discharge—are

b. Pinworms;

c. Viruses and bacteria which normally infect the throat and lungs;

d. Candida or thrush—a less frequent cause in little girls;

e. Trichomonas and gonorrhoea—almost never contracted unless the child has been sexually assaulted;

f. Foreign bodies which the child herself has placed in the vagina. (See No. 7 below)

g. If a child complains of itching and the vulva appears red or irritated, suspect bubble baths, detergents used to wash clothes, or harsh, perfumed soaps.

h. In the summertime, the chemicals in swimming pools or the damp and grit of sandboxes can also cause the symptoms of vulvovaginitis.

7. It is normal for a little girl to place something in her vagina

Between the ages of four and six, little girls are sometimes very curious about their genitals and may place something in the vagina—usually toilet paper or tissue but sometimes a paper clip, a peanut, a piece of crayon—as part of the exploration. (Does this hole in me have a bottom? Does it go all the way through me?) A foreign body placed in the vagina will usually cause heavy discharge and a very foul odour; the odour will distinguish between this cause and, say, a bubble-bath-induced vaginitis.

8. Treatment for foreign objects in the vagina

If a very foul odour makes you suspect that your daughter has placed something in her vagina, see the doctor, who should be able to wash it out painlessly. She will have to be examined, but this will not be painful; a tiny speculum will be used, if any is at all. A large foreign body which has lodged well up into the vagina may have to be removed under anaesthesia.

As preventive medicine, talk to your little girl and satisfy her curiosity about her vagina; simply tell her, calmly but firmly, not to put anything into it because this may hurt her.

9. Treatment of vulvovaginitis in little girls

Eighty per cent of cases are caused by faecal contamination. Assume this is the cause and start treating it yourself. Making the child soak three or four times a day in a warm water bath for ten to twenty minutes will clear the irritation. Use *only* a mild soap without perfume. After she has a bowel movement, wash her yourself with soap and warm water. Plain petroleum jelly will soothe a lot of irritation on the outside of the vagina.

If the symptoms persist for more than two days, or if there is any bleeding or pain, consult a doctor. Meanwhile, as preventive medicine, get rid of the bubble bath for good; use only mild soaps all the time; use a gentle detergent on her clothes, even if you have to wash them separately from everyone else's.

For other infections, such as candidiasis (thrush), special preparations will be given by the doctor. If there is any chance at all that your daughter has been molested (a trichomonal or gonorrhoeal infection is almost a sure sign), seek professional psychological help and legal aid immediately.

10. Labial agglutination (closing of the lips of the vagina)

Related to vaginal infections in children is labial agglutination (ag-GLUE-tin-ation) or fusion in which the small lips of the vagina seem to get stuck together so that the vagina looks as though it has closed up.

This is not serious: it is a side effect of vulvovaginitis, and is only cause for alarm if accompanied by bleeding or if the child has difficulty urinating.

Try hip bath treatments; dry your daughter after each one and apply petroleum jelly. After a few days, try to *gently* separate the lips. If they do not separate, consult a doctor who may prescribe a steroid or oestrogen cream to thicken the lips and make them more resistant to infection. Oestrogen should be used only in very small doses and for short periods of time. Applied lightly for one to two weeks, the cream should make the lips part by themselves.

In severe cases the doctor may have to part the lips of the vagina. *This should be the last resort, because it is painful to the child.* Never let a doctor do this as a first step, and if it is suggested as a first step, get another opinion.

11. Urinary infections
These are common in young girls, sometimes caused by faecal contamination and irritating soaps and bubble baths. The symptoms are plain: pain on urination and frequency. The diagnosis and treatment involve a urinalysis and, if positive, treatment with sulphonamides or some other antibiotic.

Sometimes, doctors suggest dilation of the urethra. This is a painful treatment, potentially traumatic psychologically and usually unnecessary. Get a second opinion.

12. Vaginal bleeding in little girls calls for prompt medical attention
This can be caused by injury (a fall off a bike), infection, a foreign body, serious illness such as a tumour, or sexual assault. Go to the doctor right away, for diagnosis and treatment.

13. How to prevent vulvovaginitis and urinary tract infections in little girls
a. Teach your daughter to wipe from front to back after a bowel movement, and teach her to keep wiping with successive pieces of paper until the paper is clean.

b. Don't use harsh detergents on her laundry.

c. Don't allow her to use strong, perfumed soaps. Stick to the mildest soap available. Don't use bubble bath or bath oils.

d. Don't let her sit around in a wet bathing suit. Make sure that she washes herself in plain water after swimming in a chlorinated pool.

e. Make sure she wears cotton underpants. If she wears tights, make sure she wears them *over* her pants.

f. Teach her not to put things inside her vagina, if she has done so in the past. If she has never done so, don't give her the idea by bringing up the subject.

14. Virginity

Virginity is a very vague and unimportant concept, notwithstanding the great obsession, which male-dominated cultures have had with it over the centuries.

Physically, a girl is a virgin until her hymen is broken. This usually happens either through the use of tampons or by sexual intercourse. The size of the opening in the vagina varies. Bleeding does not always occur at the time the hymen is broken. It depends whether a blood vessel has been ruptured or not. Excess physical activity does not cause the hymen to be broken.

Experientially, a girl is a virgin until she has had sex. It is best not to burden your little girl with any notion of the importance of physical virginity. It should be her sexual activity, not the state of her hymen, that should be of interest to her.

15. Masturbation is common among young girls

Masturbation affords sexual pleasure, if not full orgasm, to young girls, and many of them do it. There is nothing abnormal about this. There is nothing abnormal if they don't do it. Masturbation may cause irritation of the genitals. Treat it as you would vulvovaginitis, with vaseline and baths, but don't make too much of it or you may be inviting your daughter to continue with her masturbation obsessively, just because she gets so much attention that way.

10

CHANGE OF LIFE

The word "menopause" is commonly misused to refer to all the symptoms, side effects, crises, and discomforts associated with that time in her life when a women's ovaries cease to produce eggs and she stops menstruating. Specifically, *menopause* refers only to the end of the menstrual flow—which is but one aspect of a time more properly called the *climacteric* (kly-MAC-teric) or change of life.

Change of life can occur usually in women between the ages of forty-three and fifty-five; normal cases exist beyond that range. Some doctors and women think of change of life as a deficiency disease of the ovaries and prescribe medicines from the onset. They are overstating the case quite excessively. *Change of life is not a sickness.* It is a normal process through which all women pass.

Much of the anxiety about change of life is due not to its actual physiological effects but to the deep-rooted, negative attitudes we have towards ageing. People who treat change of life as though it were a sickness are often treating nothing more than their own fears of growing older. In Britain where close to 15 per cent of the population are over sixty-five, it should be a national priority to develop a new attitude about ageing. Change of life does not finish a woman any more than some company rule about retirement actually ends the working capacity of any individual. In fact, women who manage to become attuned to their bodies rather than listen to the propaganda of the youth culture may feel better *after* change of life than they did before.

Remember that the men around you are growing older too; remember that if you were twenty-two again, you wouldn't know anywhere near as much as you do now; remember that the average British woman lives to be 74 years old and that at least one third of your life is still ahead of you.

270

In fact, even with symptoms and discomforts, change of life is a sign of good health and normal progress—just as menstruation was when you were a girl.

BIOLOGICAL CHANGES DURING CHANGE OF LIFE

1. Normal change of life

Biologically, during the last four or five years of menstruation, the menstrual cycle gradually comes to a halt. The number of eggs in the ovaries declines and no ovulation occurs. The ebb and flow of oestrogen and progesterone production stops. The hypothalamus and pituitary continue functioning, however, producing the releasing hormones and follicle-stimulating hormone (FSH) and luteinizing hormone (LH). These latter two hormones are secreted in very high levels after menopause because the ovary is not responding in the way it did before. By the time women reach their sixties, the hormones have fallen considerably although FSH remains higher than during reproductive life.

The most common menstrual pattern in change of life is this: gradually, the number of days between menstrual periods increases, interspersed with regular cycles of normal length. *Most women cease ovulating gradually: you cannot be sure of your infertility until menstruation has ceased for good.* Sometimes, menstrual bleeding is normal; sometimes light, next to nothing. Menopause occurs when the monthly flow ceases.

Since the moment that the menopause has occurred is difficult to ascertain, women going through change of life should still be careful about contraception, heeding the following guidelines, recommended by the Family Planning Association: if the woman is *under fifty* and periods have stopped for *two* years, then contraception can be discontinued; if a woman is *over fifty* and periods have stopped for *one* year, the contraception can also be stopped.

Usually, the whole change-of-life process takes a year or two. Some women have discomforting symptoms because of the new hormonal supply pattern that is establishing itself—*but only about 10 per cent have severe symptoms of any kind.*

At their worst, the discomforts of change of life can be very unsettling—but like dysmenorrhoea, they are the upsetting side effects of a *normal* process. Even when you are suffering from bad hot flushes, for example, *you are still healthy. These are not symptoms of disease.*

271

2. Hormone production system at change of life

Change-of-life discomforts are caused by hormonal changes, particularly oestrogen loss. But the body anticipates these, and has other machinery to *naturally* replace the hormones that are no longer being produced in as great quantity by the ovaries.

a. *The adrenal glands* continue to produce some oestrogen as well as large amounts of androgen (male hormone) which are converted to oestrogen in fatty tissue and other parts of the body.

b. *The ovaries themselves* continue to produce very small amounts of oestrogen as well as androgen that is converted to oestrogen.

What makes women differ so greatly in their physiological reaction to change of life is that *the capacity to metabolize androgen into oestrogen varies widely among individuals.* About 40 per cent of postmenopausal women have blood levels of oestrogen which are just as high as the levels in the first half of their menstrual cycles before change of life. (Ref. 1)

3. Physical symptoms of oestrogen decline which may occur at change of life

These include:

a. Hot flushes;

b. Thinning of the vaginal lining.

The physical symptoms of oestrogen decline *do not* include such problems as hypertension, heart attacks, obesity, reduced vision or hearing, and the many other diseases which increase with age, not just with menopause.

4. Hot flushes

A hot flush is a discomforting sensation of being suddenly roasted, heated up from within. The hot flush usually begins in the chest, spreads to the neck and head; it will make a woman turn very red, and may make her perspire heavily. Sometimes a hot flush begins in the toes and spreads over the entire body. It lasts from several seconds to several minutes, and may leave the woman with a chilled feeling. Hot flushes may start before menopause but more frequently begin in the years afterward. At least 75 per cent of women have some hot flushes during change of life, but in only 10–20 per cent are these so severe that treatment is needed. Remember that these are often unnoticeable to an observer.

5. What causes hot flushes

No one really knows. For no apparent physiological reason, the blood vessels have suddenly become more sensitive to changes in

272

the nervous system. They dilate involuntarily; blood rushes to the skin surface, heating up the body; then the vessels revert to normal size. Some say this is due to oestrogen deficiency; others say it is due to high levels of FSH and LH.

6. Treatment of hot flushes

Unless the hot flushes are very severe, prolonged, or frequent, there is no need for treatment. In time, they will end—and most women learn to cope with them until they do.

Try to avoid stressful situations for these aggravate the condition. By this time, you're old enough to know if city traffic or business negotiations or your son's rock group try your nerves in the best of times. Change of life may be the best of times, therefore, to avoid them.

If you are bothered by frequent, prolonged, extremely severe hot flushes, or if your sleep is being disturbed mercilessly, you may consider medical treatment, which will usually relieve the symptoms. (See No. 23 below).

7. Thinning of the vaginal lining

Normally at change of life, the vaginal surface, which formerly consisted of ten to twelve layers of cells, begins to thin to about two to three layers, a symptom of oestrogen decline. Previously, the thick vaginal lining protected the vagina from infection. Vaginal lubrication—one of women's responses to sexual excitement—is not affected by this thinning. If this thinning is severe and an infection does occur, a woman may experience pain or burning during intercourse, vaginal discharge, and a tight feeling in the vaginal area. These symptoms, if they occur at all, do not usually occur until several years after the periods have stopped.

Only 25–35 per cent of women experience so much thinning in vaginal lining that they are made uncomfortable; this is called *atrophic vaginitis*.

8. Diagnosis of thinning in the vaginal lining

Examination of the vagina will confirm whether severe vaginal thinning has occurred. A vaginal swab is sometimes taken to see if the woman has candida or trichomonas. Sometimes vaginal smears may be used to check the hormone levels, although the usefulness of this investigation is disputed. Sometimes the inflammation (or vaginitis) may be severe enough to cause some bleeding from the vagina, but never assume that this is the cause of bleeding after the menopause, which should always be investigated thoroughly.

9. Treatment of thinning in the vaginal lining

Treatment can begin with the over-the-counter lubricating jellies (*never* Vaseline) often used during intercourse. If these don't relieve the symptoms, small amounts of oestrogen cream may be prescribed. These creams, applied directly to the vagina, act to thicken the lining. Since the oestrogen may be absorbed into the body through the vagina, only the minimum amount needed to keep the symptoms under control should be used. Usually the woman applies the cream daily for a week; then she can cut back gradually to as little as once or twice a week. (See No. 23 below)

10. Pelvic relaxation symptoms often appear after menopause

After menopause, some women may experience symptoms of pelvic relaxation for the first time, or the symptoms may become severe. These include bulging of the vaginal walls (cystocele and rectocele) and the loss of urine during coughing and sneezing. (See p. 308) In some cases, pelvic floor exercises to improve vaginal tone (see p. 153) will greatly alleviate these symptoms. Try these methods before considering surgical repair and/or hysterectomy, which may be suggested. Vaginal repair operations need not include a total hysterectomy. The need for this should be discussed with your doctor.

11. Skin changes at change of life

After menopause, oestrogen decline *may* contribute to a thinning and drying of the skin all over the body, most notably on the face, arms and breasts. It is very hard indeed to tell what part of the skin change is actually due to lower oestrogen levels, and what part is due to the simple passage of time, to weathering. Women who have spent a lifetime in the sun and/or the wind tend to become more wrinkled than other women as they grow older.

OPINION: Because of fanaticism about youth and beauty, which has little to do with health, oestrogenic compounds may be prescribed for these normal skin changes. *Don't use them! Hormone replacement therapy is not a safe treatment for wrinkles!* Even oestrogen-containing creams may be dangerous if used excessively, since oestrogen is absorbed through the skin into the body. And in most cases, the oestrogen has little effect on the skin.

Remember: you are old enough now to deserve a mature redefinition of beauty—and it starts, as always, with your own acceptance of your own particular flesh.

12. Glandular tissue of the breasts diminishes during change of life

This may mean that your breasts will lose some of their fullness, and firmness and may change shape, but since most of the breast is composed of fatty tissue, these changes are small and are often not noticed, especially by women with big breasts. Hormone treatments will not help. Now as always breast shape depends on good posture, regular exercise, good muscle tone, and the distant signals of heredity. Some women at change of life may experience tenderness of the breasts.

13. Hair changes during change of life

Some women experience thinning of the pubic hair as well as the hair on their heads, or may note a slight increase in body hair, especially on the face. This is due to the relative increase in androgens; don't worry about it. If you have a few more hairs on your face because of androgen increase, remember that much of that same androgen supply is being turned to oestrogen, thereby naturally replacing that critical female hormone you may have lost when you stopped ovulating.

If hair growth is excessive (on the chest, or all over the face), then the woman should be examined for some other endocrine disorder. *This is not normal* for menopausal women.

If you find you have a few obvious hairs which embarrass you, you can have them removed by electrolysis. This is a simple technique in which the hair follicle is destroyed by a small electric current passed through a needle inserted into the follicle. Have it done only by a qualified beautician.

14. Weight gain is not a side effect of change of life

The biological processes of change of life *do not* cause the weight gain many women experience in these years. What creates the weight gain is a decrease in activity with no concurrent decrease in food intake. It has been proved that lying in bed doing nothing increases the loss of calcium from the bones (osteoporosis) and it may be that regular exercise has the opposite effect.

A woman at this time may not experience a gain in pounds but rather a change in body proportions, making her *look* fatter even if she doesn't weigh more. For example, the upper arm may grow heavier; the waistline may thicken. If you are not actually gaining weight, don't worry about these changing proportions; regular exercise will go far to control them, *especially if you have been doing it all along.* A new change-of-life exercise routine is great for your circulation, but don't expect it to reverse the proportions of your body back in time.

15. Sex drive and sexual activity in change of life

Men—not women—have the greatest problems with decreased sex drive with ageing. There is no physiological reason for a woman to experience a letdown in libido or sexual pleasure. The major hormone factors are poorly understood but the hormones continue to be produced by a woman's body in sufficient quantity well into old age.

Many women note an *increase* in sex drive after menopause, when pregnancy is no longer a risk. (This is comparable to the soaring libido some women report after surgical sterilization, for exactly the same reason.)

Psychological problems with sex at this time are often caused by men, who may be bewildered at their loss of power and somehow shift the blame on to partners; and by women who allow themselves to be traumatized by feelings that they are no longer attractive because they are no longer menstruating and cannot have children.

16. Severe premenstrual tension is a sign of progesterone deficiency at change of life

During the years immediately prior to menopause, many women experience a severe increase in premenstrual tension including breast tenderness, a feeling of fullness in the pelvis and lower abdomen, and weight gain. This has nothing to do with oestrogen decline. It is thought to occur because of the imbalance between oestrogen and progesterone. One in three women respond well to progestogens given orally in the second half of the cycle, and one in three responds to pyridoxine (Vitamin B6).

17. Normal patterns of menstrual bleeding during change of life

There are two *normal* patterns:

a. A gradual decrease in the amount of flow; gradually longer times between periods, interspersed with regular periods; occasional skipping of a period until, gradually, it just doesn't come back.

b. Regular menstruation straight through to a total stop.

18. Suspicious patterns of menstrual bleeding during change of life

a. Women should not experience heavy or gushing flows;

b. The period should not last *longer* than usual;

c. Periods should not occur any more frequently than every twenty-one days;

d. Once bleeding has ceased for twelve months it should not recur.

Any of the above patterns may indicate just an unusual hitch in normal menopause. However, these patterns may also suggest a problem—so a woman should have herself checked.

19. Diagnosis and treatment of unusual bleeding patterns around the change of life

If an unusual pattern occurs, a D & C (see p. 317) is the best course for diagnosing the cause and, in a few women eliminating it. Some of the more serious causes, *occurring in a minority of women,* are hyperplasia of the endometrium, and cancer of the endometrium, cervix or ovary. (See p. 348) A cervical smear (taken from the cervix, the neck of the womb) should always be done before a D & C, to diagnose or rule out cancer.

Endometrial biopsy and endometrial washings are procedures performed to obtain small samples of the uterine lining in cases of minor bleeding problems around the time of menopause. If the washings or biopsy show no abnormality, if the bleeding problem is minor and if bleeding patterns subsequently return to normal, a D & C can sometimes be avoided. (See p. 354) As yet, endometrial biopsy and endometrial washings are mainly done for research purposes, but they may be accepted as an alternative to D & C in the future.

20. Other symptoms of menopause

Some non-specific problems, such as dizziness, headaches, nervousness and numbness in the fingers are commonly attributed to change of life. Some studies show that these symptoms are more common during change of life, others show that they are not. (Refs. 2, 3). *There is absolutely no proof that these symptoms are caused by oestrogen decline, so oestrogen is not an appropriate treatment.*

Don't blame everything on change of life! You may succeed in convincing yourself that it is making you sick when it is not; you may end up taking drugs which are worse for you than change of life itself, drugs which may not alleviate your symptoms in any case.

21. Premature change of life

In a very few women, menopause occurs at an early age—in the twenties or thirties—for several reasons:

a. *Heredity.* In this case the menopause is not a sign of ill health but simply due to genetic factors.

b. *Ovarian failure.* Reports suggest that mumps infection of the ovaries may be another cause of premature menopause. (Ref. 4)

Still other women may develop antibodies to ovarian tissue, in an auto-immune reaction as in rheumatoid arthritis (Ref. 5 and see pp. 360-62)

c. *Surgical removal of the ovaries.* This is the most common cause of premature menopause. Loss of *one* ovary will not lead to change of life, but removal of both will cause this. *In young women, removal of both ovaries should be carefully guarded against unless absolutely necessary!* (See p. 321) Premature menopause can be distinguished from other causes of amenorrhoea (loss of periods) by a test for blood FSH and LH levels. These are elevated after the menopause.

22. Menopause and oestrogen withdrawal are more difficult for young women

The metabolism of androgen into oestrogen happens naturally in older women who have *gradually* approached change of life. But this form of oestrogen replacement is nowhere near as reliable among young women who have *suddenly* encountered change of life because of surgical removal of the ovaries or ovarian failure. The resultant sudden oestrogen loss may inflict severe symptoms, aggravated forms of all the ordinary side effects. The shock for some women of hearing that they have lost their ovaries in what they expected to be a less major or investigative operation makes matters worse.

RECOMMENDATION: *Premature menopause is one of the very few situations in which hormone replacement therapy is recommended routinely.* A woman should continue the therapy until she is forty-five to fifty years of age and then gradually reduce the dosage to nothing. (See No. 26) By this time the body's auxiliary hormone-supply systems may catch up with her situation. Another reason for hormone replacement therapy in this instance is that prematurely menopausal women who do not receive it seem to experience a greater tendency toward osteoporosis and heart attacks. (Refs. 1, 6)

HORMONE REPLACEMENT THERAPY

23. Hormone replacement therapy (HRT)

HRT means giving hormones after the menopause to relieve severe symptoms. These used to be oestrogens given continuously, but today both oestrogen (natural or synthesized) and progestogen (synthesized progesterone) are usually given in a cyclical fashion. With the addition of progestogen, most women will recommence having periods so that the endometrial lining is periodically shed to reduce the possibility of hyperplasia which may lead to endometrial cancer. (See p. 353) There is still a certain amount of controversy about this therapy. The use of HRT has been quite commonplace in the USA for many years, but in Britain GPs have been reluctant to prescribe HRT, partly through conservatism and caution, and partly because they feel women should put up with these things. HRT has been available privately for some years, but recently the British National Health Service has set up menopause clinics in several areas. If your own doctor is unhappy about prescribing HRT, ask him to refer you to one of these clinics. Sometimes doctors at family planning or well woman clinics give helpful advice.

24. Who should use hormone replacement therapy?

HRT should be available from your doctor if you suffer severe symptoms such as:

a. Prolonged hot flushes;

b. Severe vaginal dryness and thinning after menopause;

c. Premature menopause, resulting from ovarian removal or failure before age forty (to be taken only until age forty-five to fifty).

25. The safest method of taking oestrogen, for women who must have it

a. Always take the lowest possible dose which will relieve the symptoms (this applies to pills and creams).

b. Take the therapy for the shortest time possible.

c. Take the oral doses in a cyclic fashion with progestogen.

These rules should be followed whether the woman has her uterus or not. The major reason for the cyclic administration is to avoid continuous unopposed oestrogen effects on the endometrium and the breasts. Oestrogen alone, continuously given, is more likely to be a cause of endometrial cancer and may have a similar effect on the breasts.

RECOMMENDATION: One of the best methods of oestrogen replacement is to take oestrogen daily for the first two weeks of the month and then take it with a progestogen tablet each day during the third week. The last week of the month, take nothing. This method of taking the pills may help to reverse any changes which the oestrogen may have caused in the endometrium or breasts. Discuss this cyclic method of taking the oestrogen with your doctor. It mimics the natural cycle and is now available in pack form, just like oral contraception.

26. Once symptoms are under control, start decreasing the oestrogen dosage

Women taking oestrogen to alleviate hot flushes should usually start on a fairly high dose and gradually cut back; after being on the drugs for one or two months, take a lower dose or take the pill every other day. Let your doctor know you are doing this. Always go one week a month without any oestrogen at all. After several months, you may be able to withdraw from the treatment completely. Try not to use it for more than six months except in premature menopause.

27. Which type of oestrogen?

Most doctors in Britain believe that natural oestrogens are less likely to cause blood clots than synthetic oestrogens. However, synthetic oestrogens are much cheaper, and the dosage can be adjusted more easily, so doctors may prescribe these.

28. Alternatives to oestrogen in the control of hot flushes

Options do exist for women who are severely bothered by hot flushes.

a. Some drugs, such as cloridine, which act to stabilize the nerve endings around the blood vessels are suggested by some doctors, but they are not effective in all women.

b. *Progestogens may control hot flushes* to a large extent and are probably much safer for many women, especially those with complicating problems such as obesity, hypertension, cystic breasts, heart disease and diabetes.

c. If the symptoms are particularly severe at certain times of the day or under certain stressful conditions, *sedatives* or *mild tranquillizers* may be helpful for *short* periods of time.

d. *Ginseng extract* and *vitamin E* work for some women and certainly hold little risk in *moderate* doses. This may just be a placebo effect.

29. Other side effects of hormone replacement therapy

a. Breast tenderness is a frequent side effect, most pronounced in those women with a tendency towards cystic mastitis. If this happens, lower the dose, or take the pills every other day, and take progestogen two weeks during the month.

b. Oedema and weight gain may also appear as side effects. If these side effects are excessive, either go off the drugs, lower the dosage, or switch to another type of oestrogen.

30. Bleeding during hormone replacement therapy

If women are still menstruating when oestrogen therapy is begun, the usual menstrual pattern should continue. Sometimes women on combined oestrogen and progestogen replacement have continued to menstruate into their sixties, an undesirable result for many women. Women who have stopped menstruating before oestrogen administration will usually experience no return of bleeding as a rule.

Bleeding in the middle of the cycle, prolonged bleeding, or bleeding after the periods have once stopped are all abnormal patterns (see No. 18 above) and must be evaluated by endometrial biopsy, endometrial washings, or D & C.

31. Testing for changes in the endometrium and breasts should be routine during hormone replacement therapy

Some doctors perform endometrial biopsies or washings before starting women on oestrogen if they are at high risk for endometrial cancer. (See p. 353) Never take oestrogen without checking routinely for possible side effects!

Your breasts should be examined once a year by your doctor and monthly by you.

32. Who should avoid oestrogen-replacement therapy?

Women with:
a. Breast cancer or severe cystic disease of the breasts
b. Endometrial cancer or hyperplasia
c. Ovarian cancer
d. Large fibroid tumours of the uterus
e. History of phlebitis or other clotting disorders
f. Severe heart disease, kidney disease, diabetes, or hypertension

33. Hormone replacement pills are not protection against pregnancy

Other birth-control methods should be continued if a woman is still menstruating. Birth control pills are not recommended for women over forty. (See p. 45)

34. Hormone replacement therapy does not protect against cardiovascular disease

The incidence of heart attack, stroke, or hardening of the arteries is lower in women under fifty than in men. After that age, women apparently catch up with the men in the incidences of these diseases. For this reason, it has long been thought that oestrogen, present before menopause, had a protective effect against these diseases. Oestrogen replacement was believed to be effective in guarding against these diseases after menopause.

This theory is generally discredited.

Cardiovascular disease has now been related to other factors, like overwork, smoking, high cholesterol and triglyceride levels—any one of which complicates your chances of a heart attack more than oestrogen. In addition, now that extensive autopsy data is in for men and women older and younger than fifty years, the rates of coronary artery disease appear to be identical. (Ref. 1)

35. Osteoporosis—the role of oestrogen is unclear

Osteoporosis (oss-tee-oh-por-OH-sis) is a thinning of the bones and actual loss of bone matter which occurs in postmenopausal women more frequently than in premenopausal women or in men at any age. It is usually not a problem for women at change of life, but seems to start then and grow serious in elderly women. It can lead to hump back; to a softness in the hip bones and in the vertebrae (the connected sections of the spine) so that these may break very easily in old age.

36. Causes of osteoporosis

There is considerable debate over the role of oestrogen in the prevention and treatment of osteoporosis. Some studies show that bone density is considerably higher in women who have been on replacement oestrogen and that bone thinning can be prevented by giving oestrogen after menopause. (Refs. 6, 7) These are very promising studies, but so far do not tell us whether there are some women who will benefit from oestrogen therapy and others who will not. Since only one in four women suffer from osteoporosis, this means that a lot of women would be exposed to the dangers of oestrogen to prevent fractures in a small group.

On the other hand, there is no proof that osteoporosis is *caused* by oestrogen deficiency. It results from an alteration in the body's ability to metabolize calcium (the major bone mineral) and phosphorus, which comes with age. Men and women seem to metabolize these minerals differently; in women, the metabolism which supports bone formation tends to fall off more greatly as the years pass. This may be caused by a change in kidney function; a change in the ability of the intestinal tract to absorb these minerals; or from a hormonal imbalance (having nothing to do with sex hormones) from the adrenal gland that affects the metabolism of bone. (Ref. 8) Even more simply, it may be that women need to supplement their diets with calcium more than men do, just as younger women have to supplement their diets with iron on occasion.

Other factors which *increase* the risk of osteoporosis are heavy smoking, thinness, inactivity, and heredity. Excess consumption of antacids containing aluminium hydroxide may contribute to the thinning of bones by interfering with calcium and phosphorus metabolism. (Ref. 9)

37. Diagnosis of osteoporosis

Ordinary X-rays will not detect a thinning of the bones until osteoporosis is relatively far advanced. Special X-ray density studies can detect this condition at an earlier stage. LOOK AHEAD: In the future, testing to determine the density of your bones as change of life nears may become routine to treat early stages of osteoporosis. (Refs. 6, 7)

38. Good diet and exercise can prevent and control osteoporosis in most women

Starting at age thirty, make sure you are getting at least 800–1200 mg of calcium per day: it is available in milk, cheese and other dairy products. Exercise daily; that increases your body's ability to metabolize calcium and phosphorus, and most important, good muscles can shore up weakening bones considerably. Take the minimum daily requirements of Vitamin D but *be careful not to take more; excess Vitamin D can actually aggravate osteoporosis*

Fluoride in the water supply may help to delay osteoporosis. If your community's water supply is not fluoridated, take supplementary tablets. (See p. 243)

39. Routine hormone replacement therapy is not recommended treatment to prevent osteoporosis

At the present time, the risks of oestrogen therapy are too great to warrant its routine use to prevent osteoporosis in all women. Oestrogen can be used to treat osteoporosis, but it seems advisable to wait and see if high-risk women can be more accurately identified before the drug is used routinely as a *preventive* measure. If you are at high risk (see No. 36 above) discuss this with your doctor.

The important exception to this is young women with premature menopause (either surgical or spontaneous) in whom oestrogen has a definite effect in preventing osteoporosis (Ref. 1)

EMOTIONAL CHANGES

40. Emotional and psychological aspects of change of life

An elaborate mythology in many cultures suggests that women go crazy at change of life. This has been the rationale for denying mature women, at the peak of their powers of judgement, real power in politics, for example. In the USA it has been the cause of thousands of unnecessary hysterectomies and millions of unnecessary oestrogen prescriptions. It has its impact on family life, giving teenagers an excuse to disregard their mothers and men a sorry tale to tell to younger women. It is a kind of madness of its own. Women do not go crazy at change of life. Some go through, at worst, a difficult time.

a. *Endocrine changes may cause emotional problems.* The change in hormonal cycles, the switchover from an endocrine machinery whose centre is the ovaries to an endocrine machinery whose centre is the adrenal glands, often affects the hypothalamus, the endocrine centre in the brain which controls a number of chemical reactions in the body, including some emotional reactions. This means that a woman at change of life may feel more tense; may be moved to tears more easily; may experience sensations of great well-being. How strong these impulses are depends to a great degree on *the other emotional strains* that operate in a woman's life at this time. (See 'b' below) If her life is calm and she is feeling happy, the endocrine changes will not be much of a problem.

Avoid long-term drug therapy for the emotional crises of change of life.

Just because you find yourself weeping easily does not mean that you must be treated with tranquillizers. Dangerous drug habits are often formed at this time because of the tendency to overprescribe for symptoms that are normal and will surely pass. Try tennis instead; thousands have. Try a new job, a long holiday, going to classes, painting watercolours, standing for election, anything that diverts and refocuses your energy. Your children may laugh at you, but at *their* age, they should be laughing at themselves.

b.*Outside pressures deepen the tensions of change of life.* Between the ages of forty-three and fifty-five, a number of events may be complicating a woman's emotional environment. Her parents may be old and sick; their imminent death is a forewarning of hers, frightening and draining. Her children may be leaving home, creating a great empty space around her. Careers, in which so much time and money have been invested, have a tendency not to be so satisfying now that you have been working at them for twenty years. Likewise for relationships. It is not oestrogen that must be replaced now, but the splintering pieces of a lifelong environment.

The worse these outside pressures are, the more likely a woman is to suffer emotionally at change of life. The feminist movement has been a great help in giving women a sense of their possibilities for *renewal,* and even if you have never read feminist literature before, you should take a look at it now; it suggests plans of action that can help a woman change her environment, rework her attitudes towards herself; it is preventive medicine for the awful feeling that you are suddenly in the dénouement before the end of the play; you are not in any such thing; on the average you have thirty to forty years to go, and there are millions of women who can by their example suggest the ways you may go with it.

c. *Change of life happens to men too—and that is part of a woman's problem.* Obviously there is no male menopause, because menopause refers specifically to the cessation of menstrual flow. But men do experience the crises of change of life and often actually have fewer resources to deal with them. If there were such a thing as testosterone-replacement therapy, they would probably be taking it with abandon (and quite uselessly)—to thicken their thinning hair, quicken their slowing sex drives (some do use testosterone for this), smooth out their wrinkles, shore up their overworked hearts and stiffening bones. Change of life may be a bad time for some women, but it is in itself *not a disease, merely a natural phase of life.*

11

DISEASES OF WOMEN

A number of diseases afflict women specifically; some relate to age and stage of life; some stem from pregnancy and childbearing; some relate to sexual activity; some, arthritis, for example, are apparently unrelated to sexual and reproductive character, but select women as their primary targets anyway. The best way to avoid a disease is to know about it before it happens, or to know what it looks like at the earliest stages, so that if it happens to you, you can get to work right away on a treatment. Knowing about a disease means talking about it, even if it is a disease that society would prefer not to discuss.

The taboo on talking about breast cancer, for example, was broken by wives of political leaders, like Betty Ford in America, who openly discussed their surgery. As a result, millions of women who might not have dealt with breast cancer until it was far advanced, went to early detection clinics. These women practise *preventive* medicine against a disease which had previously been so hushed up that few people understood that it could be detected at a curable stage.

Younger women are fortunate to be growing up in a society where public discussion about women's health is the rule, not the exception, and they should never allow the quiet to set in again. Shyness and secrecy are the twin demons that, for centuries, kept women sick or thinking they were sick when they really weren't. What is true for public communication is true for communication between mother and daughter, between friends, between doctor and patient as well. Talk to the women around you; talk to your doctor; talk to the men around you. The more people talk to each other about their health, the more they can do to keep each other healthy.

VAGINITIS AND VENEREAL AND SEXUALLY TRANSMITTED DISEASES

1. Types of vaginitis

Vaginitis (va-gin-EYE-tis) refers to all inflammations, irritations and infections of the vagina. Some of its non-specific symptoms include discharge, itching, burning, and odour. These same symptoms may be caused by infectious agents such as trichomonas (TRI-ko-mo-nas), candidiasis, bacteria, or by allergies to sprays, douches or tampons. (See p. 225)

Vulvitis (vul-VYE-tis) redness and itching of the skin—often accompanies vaginitis.

2. Vaginal discharge is not always a sign of vaginitis or any illness at all

The vagina is a moist and constantly changing environment, responsive to every step in the menstrual cycle, and to sexual arousal. Most women experience a certain amount of vaginal secretion at all times. You can tell that the discharge is not normal if it is foul-smelling, if it causes itching or burning, or if it is accompanied by any other symptoms of illness like fever, headache, extreme fatigue. A feeling of wetness or a light yellow to white smear on your underwear is in itself nothing to worry about. In fact, it signifies that you are functioning normally.

3. Vaginal odour is not always a sign of vaginitis

Some drug and cosmetic companies, always in search of a new "problem" that requires a new product to conquer it, have attempted through advertising to make vaginal odour much more of a problem than it really is. Because the power of suggestion is so great, a woman who never thought she smelled bad can read a magazine and conclude that she must have smelled bad all along, and run out to her chemist to purchase a spray that will make her and her underwear smell like a field of flowers. (See pp. 223-4)

Don't be fooled!

Of course, vaginal secretions and sweat glands in the pubic area cause a smell. But it is almost always not unpleasant and it is almost always undetectable to anyone except you. If you are concerned about offending a sexual partner, then wash with soap and water. Only if vaginal odour is very strong should you worry about it and be checked for vaginitis.

4. What to do if you think you have vaginitis

If the normal vaginal discharge increases and you think you are developing vaginitis, try several things before going to a doctor:

a. If you have been wearing underpants made of synthetics, switch to cotton. It is more porous, allows greater circulation of air in the vaginal area, and absorbs moisture. Synthetic materials tend to trap moisture so that it persists and causes irritation.

b. If you have been using bubble bath, stop—and use plain soap and water. Maybe your body is just reacting adversely to the application of chemicals.

c. If you have been using harsh, perfumed soaps around the vulva, switch to a milder soap.

d. If you have been using a biological detergent, try a milder laundry product or try rinsing out your underwear by hand with a mild soap.

e. Take frequent baths. Add 1 cupful of vinegar to the bath water.

If symptoms persist for three to four days, get worse, or are accompanied by fever, abnormal bleeding, or severe pain, *see a doctor at once.*

5. Diagnosis of vaginal infection

If you have a vaginal infection, or the symptoms of one, you can expect your doctor to:

a. Take a complete history.

b. Do a complete pelvic examination (see p. 391), including a culture for gonorrhoea if appropriate.

c. Take a cervical smear, if this was not recently done.

d. Do cultures for candida and trichomonas (HVS) and a wet smear. These tests will be done routinely in a VD or 'special' clinic (also sometimes called an STD—'sexually transmitted diseases' —clinic).

e. Take a smear of the suspicious vaginal discharge, to be analysed in the laboratory.

INSIST THAT ALL THESE SMEARS BE DONE! Your best chance of getting them done thoroughly is to go to a VD clinic. Half of all those who attend these clinics do not have VD, but have learnt that this is the best way to get quick and efficient treatment. Discharges from the various vaginal infections mimic each other, so that it is very frequently hard to diagnose them just from observation. You will increase your chances of a cure if you insist that your doctor does the tests.

6. Candidiasis or thrush

Candidiasis (can-di-DI-a-sis)—thrush or moniliasis (mow-NILL-eye-a-sis)—is the most common form of vaginitis. Sometimes called thrush or a "yeast" infection, it is actually caused by a fungus called *Candida albicans* (in Latin, *candida* means dazzling white, *albicans* means white).

The symptoms of candidiasis are:

a. A thick, white discharge that often has the consistency of cottage cheese;

b. Severe itching in the vaginal area;

c. Irritation and redness around the vulva and sometimes around the anus.

7. Who is likely to get candidiasis?

Women in the reproductive age group are most likely to get candidiasis. Premenarchal girls and postmenopausal women rarely find it a worry. However, several factors predispose women to candidiasis beyond general chronological factors.

a. If a woman is taking steroids like cortisone to counteract another illness, that may upset the bacterial balance in the vagina and favour the growth of candida.

b. The same is true of antibiotics. You may contract candida while taking broad spectrum antibiotics to cure a streptococcal throat or urinary infection. The antibiotics kill off the bacteria which usually keep the fungus in check.

c. Women with diabetes are prone to candidiasis. When the diabetes is under control, the candidiasis is usually under control. It tends to become a problem when blood sugar gets high or when sugar builds up in urine.

d. Any state which produces high levels of hormones or lowers vaginal acidity favours candidiasis. Therefore, women taking birth control pills (see p. 43) and pregnant women may be bothered by it. Using Dettol or bath salts in your bath may encourage candida.

8. The treatment of candidiasis

WARNING: Whatever you do to treat candidiasis, *don't scratch!* The itch may be driving you crazy, but scratching will only make it worse. Several preparations can give almost instant relief—gels, creams, pessaries which can be applied directly to the vagina once or twice a day. STOP PRESS: Impregnated tampons are now available on prescription and seem promising. So far only one brand, called Gynodaktarin, is available.

For a new case of candidiasis, treatment should last seven to fourteen days. Keep using the medication even after the symptoms are gone, as long as your doctor or clinic has told you to use it; that will increase the chances that the candida will not return. When itching is very severe, some doctors prescribe a low-dose steroid cream or lotion to be applied directly to the vulva to relieve the discomfort.

Most candidiasis preparations are available only by prescription.

RECOMMENDATION: *Over-the-counter drugs that claim to relieve vaginal itching are not ideal for this condition.* They will not eliminate the fungus. There are treatments you can buy yourself in the supermarket: yoghurt and plain white vinegar. Live yoghurt— the plain kind (without fruit!)—appears very effective for mild cases. Put the yoghurt into a plastic squeeze bottle or a pastry tube and apply it directly to the vagina. It contains a *lactobacillus* (lac-toe-ba-SILL-us), a bacteria derived from milk, which is similar to that normally found in the vagina. This bacteria blocks candida naturally. Some women prefer to use the yoghurt starter material (which also contains lactobacillus)—available in health food stores —as a douche ingredient. Two tablespoons of vinegar to a pint of water is also a helpful douche; although it may not cure the candidiasis by itself, it is very helpful as a companion treatment with medical therapy. Like the lactobacillus in yoghurt, the acid in vinegar helps to make the vagina inhospitable to candida (and to other infective organisms). Boric acid can also be used. The chemist will tell you how much to use.

9. What to do if candidiasis is chronic

Some women get candidiasis so frequently that they begin to feel it has never gone away. Usually, some environmental factor is to blame. If you can isolate it and banish it from your life, you can probably control the candidiasis.

If you have contracted candidiasis as a result of antibiotic treatment in the past, get some candidiasis medication and use it as *preventive* medicine *every time* you must take antibiotics. Sexual partners, male and female, should be treated if the disease persists. Ask your doctor what medicine they should use.

Many women with recurrent candidiasis harbour the fungus in the bowel; reinfection occurs chronically from the anus. Nystatin, a prescription drug taken orally, can clear the bowel of the disease. Sometimes, diaphragms are contaminated with candida: if you think this is the case, replace the diaphragm or soak it in antiseptic solution.

If you are taking the pill, switch to a brand with lower oestrogen or find another form of birth control. If you have a family history of diabetes, suspect diabetes as the cause and get a blood sugar test.

Another way to treat chronic candidiasis is to anticipate it. If you often develop the infection in the last phase of your cycle, treat yourself prophylactically with anti-fungal preparations several months in a row.

Rarely, reinfection can occur from candidal infections of the finger nails or even from infection of dentures. Occasionally the sexual partner may be a symptomless carrier, or may be passing the infection on from another woman.

10. How candidiasis is diagnosed

Most women get to know the symptoms of thrush and are quite sure when they have it. If you have had the infection verified at least once by a doctor, if predisposing illnesses have been ruled out, and if you can learn to make the infection go away on your own (see No. 8 above), you certainly do not have to visit a doctor each time.

The initial diagnosis is usually made in the laboratory. VD clinics can test for it straight away. A sample of the discharge is placed on a microscopic slide with some 10 per cent potassium hydroxide. This solution kills off the other cells present and allows the candida to stand out. GPs or gynaecological clinics usually send a swab away for culture tests to verify the diagnosis. This takes two or three days.

Sometimes a routine cervical smear will turn up evidence of candidiasis that has given no symptoms. If you have no discomfort, these cases do not have to be treated.

11. Side effects of anti-fungal drugs

If the problem seems to be getting worse, it may be that you are having sensitivity reactions (itching, swelling) to the treatment. Relief from the symptoms of candidiasis should be expected within two to three days. If you don't get it, suspect the drug and switch to one of the many alternatives.

12. Trichomoniasis

This form of vaginitis is caused by a one-celled organism called *Trichomonas vaginalis*, which lives in the vagina, cervix, urethra, and bladder of women and the urethra and prostate of men. This organism can cause an inflammatory reaction that is very uncomfortable.

13. What are the symptoms of trichomoniasis?

a. A thin, frothy, yellow-green discharge sometimes with a foul odour;

291

b. Itching or vaginal irritation, usually worse just after the menstrual period.

c. Burning and frequency of urination. The "trich" organism can be seen in a wet smear of the discharge mixed with saline solution—it is alive, swimming around on the slide. It may also be detected on the cervical smear. Some doctors will suggest treatment even if you have no symptoms to prevent trouble later. (See No. 16 below)

14. Who is likely to get trichomoniasis?

With very few exceptions, only sexually active women get "trich" or TV. For this reason it is considered sexually transmitted. Men do not usually have symptoms when they harbour TV, but they may have a slight discharge from their penis and some burning on urination. They usually think they have gonorrhoea, and unfortunately some doctors will treat them for gonorrhoea without checking for trichomonas. Since 90 per cent of the sexual partners (male or female) of infected women harbour trichomonas, they must be treated to keep from reinfecting the women.

15. Trichomonas can cause dysuria

These organisms can invade the urinary bladder and urethra and cause pain on urination (dysuria) which does not resolve until the trichomonas is treated. (See No. 46 below) In a severe infection when the vulva and the urethra are swollen, the pain may prevent urine being passed, leading to urinary retention.

16. Treatment of trichomoniasis

Metronidazole (Flagyl) is the drug most commonly used which kills the trichomonas organism. Both partners usually take one 200 mg tablet three times a day for 7 days. More recently, studies have shown that one dose of two grams for each partner also gives a good cure. (Ref. 1) This may be preferable because of the side effects of Flagyl. (See below) Naxogan is an alternative drug. Unless both partners are treated, the problem of reinfection remains.

17. Watch out for the side effects of Flagyl

Flagyl can irritate the throat or stomach, and should, therefore, always be taken *with meals.* Avoid alcoholic beverages while you are taking Flagyl; the combination causes nausea. Some women find that the drug (like many anti-bacterial agents) leaves them with a strange taste in their mouths, a feeling of furriness on the tongue.

Urine sometimes turns dark. WARNING: *During early pregnancy, when it is quite possible to contract trichomoniasis, Flagyl should not be used at all.* There is a possibility that it would affect the embryo as the drug passes through the placenta.

18. Side effects of the drugs used to treat vaginitis

Allergic reactions are possible with any drug and those used to treat vaginitis are no exception. Some pessaries, especially the foaming type, increase irritation.

19. Gonorrhoea as a cause of vaginal discharge

All sexually active women with vaginal discharge should be tested for gonorrhoea, which frequently causes infection in the cervix and may cause a dischage. (See No. 33 below)

20. Other causes of vaginal discharge

Several other organisms have been suspected of causing vaginitis, cervicitis or pelvic infection.

a. *Chlamydia.* This organism, intermediate in size between bacteria and viruses, has been found to be present in one third of women whose sexual partners have non-specific genital infection and in up to two-thirds of men with this complaint. It may cause a slight colourless and odourless discharge and may be associated with a urinary tract infection. Swedish workers have isolated, by laparoscopy, the organism from the Fallopian tubes in women who have acute salpingitis (infection of the Fallopian tubes), and they consider it may be more dangerous than the organism responsible for gonorrhoea in terms of future fertility. (Ref. 2)

The best treatment is considered to be 250 mg of tetracycline or erythromycin every six hours for three weeks, although some doctors give shorter courses of antibiotics. Others think it is almost impossible to eradicate the infection once acquired.

b. *Mycoplasma* was considered an important cause of pelvic infection in the 1960s and there is still controversy about its role in non-specific genital infection (NSGI) and pelvic inflammatory disease (PID). It may be found in healthy men and women and it is possible that it only causes harm after damage has been started by another organism.

c. *Haemophilus vaginitis.* This is also called *corynebacterium vaginitis.* It shows itself as a foul-smelling greyish irritating discharge and is found very commonly in the USA. In Britain it is rarely diagnosed, even in V.D. clinics, and this may have some relationship to the lesser use of douching in this country. Douching may upset the vaginal acidity, and flora (the normal germs that live there) and thus haemophilus starts to grow. The man is not affected, but is thought to act as a carrier. Treatment is with metronidazole or ampicillin for a week.

The best way to get a quick and accurate diagnosis is to go to a V.D. clinic where the proper tests will be done. Few GPs have access to the laboratory facilities required, and the wait for a gynaecological appointment is too long.

21. Venereal warts (condylomata acuminata)

From the Greek word *kondyloma* (a knob) and the Latin *acumino* (to sharpen) condylomata (con-dill-OH-mat-a) acuminata (ak-KU-mi-na-ta) are increasing in frequency among women and men. In women, small warts grow on the vulva and vagina, sometimes on the cervix. The disease is caused by a virus similar to that which produces such warts on other parts of the body, usually spreads through sexual contact and is usually associated with other vaginal infections.

STOP PRESS: Recently doctors have found that women who develop cancer of the vulva and men who have cancer of the penis are more likely to have been treated for venereal warts 30 to 40 years before. This may not be cause and effect. Watch for further reports.

22. Treatment for venereal warts: Trichloracetic acid and podophyllin

For men and for women the treatment is the same. Small areas of warts are touched with these chemicals which kill the virus that caused them. Trichloracetic acid is a caustic substance. Talcum powder is usually applied to soak up moisture and prevent the medication spreading to normal skin. The treated area is rinsed with lots of water within two hours after the application. The process is repeated every 3–4 days until the warts disappear. This is usually done by a doctor, either your GP or at a VD clinic.

WARNING: *Pregnant women with large areas of warts must not use podophyllin because the medication may hurt the fetus, if large amounts are absorbed into the woman's blood stream.*

23. Treatment for venereal warts: liquid nitrogen or carbon dioxide snow

Small areas of affected tissue are killed by application of a solution that freezes them and removes them for good. Although the treatment sounds cold and uncomfortable, it is in fact almost painless. It can be used on warts *inside* the vagina, and has the added advantage of being fast and can be done at an outpatient clinic. This treatment is also being used extensively to treat cervicitis (see No. 30 below) and chronic severe haemorrhoids.

STOP PRESS: Lasers are now coming into use for the treatment of venereal warts. This is very expensive, but is said to be painless and healing is quick.

24. Folliculitis

Folliculitis (fol-lick-you-LIE-tis) is a very common disorder, in which the pubic hair roots become inflamed, starting as small red bumps that can grow large and painful like a boil. Hot soaks and frequent scrubbing are the recommended treatment. Folliculitis can happen to anyone and commonly recurs premenstrually. Cloxacillin is the preferable drug for women who get recurrent large boils, if these are due to a staphylococcal infection.

25. Herpes simplex and genital herpes

Herpes simplex is a commonly occurring virus of which there are two types. The first type usually infects the mouth and lip but can be transmitted to the genitals by oral sex. So if you or your partner get cold sores or other mouth infections, avoid oral sex. Also avoid sex with anyone with genital sores. The second type of herpes simplex virus is usually the one which affects the vulva, the vagina and the cervix and causes genital herpes. Women who have had the first variety seem to develop some resistance to the second.

Genital herpes comes in varying degrees of severity, but can be extremely painful and incapacitating, especially during the first bout. It is transmitted primarily through sexual contact, and has been on the rise like other forms of venereal infection. *Most serious, this virus may have a role in causing cervical cancer.*

26. Symptoms of genital herpes

After a three to seven day incubation period, a woman will note many small blisters in the genital region. The blisters burst rapidly and leave a multitude of small but extremely painful ulcers with red edges. The first episode of genital herpes may last up to three to six weeks, accompanied by fever and swelling of large lymph nodes in the groin. Urination is extremely painful, for the burning caused by the ulcers is irritated by the passage of the urine over them. Sometimes the disease does not come back. Sometimes it recurs, every six to eight weeks, usually with a decline in severity and the number of ulcers each time.

27. Treatment of genital herpes

Viruses, in general, have eluded cures by medical science, so, at this time *only the symptoms, not the source of herpes can be treated.* See a doctor for diagnosis. This can be made by culture or smear of the lesions. Sex is taboo if either partner has active herpes; it will probably be too painful to be pleasurable anyway.

a. Antiviral agents are available from your doctor. The most common is 5-iodo-2-deoxyuridine. It comes as an ointment or as drops (Liquifilm).

b. Apply ether or chloroform to the lesions to relieve the stinging and pain.

c. Bathe in cool salt water several times a day.

d. Relieve the pain of urination by pouring cool water over the area while you are urinating, or urinate in the shower.

e. Take a mild analgesic every four hours.

WARNING: In past years, various dyes—Congo Red, Acridine Orange—were applied to the herpes lesions and then subjected to ultra-violet light. This treatment is now discredited.

28. Relationship of genital herpes and cervical cancer

In several large studies of women with cervical cancer, blood testing showed that a much larger number of them had had herpes virus type II than a group of women with no evidence of cervical cancer. (Refs. 3, 4) There is no absolute proof, just a suspicion that the two are often linked. One theory suggests that women with cervical cancer are more prone to sexually transmitted diseases than others.

This means that all women who have had genital herpes must be absolutely religious about getting a cervical smear every year, even if she has to pay for this, for only in this way will cervical cancer be detected at an early, curable stage. (See No. 175 below)

29. Vaginitis and vulvitis not caused by infection

a. Menopausal women (See p. 273) may suffer from *atrophic vaginitis*—a discharge and itching caused by the decrease in oestrogen and a mild infection.

b. Allergy can cause vaginitis-vulvitis symptoms. For example, you may be allergic to clothing material, soap, detergents, vaginal sprays, contraceptive jellies, anything that, when applied to the area, creates a "contact dermatitis", an itching and skin reaction. If examination and lab tests indicate no infection, look for an allergy, eliminate the offending material and you will feel fine again.

c. Overuse of sprays or vaginal medications can create the symptoms of vaginitis. *Do not use prescribed vaginitis creams after the condition is cured;* the treatment itself may become counter-productive.

d. Forgotten tampons and ring pessaries can cause symptoms similar to those of vaginitis.

30. Cervicitis

This is an inflammation of the cervical glands, frequently accompanied by vaginitis.

Acute cervicitis due to gonococcal infection or, rarely, herpes causes pain on intercourse and an associated vaginal discharge, which is minimal in the case of gonorrhoea, but profuse in herpes infection.

Chronic cervicitis was much more common 20 years ago when prolonged labour and difficult forceps deliveries led to a damaged, torn cervix which could easily harbour infection. This was treated by cervical cautery (the damaged or infected cells being burned off electrically), but the need for cervical cauterization today, whether done by diathermy or cryocautery, is much less.

The role of *chlamydia* (see No.20a above) in causing a low grade cervicitis which may cause bleeding after intercourse is not widely known to doctors. The diagnosis can be made by culture of the organism at research centres, or presumed in a woman in which the cervix looks unhealthy if her partner is examined and found to have non-specific genital infection. It is best treated with tetracycline or erythromycin.

31. Cervical erosion or ectopy

This is a *cervical eversion*, in which the lining of the cervical canal is turned outward, becoming visible in the centre of the cervix and making the cervix more susceptible to infection and irritation. Sometimes there is an excess mucous discharge that cannot be controlled except by cautery. (See No. 30 above) This is also called a cervical *ectropion* or *ectopy*.

32. Psychosomatic vaginitis: Is there such a thing?

In very rare instances, a woman may have all the symptoms of vaginitis with no infection or irritation to cause it. After careful evaluation and discussion, her doctor may conclude that some psychological problem is expressing itself this way. It is possible. If other diseases such as ulcer, colitis, and migraine headaches can have psychosomatic causes, so can vaginal discharge. If you have a problem with your sex life, spell it out to your doctor. *The problem with this diagnosis is that it is used too often as an excuse for not evaluating a discharge completely.* Make sure that smears and cultures are done before accepting the conclusion, and verify it with a second medical opinion.

VENEREAL DISEASE

33. Gonorrhoea (gon-nor-REE-a) ("clap")

More people get gonorrhoea from each other than any other disease except the common cold. The disease is most common among people under 25 and people who have many sexual partners. After something of an epidemic, the incidence of gonorrhoea seems to be levelling out, perhaps because of increased public awareness, and renewed interest in VD-preventing condoms and foams. (See p. 72)

Gonorrhoea is caused by a bacterium, *Neisseria gonorrhoea*, named after the scientist, Albert L. S. Breslau Neisser, who discovered it in Germany in the late nineteenth century. It can infect the mucous membrane of the vagina, the cervix, the urethra, Bartholin's glands (see No. 129 below), rectum, and throat. The gonorrhoea organism dies very quickly if it does not lodge in these places. It is therefore next to impossible for it to be transmitted by any means except sexual contact. You cannot, for example, get it from a toilet seat. Unless your GP has an interest in VD and access to laboratory facilities, always go to a VD clinic for tests.

34. The vast majority of women with gonorrhoea (80 per cent) have no symptoms at all

They may have the disease, may be transmitting it to others who are transmitting it to others. It may be infecting the tubes and ovaries, without the woman herself ever knowing it.

a. RECOMMENDATION: For this reason, sexually active women should have routine tests for gonorrhoea. Only the lab can tell for sure. A culture is taken from the cervix, and sent to the lab for verification, as part of the regular gynaecological examination. *Do not let a doctor tell you that you have gonorrhoea without verifying the diagnosis with a culture.* This takes about forty-eight hours and *must* be done because other organisms in the vagina are very similar to the gonorrhoea bacterium and may be confused with it. The culture misses the disease in 20 per cent of cases because the bacteria are so difficult to grow. If you are worried have a second test.

b. Another way to be quite sure that you have gonorrhoea is when your sexual partner develops it. In this case, seek treatment (not just testing) immediately.

c. If a woman has symptoms of tubal infection—fever, severe abdominal pains, heavy vaginal discharge—gonorrhoea may be the cause. She should be started on treatment at the same time that she gets the gonorrhoea test. (See No. 37 below)

Other possible symptoms of gonorrhoea include a discharge from the urethra; burning on urination (this symptom, shared by men and women, accounts for the common reference to the disease as "getting burned"); irritation of the vulva; vaginal discharge; proctitis (prock-TIE-tis)—pain on defaecation, a foul-smelling discharge from the anus. These things may not always indicate gonorrhoea, but they are all signs of ill health and require medical attention.

35. Symptoms of gonorrhoea in men

Frequently a man will experience a discharge from his penis, a sign that the urethra is infected. Another symptom is a feeling of burning during urination. However, up to 10–20 per cent of men have no symptoms at all, contrary to the once popular view that men *always* have symptoms. (Ref. 5)

If your partner has a discharge from the penis, don't let him delay in being checked by a doctor. Also, don't believe him if he says that the discharge is due to "straining" (a common rationalization.) He may be kidding himself; don't let him kid you. Make him use a condom if you have intercourse.

36. Effects of gonorrhoea in women

The Bartholin's glands may be affected; the ovaries and Fallopian tubes may be infected, causing infertility. In both sexes, generalized gonorrhoea can cause skin rashes, hepatitis (liver infection—Fitz-Hugh-Curtis Syndrome) and arthritis. (See No. 237 below)

If a baby is born vaginally to a mother with gonorrhoea and antibiotic drops are not placed in the eyes, the baby may get conjunctivitis. Left untreated before penicillin was available, this led to blindness.

WARNING: *Women having their babies outside hospital should take care not to overlook this treatment.*

37. Treatment of gonorrhoea

When the disease has no symptoms, there are several alternative treatments.

a. Procaine penicillin injection, one dose of 2.4 megaunits, can be given along with Probenecid, a drug which heightens the level of penicillin in the blood.

b. Or ampicillin (3.5 grams) along with probenecid can be given orally.

c. For people allergic to penicillin, tetracycline, erythromycin or spectinomycin can be given.

d. When gonorrhoea has caused *severe pelvic inflammatory disease* (PID) (tubal infection), a woman must be treated in hospital with penicillin by injection.

Since some strains of gonorrhoea resist penicillin, cultures must be done at one to two weeks and at six weeks to make sure that the drug has worked. This also tests that a woman has not become reinfected. (Other bacteria cause pelvic infections as well— chlamydia, mycoplasma or TB.)

e. *Sexual partners must always be treated.* If you find that you have gonorrhoea, don't be embarrassed to tell the people you've been sleeping with: you are endangering them and their sexual partners if you don't.

38. How to prevent gonorrhoea

Know your sexual partners as well as you possibly can. Not knowing a man is reason enough to suspect that he may be carrying gonorrhoea, so insist that he use a condom. Vaginal foams and jellies have been shown to have a preventive effect, so use them. (Ref. 6) If the man has any discharge from his penis or any sores in the genital area, don't have intercourse; these are very likely symptoms of VD.

Have regular checkups and gonorrhoea cultures at least every six months, more often if you have had possible contact.

39. Syphilis ("the pox")

Syphilis, less common but much more serious than gonorrhoea, spreads in exactly the same way—by sexual contact. If left unchecked, it can affect the brain and the heart; it will destroy the sufferer long before it kills, and the children of syphilitic parents will be grievously affected if they survive. Like gonorrhoea, syphilis has been on the rise again, a price we are paying for the sexual revolution and the decline in the use of condoms. In the UK 90 per cent of new cases are in homosexual men, so beware the casual encounter with a bisexual male!

40. The four stages of syphilis

a. Stage one: Primary syphilis occurs 10 to 90 days after sexual contact in the form of a chancre, a *painless* ulcer with an elevated edge usually around the genitals. If the man you are with has an ulcer on his penis, be suspicious. Send him to a doctor and avoid sexual contact. Frequently, a woman does not notice this stage in herself because the ulcer may be inside the vagina. The chancre may also occur on the labia, the tongue, lips, or nipples and lasts from three to nine weeks.

If you have any sore that does not heal after a matter of days, get it checked. Even if it isn't syphilis, it may signify another disorder.

A blood test will verify the first stage of syphilis about three to four weeks after is has been contracted. However, it can be detected earlier if the chancre is found; a scraping from it is taken and tested for the presence of the syphilis organism, a long, thin bacteria virus called *Treponema pallidum.*

b. Stage two: About three months after contact, warty growths may appear around the vagina. Called *condyloma lata*, these are flatter than condyloma acuminata (venereal warts) (See No. 21 above). A spotty rash may show on the palms and soles, and sometimes all over the body.

A blood test during this phase will always be positive. The disease may have no obvious secondary stage but may pass directly into the latent phase.

c. The *latent phase* of syphilis has no symptoms and may last from two to 20 years. During this phase the blood test is always positive. This stage may not occur at all and the disease may pass directly to the tertiary stage.

d. It is during the *tertiary stage* of syphilis that the heart and brain may be affected. It may start any time after stage two, so that early detection of the disease is vitally important.

41. How syphilis is detected

Routine screening blood tests are very accurate in detecting syphilis. They should be obtained every year without fail by women who have had more than one partner.

If the screening test (RPR or VDRL) is positive, the blood is sent for more exact tests. This is because the first test can sometimes be falsely positive: some viral illnesses and other medical problems such as lupus (See No. 230 below) can cause the same blood results as syphilis.

Once the specific test shows positive, treatment should begin immediately for *all* the sexual partners of the person on whom the test was done. Clinics always record the occurrence of cases of syphilis. In most localities investigation of sexual contacts is undertaken immediately.

You will be asked to cooperate in naming sexual contacts so that they can be traced and treated. Confidentiality is always maintained.

42. Blood tests for syphilis during pregnancy
Blood tests for syphilis should be given in pregnancy, for untreated syphilis can cause serious congenital deformities if not the death of the fetus. These are done routinely in NHS antenatal clinics.

43. Treatment of syphilis
Procaine, a long-acting penicillin, is given by injection intramuscularly.

a. For early cases daily shots of 600 mg are given for 10 days.

b. If the disease has reached the secondary or later stages, injections of up to 1200 mg are given for 20 days.

c. If a person is allergic to penicillin, erythromycin or tetracycline can be used for 15–20 days.

Generally, tests for syphilis remain positive after treatment but the titre (or concentration of antibody) in the blood decreases. It is important that routine blood tests continue because a person can catch syphilis again, and if so, the titre in the screening test will rise again.

This is a task for a specialist. Your family doctor should not try to treat you himself, but should refer you to a VD clinic.

44. Other venereal and sexually transmitted diseases
Some other diseases—chancroid, granuloma inguinale and lymphogranuloma venereum—occur rarely in the western world. They strike mainly in tropical countries and are all characterized by sores or lesions on the vulva and swollen lymph nodes in the groin. If you have any of these symptoms, seek medical treatment immediately, for these can be chronic debilitating diseases if allowed to continue for any length of time.

WARNING: Other non-venereal diseases, such as hepatitis, can be transmitted by sexual contact. If your partner develops hepatitis, ask your doctor for a blood test.

45. Pubic lice and scabies
Pubic lice, tiny bugs which burrow into the roots of the pubic hair and cause intense itching, can be transmitted from a sexual partner and also from bedclothes, towels, toilets. Treatment is a shampoo (Prioderm), which is washed into the pubic hair. Reinfec-

tion is a danger unless sexual partners, all linens and bathrooms are disinfected as well. If the disease recurs and doesn't go away, pubic hair may have to be shaved.

This has long been thought of as a disease of poverty. But it has been known to strike the unwary traveller, even in not-so-impoverished hotels, particularly overseas.

Scabies is also caused by a small bug, which typically burrows into the skin around the elbows, wrists, buttocks, and genitals, causing a track of red dots and intense itching. It is passed sexually, as well as by any close contact, and has been on a dramatic upswing over the past few years. The treatment is the same as for pubic lice—except that the sufferer uses a lotion, not a shampoo.

CYSTITIS AND URINARY TRACT PROBLEMS

46. Cystitis
Cystitis (siss-TIE-tis) is a general term for inflammations of the urinary bladder. It is much more common in women than in men, because women have a very short urethra—the tube leading from the bladder to the vagina. Most infections which cause cystitis are caused by introduction of organisms from the outside, from the vagina or anus; these then spread up through the urethra and into the lining of the bladder. In some cases, the symptoms of cystitis can occur without any disease process—for example, through an allergic reaction. This is cystitis at its best—a temporary annoyance, not threatening to general good health. At its worst, cystitis is caused by an infection of the bladder which can spread to the kidneys and cause pyelonephritis, which may seriously impair kidney function. Thus, the symptoms of cystitis, if they persist for two or more days, must always be evaluated by a doctor.

47. Symptoms of cystitis
These include:
  a. Frequent need to urinate (see No. 48 below)
  b. Pain on urination (dysuria)
  c. Having to get up at night to urinate (nocturia)
  d. Occasionally blood in the urine; if present see a doctor as soon as possible (haematuria)

48. Causes other than infection of urination frequency with or without pain
  a. Pregnancy. The frequency experienced by women early or late in pregnancy may be due to the pressure of the baby's head on the

bladder, not to infection.

b. Allergic reactions from rubber in sheaths, spermicides, scented or perfumed soaps, bubble bath, talcum powder or biological detergents in underpants.

c. Oestrogen deficiency in post-menopausal women (atrophic cystitis).

d. Irritation from a poorly fitted diaphragm.

e. Anxiety may cause frequency. The woman passes small amounts of urine every few minutes.

f. Excessive fluid intake, especially tea or coffee, causes frequency, with large amounts of urine every hour or so.

g. Diabetes mellitus (sugar diabetes) may first be detected by excessive thirst and frequent urination.

h. Diabetes insipidus also presents in this way, due to the lack of anti-diuretic hormone (ADH). It may follow a serious skull fracture.

49. Major causes of cystitis

It is often impossible to detect the underlying cause of an isolated case of cystitis. Recurrent cases are often caused by, or at least associated with, the following:

a. Increase in the frequency of intercourse, especially when this occurs for the first time, for example in "honeymoon cystitis".

b. Poor personal hygiene and improper toilet habits.

c. Uterine prolapse, including cystocele in older women. (See No. 64 below)

d. Sexually transmitted diseases, especially non-specific genital infection.

e. Insertion of a catheter into the bladder during labour or after abdominal operations. Routine catheterization prior to D and C or abortion is unnecessary if the woman empties her bladder before going to the theatre.

50. Improper toilet habits as a cause of cystitis

Faecal contamination can cause cystitis when a woman who has moved her bowels wipes from the back to the front. Always wipe the anal area separately from the vaginal area. Teach your daughters to do so at the beginning of toilet training. Women should try to urinate regularly, at least every three or four hours. Holding urine in the bladder for many hours predisposes to infection. This is particularly likely if the woman has diarrhoea.

51. Diarrhoea as a cause of cystitis

A woman who is suffering from diarrhoea may contract cystitis because of contamination of the urethra from the frequent bowel movements. So, if you have diarrhoea, take extra care in cleansing the genital area.

52. "Honeymoon cystitis"

This cystitis, usually associated with a sudden increase in the frequency of coitus, probably comes from irritation at the base of the bladder during repeated penile thrusting and from the deposit of organisms at the opening of the urethra during intercourse.

Women who find they contract cystitis after times of intense sexual activity should

a. urinate *before and after* intercourse, since the urine may wash away the organisms that have been deposited in the urethra;

b. use a vaginal lubricating jelly (*not* Vaseline), which may minimize irritation at the base of the bladder.

Some practitioners suggest that, when the condition is recurrent, antibiotics be taken for short periods of time before and after intercourse.

53. The urethral syndrome (recurrent cystitis)

Most women who experience "honeymoon cystitis" recover with rest, fluids and antibiotics and have no further problems. However a few continue to have cystitis associated with intercourse, even though sexual activity is not excessive. It is thought that they are particularly susceptible to bruising in the vulval area and to the organisms which live around the anal area and enter the urethra during sexual activity. Angela Kilmartin's book *Understanding Cystitis* is recommended to women suffering from this condition.

The following steps may help (Ref. 7):

a. Pass urine before and after intercourse, firstly to prevent organisms multiplying, and secondly to wash them out of the urethra.

b. If vaginal lubrication is insufficient even after adequate stimulation, you can use KY jelly to help the insertion of the penis.

c. Clean the vulva before and after intercourse with a specially boiled flannel.

d. Make the urine alkaline by drinking plenty of water with sodium bicarbonate if symptoms occur.

e. Take a mild antibiotic such as Furadantin (nitrofurantoin) prior to intercourse and on the following day.

f. Avoid anal intercourse or stimulation.

54. Catheter placement as a cause of cystitis

After surgery or childbirth, if a woman is unable to empty her bladder naturally, a catheter (KATH-eh-ter)—a long plastic tube—may be placed in the urethra to help urination. The simple presence of the catheter may cause cystitis by allowing bacteria to get into the urethra.

OPINION: *Catheterization, therefore, should never be a routine procedure.* It should only be done when a clear urine specimen is otherwise unobtainable, or in urological and gynaecological tests that absolutely require the procedure.

55. Cystitis in association with sexually transmitted diseases

Women infected with gonorrhoea or non-specific genital infection may notice pain on urination and in the latter case may develop a bacterial urinary tract infection. If you develop cystitis after intercourse with a new partner, it is important to have the whole range of tests for sexually transmitted diseases. These are not usually available from your general practitioner, but will be done in a VD clinic. (To find a clinic, look under VD or STD in the phone book or ask your local hospital where the "special clinic" is.)

56. A respiratory infection may cause cystitis

A viral or bacterial infection of the throat may also lead to cystitis—inflammation of the urinary tract by the same organisms —especially in children.

57. Chronic cervicitis as a cause of cystitis

Some doctors believe that when a cervix is chronically infected, bacteria that are causing the cervicitis (see No. 30 above) can pass through the lymph channels into the bladder, causing cystitis as well. A woman with cervicitis who has recurrent episodes of cystitis should have both treated. Trichomonas organisms are found in the bladder but are not thought to infect the bladder. (See No. 15 above)

58. A large cystocele can lead to cystitis

A cystocele (SIS-toe-seal) or hernia in the bladder wall can prevent complete voiding and lead to stagnation of the remaining urine in the bladder. This in turn can create an infection and cystitis. The cystitis can be relieved through medication until the cystocele is corrected. (See No. 64 below)

59. Factors other than infection which can cause cystitis symptoms

Some women are allergic to foods (lobster, for example) and urinate frequently as a result. Others get these symptoms because of irritations from soaps, bubble baths, detergents and sprays. Pelvic congestion before menstruation (see No. 89 below) can sometimes have the cystitis side effect. Anxiety leading to frequent urination produces at least this one effect of cystitis, as does excess intake of coffee, tea or other liquids.

If you use a diaphragm, have the size checked.

60. Cystitis is more common in pregnancy

Because of pressure of the growing fetus on the bladder, pregnant women are susceptible to relative stagnation in the urinary system. Therefore, the incidence of cystitis is somewhat higher. Some symptoms, such as frequency of urination in early pregnancy, are just due to pressure.

61. Kidney disease (pyelonephritis) and cystitis

Pyelonephritis (pie-low-ne-FRY-tis), an infection of the kidneys, can result if cystitis infection spreads from the bladder to the kidneys. *This may be a serious, debilitating disease and should never be allowed to develop from cystitis, which can be stopped at a much earlier stage.* The symptoms of pyelonephritis are fever, back pain just under the ribs, and the symptoms of cystitis. A woman can frequently be very sick with abdominal pain and vomiting as well.

62. Diagnosis and treatment of cystitis

If you get the symptoms of cystitis (pain on urination and frequency) start to drink plenty of water right away and go to your doctor as soon as possible. Ideally he will send a mid-stream specimen of urine (MSU) to the laboratory before treatment is started. This involves cleaning the vulva and catching the urine in a sterile pot after passing a small amount into the toilet.

If you are uncomfortable but not sick, the doctor may prescribe potassium citrate or sodium bicarbonate to make the urine alkaline and await the result of the urine culture to confirm that you have an infection before choosing the best antibiotic.

If you are in pain or unable to work because of the frequency, your doctor may start you on medicine straight away. A sulphonamide such as septrin or ampicillin is usually chosen. They bring about an improvement in 80 or 90 per cent of urinary tract infections. Check with your doctor two or three days later that the bacteria are being killed by the antibiotic prescribed. It is important to complete the course of tablets even if you feel better quickly. Otherwise there may be a few bacteria left which will cause trouble later.

If it is a second or third infection, insist on an MSU being tested even if your doctor does not suggest it. If you suspect that you could have picked up a sexually transmitted disease, go to your nearest VD clinic. They will take all the necessary tests and send an MSU for culture.

If the attacks continue, referral to a urologist for complete investigation of the urinary tract should be requested.

PELVIC RELAXATION

63. "Pelvic relaxation": tissue injury in the pelvic area

Pelvic relaxation is a general term referring to disorders of women caused by the tearing, stretching, or loss of tone in the pelvic muscles and fibrous tissue. Often called prolapse or hernias, these disorders usually occur after a number of pregnancies, and tend to be aggravated postmenopausally. Obese women and women engaged in hard labour that puts a great strain on the stomach muscles are also susceptible to pelvic relaxation. Sexual activity, no matter how strenuous, can never cause this problem.

64. Cystocele

A cystocele (SISS-toe-seal) is a bulging of the bladder which amounts to a hernia in the upper wall of the vagina. The size can vary depending on how badly the tissue is damaged. A large cystocele can put painful pressure on the vagina or actually protrude through it. Women with large cystoceles have a predisposition to urinary tract infections.

Another frequent association with cystocele is *urethrocele* (yur-EETH-roh-seal) in which the urethra bulges down below the pubic bone. Sometimes, the ligaments which normally hold the uterus in place are so stretched that the uterus descends into the vagina and sometimes even to the opening of the vagina. This is called uterine prolapse or dropped womb.

65. Rectocele

A rectocele is a weakening in the muscular support of the rectal wall so that the wall bulges into the vagina. When a woman is moving her bowels, the pressure will be most uncomfortable; she may be unable to defaecate without placing a finger into the vagina to give support to the wall.

66. Enterocele
This is a hernia where the top of the vagina bulges into the lower part. In effect, the vagina is doubling over into itself.

67. Symptoms of pelvic relaxation
a. A woman may feel unusual pressure in the vaginal area, or just general discomfort in the pelvic area often accompanied by backache.

b. She will feel tired will find that she wants to put her feet up, or that she is more comfortable wearing a panty girdle.

c. Pain on intercourse. The simple pressure of the penis on the descended uterus may make sexual relations uncomfortable.

d. Because of pressure in the pelvic area, a woman may lose a little urine, especially when she coughs or sneezes or does anything else to increase the pressure, even momentarily. This is called *stress incontinence.*

A woman and her doctor should have a careful discussion and a thorough examination should be made to distinguish stress incontinence from the several other causes of urinary incontinence. The woman with stress incontinence loses her urine only on coughing or sneezing or other such exertion. This is the only form of incontinence which responds to surgery. The other forms may in fact be made worse, so make sure tests are done. A cystometrogram (See No. 71 below) and other neurological tests can rule out most of the other disorders, many of which can be treated medically with antispasm drugs. A more continuous dribbling is more typical of this type of urinary problem. In addition, certain drugs such as some of the antihypertensive drugs may cause a bladder dysfunction and leaking. Discuss changing medicine with your doctor.

68. What causes pelvic relaxation?
We still don't really know, but it is much more likely to occur in women who have had children. Damage to the supports of the uterus may occur during the second stage of labour if this is very long or if a forceps delivery is to be performed. Hard physical work right up to delivery and immediately after may predispose to later prolapse. Obesity and chronic cough aggravate the condition.

69. Episiotomy cannot prevent pelvic relaxation
Episiotomy (eh-PEEZ-ee-ot-omy)—a surgical procedure by which an incision is made to widen the birth canal during delivery (see p. 141)—may prevent tearing of the perineum and the urethra as well. It is *not* effective in preventing cystocele or rectocele, or

enterocele (the tearing of the tissues that support the upper vagina) which is the most common form of pelvic relaxation.

70. Ring pessaries can relieve the symptoms of pelvic relaxation in some cases

These firm plastic rings are placed in the vagina and when properly fitted can reduce the symptoms of incontinence and vaginal relaxation. They are particularly good for older women, for whom surgery is too risky. They must be periodically removed and washed.

71. Opinion: Before you decide on surgery for pelvic relaxation, do the following:

a. Try pelvic floor exercises as you were taught for post-natal recovery. (See p. 153)

b. If you are postmenopausal, try low doses of oestrogen cream for several months.

c. Stop all strenuous activity, if possible.

d. If you are fat, lose weight.

e. If you have chronic bronchitis from smoking, stop smoking.

In addition, these tests may be done before surgery:

f. A urine culture to rule out infection.

g. An X-ray of the bladder. Dye is inserted into the bladder through a catheter and an X-ray taken to see if the neck of the bladder has descended and whether the size and shape of the bladder is normal.

h. A cystometrogram, a test to determine the capacity of the bladder and the amount of pressure inside it, to rule out other disorders which might be causing incontinence;

i. X-ray of the kidneys and ureters (IVP).

When stress incontinence is severe or prolapse of the uterus is troublesome, surgery is appropriate.

72. Surgery for pelvic relaxation

The usual operation is an anterior or posterior repair (perineorraphy). This may be combined with vaginal hysterectomy if there is some other reason for removing the uterus. If there is no prolapse but the woman has stress incontinence, a Marshall–Marchetti operation in which the urethra is hitched up to the back of the pubic bone may be the best procedure.

If a woman who has had a repair becomes pregnant, she should deliver by Caesarean section: a vaginal delivery would tear down the repair.

DYSMENORRHOEA AND PREMENSTRUAL SYNDROME (TENSION)

73. What is dysmenorrhoea?

Until endocrinology (the study of hormones and body chemistry) developed as a sophisticated medical science, little was known about dysmenorrhoea (or painful menstruation) except that an enormous number of women suffered from it.

An aura of mystery surrounded dysmenorrhoea (diss-men-o-REE-a). Often it was dismissed as untreatable or psychosomatic. Your mother's home remedies hardly ever alleviated your discomfort. Your doctor often had no remedy at all and sometimes produced a complex-sounding explanation for why these menstrual miseries were "all in your head". This left you not only with stomach cramps but with ego cramps as well.

Fortunately, the mystery of dysmenorrhoea is coming to an end, although the total cure is not yet at hand.

We can now broadly classify two major types of painful menstruation:

a. Primary or spasmodic dysmenorrhoea

b. Secondary or congestive dysmenorrhoea (frequently associated with premenstrual syndrome)

74. Spasmodic or primary dysmenorrhoea affects young women

Primary dysmenorrhoea usually begins in the early years of the menstrual cycle and rarely continues after first pregnancy, or, if there is no pregnancy, after age twenty-five. It is most common among teenagers and is characterized by pain resulting from spasms of the uterine muscles.

75. Congestive or secondary dysmenorrhoea affects older women

This type of dysmenorrhoea usually occurs in women over thirty. It is more likely to be associated with some other menstrual problem, such as premenstrual syndrome and pelvic congestion syndrome, or with other pelvic problems such as pelvic infection, endometriosis (see p. 331) or, rarely, fixed retroversion of the uterus. (See below) The two types of dysmenorrhoea are sometimes not easy to distinguish, nor are the symptoms so different.

WARNING: A properly fitted IUD of the correct size should not cause painful periods in a woman who has had children. It does sometimes cause painful periods in women who have never been pregnant. If pain begins after insertion, it suggests that the device has moved into the cervical canal (and is therefore not effective) or that infection has occurred. You should consult your doctor or local clinic at once.

76. Diagnosis and treatment of dysmenorrhoea

You don't need a doctor to diagnose dysmenorrhoea. Your own body, your own menstrual cycle will tell you what you are suffering from. Fortunately for most women, the discomforts of primary dysmenorrhoea usually pass quickly, occur in mild forms, and can be lived through without special care or medicine or interruption of normal activity. The whole condition is certainly made much more tolerable by the foreknowledge that it will end within a few days.

When you are so uncomfortable that you cannot continue normal activity, treatment is in order. Just as your menstrual cycle quickly establishes a routine pattern, you should quickly ascertain a routine treatment for the symptoms of your dysmenorrhoea.

For years GPs who simply didn't know better gave women psychological diagnoses for dysmenorrhoea. How often has a doctor told a young woman that she is getting these terrible menstrual cramps because she hasn't "resolved her sexual identity" or because she "wants an excuse to get away from the pressures of life"? *Watch out:* If you believe this stuff, it may come true.

On the other hand, when a girl complaining of dysmenorrhoea is encouraged to stay home from school or stay away from sports, she is being *rewarded* for her pain—not relieved of it. If she receives lavish parental attention during her period, she is encouraged to think that it makes her a queen for a couple of days—special, exotic, unapproachable.

The sooner it is understood by everyone that menstruation is a routine physical occurrence and dysmenorrhoea an unpleasant side effect that can usually be controlled, the sooner women will be able to find relief and get on with their lives.

77. Primary dysmenorrhoea is rare without ovulation

At the onset of menstruation, when a girl's periods are still irregular and she has not begun ovulating, dysmenorrhoea is rare. Classically, the teenager develops the pain over the next few years. (This absence of pain is also common among older women who have ceased ovulating and whose menstrual periods are coming to an end.)

78. What causes dysmenorrhoea?

No one knows for sure, but there are several theories.

a. The relation of *prostaglandins* to dysmenorrhoea is only now being understood. A large class of physiologically active compounds, prostaglandins stimulate the smooth muscles of the intestine and stomach and the muscles of the uterus. Because of their effect on the uterus, they are sometimes used to stimulate abortions. (See p. 193) This usually involves side effects of nausea, vomiting, and diarrhoea caused by simultaneous prostaglandin effect on the gastrointestinal tract muscles.

The same process is at work in dysmenorrhoea; prostaglandin effect is now thought to cause cramps, nausea, diarrhoea, and vomiting. Studies have shown that 80 per cent of women are relieved of their menstrual pain if prostaglandin antagonists are taken during the crucial time. (Ref. 8)

Menstrual blood has very high levels of prostaglandins. Any factors (still unknown) which elevate prostaglandins probably increase menstrual cramps.

b. *High levels of oestrogen and progesterone late in the cycle* may cause the body to retain sodium chloride (salt) and therefore, in turn, fluid, causing increased blood flow to the pelvic area and an uncomfortable, bloated feeling. This would be especially pertinent to the pelvic congestion syndrome (see No. 89) and dysmenorrhoea associated with premenstrual syndrome.

c. Don't pay too much attention to the theory that cramps are caused by narrowing or stenosis of the cervix which prevents menstrual blood from escaping. Except in very rare cases, this theory remains unproven.

d. There is also Dr Katharina Dalton's hypothesis that dysmenorrhoea is caused by a lack of progesterone or vitamin B6 (pyridoxine).

79. How to relieve menstrual cramps

Cramps both in the stomach and the rectum usually can be relieved by mild pain-killers or muscle relaxants. Aspirin works well because it blocks the prostaglandins somewhat. If mild products which can be bought over the counter from a chemist do not work, a doctor may have to prescribe something stronger. However, addictive drugs such as pethidine or morphine or Fortral should not be used. Several instances of women becoming drug addicts have followed the thoughtless use of these strong narcotics for period pains.

80. Recommendation: Prostaglandin inhibitors are very effective in relieving dysmenorrhoea, especially spasmodic dysmenorrhoea

Theoretically, drugs which inhibit prostaglandin production should alleviate most of the pain, vomiting, and diarrhoea associated with menstruation. In fact, several medications used widely for arthritis have an antiprostaglandin effect and are excellent in treatment of dysmenorrhoea.

First try simple analgesics like aspirin. If they don't work, *insist on* antiprostaglandin drugs. These include naproxen (Naprosyn), mefenamic acid (Ponstan) and ibuprofen (Brufen). (Refs. 9, 10)

81. To prevent cramps, avoid constipation before menstruation

The constipation some women experience before their periods probably stems from the effect of high hormone levels on the smooth muscle of the bowel. The hormones cause the muscles to relax: constipation results.

Constipation aggravates menstrual cramps by distending the bowel, producing wind. If you take steps before and during your period to avoid constipation, you may be able to avoid cramping pain completely. Eat plenty of fresh fruit; try bran cereal. A mild non-prescription stool softener may help too. (See p. 235)

82. Diarrhoea and vomiting with menstruation

These symptoms are probably caused by high levels of prostaglandins in the body. A few women may have to take anti-sickness drugs during the first day of bleeding; the anti-prostaglandins (see above) may help as well.

83. Exercise may help dysmenorrhoea

Rather than believing the advertisements, which suggest you *may* exercise during menstruation, experiment with the idea that you *should* exercise at these times. Many women report that exercise, with all that it means in terms of increased blood circulation and relaxation of muscles, is a way both to avoid and alleviate dysmenorrhoea.

It may be necessary to put your feet up for an hour or so during menstrual pain, between the time you take your muscle relaxant or analgesic and the time you begin to feel better.

Try and continue the exercise pattern that you're used to. Even women athletes in competitions find that they can continue, and win, while they are menstruating. (Contrary to what some people seem to believe, bleeding does not stop during swimming or other athletic activities; but that shouldn't stop you from taking part.) Strong physical exertion may speed up the menstrual flow and thus shorten the period.

84. Orgasm may help

Orgasms during sexual relations or by masturbation decreases the amount of pain felt by many women. This is more true of congestive symptoms common in older women than the spastic symptoms affecting young girls. Orgasm during menstruation actually increases the flow of blood and relieves the pressure of pelvic congestion.

85. Progestogen treatment

Synthetic progestogens (norethisterone) given from day 15 to day 25 of the menstrual cycle may help, especially if you have congestive dysmenorrhoea. On this regime, you will still ovulate. If you require contraceptive protection, take the tablets continuously throughout the cycle. This should prevent ovulation without incurring the risks of thrombosis. Natural progesterone can be given by injection, pessaries or suppositories, or can be implanted. It is perhaps more effective than progestogen but is much more costly and less convenient.

86. Combined oral contraceptive pill

If you want contraception, the combined pill will often cure or reduce the dysmenorrhoea and reduce the heaviness and length of your periods. The risks of thrombo-embolism and other side effects have to be considered before using the pill. If you are unlikely to have sex, prostaglandin antagonists or norethisterone should be tried first.

87. Pain associated with ovulation: mittelschmerz

Many women, from time to time, note a twinge or sharp pain in one side of the abdomen about the time of ovulation. This pain is called *mittelschmerz*. Some women have the symptom every month, and a few experience severe pain for a day or two. The exact cause is unknown. It may be related to spasms in the Fallo-pian tube around the time of ovulation, or a small amount of fluid or blood may escape from the ovary at time of ovulation and irritate the lining of the abdomen. If you stop ovulation with the high dose birth-control pills, the pain will go away—but few women find the discomfort so bad that they want treatment.

88. Premenstrual syndrome: progesterone as a treatment

Many women note that as they get into their thirties they develop one or more of the following symptoms in the latter part of their menstrual cycle:

   a. Breast tenderness
   b. Nervousness
   c. Headache
   d. Dysmenorrhoea
   e. Bloated feeling
   f. Weight gain

All of these are part of the *premenstrual syndrome* so well described by Dr. Katharina Dalton in her books, *The Premenstrual Syndrome and Progesterone Therapy* and *Once a Month*.

These symptoms probably result from imbalance of oestrogen and progesterone late in the cycle, and are usually easily relieved by progestogens in low doses in the second half of the cycle.

Try gentle diuretics or sedatives first. (Over-the-counter drugs with pamabrom or caffeine produce mild diuretic effects.) If these don't work and you are absolutely miserable with premenstrual syndrome, low-dose progestogens may be used. One-third of women will be helped in this way, and some may also find their symptons relieved by taking vitamin B6 (pyridoxine).

89. Pelvic congestion syndrome

This condition may actually be part of the premenstrual syndrome or may have other causes. Some symptoms resemble symptoms of pelvic relaxation: ache in the pelvic area, low backache, and an aching in the top of the thighs, but pelvic congestion syndrome is quite a different thing. Women often feel the symptoms most keenly seven to ten days before menstruation.

The syndrome usually begins to affect a woman when she is in her thirties (as does premenstrual syndrome—see No. 88 above.) The pelvic area can be very tender during examination or during intercourse; women suffering from pelvic congestion syndrome who undergo surgery are found to have a good deal of congestion and muscle spasms in the pelvic organs and vessels.

No one really knows the source of this problem.

It can be lived with and is lived with readily by many women who suffer from it, so serious investigation has been limited.

One *theory* is that it is caused by repeated sexual stimulation without orgasm. Masters and Johnson have found that pelvic congestion occurs immediately before orgasm; theoretically, therefore, pelvic congestion syndrome is a kind of chronic, preorgasmic state. Some women do find that orgasm, either through sexual relations or masturbation, helps. (See p. 378)

Masters and Johnson showed that women with these complaints have an enlarged and tender uterus. After orgasm, the uterus is its normal size again and the pelvic exam is painless as soon as ten minutes later. (Ref. 11)

SURGICAL PROCEDURES
DILATATION AND CURETTAGE (D & C)

D & C, dilatation and curettage, is one of the most commonly performed gynaecological operations—frequently performed for diagnosis but often serving as a cure.

90. What is a D & C?

Under general or local anaesthesia, the vulva, vagina and cervix are cleansed with antiseptic solution. A speculum is placed in the vagina; the cervix is grasped with a tenaculum. The uterus is then measured for length by a sound—a long metal device with distance markings on it (a lot like the device used to check the oil level in a car). The cervical canal is widened gradually by insertion of increasingly wide dilators. When the cervix is sufficiently dilated to allow access to the uterus, the lining of the uterus is scraped off with a curette.

A local anaesthetic (usually a paracervical block) can be used. It is injected just after the cervix is grasped with a tenaculum. Women who have the operation with local anaesthetic may feel mild cramping during the scraping.

91. General usages of a D & C

a. A D & C is a cleaning of the interior of the uterus; this in itself is often a cure for various disorders. (See below)

b. A tissue scraping can be extracted during the D & C and sent for lab analysis. A report on this endometrial tissue is usually available within forty-eight hours.

c. Before the scraping, the doctor can search the endometrial cavity with a special forceps, to detect polyps, for example.

d. The doctor can also evaluate the shape of the endometrial cavity and detect any irregularities, such as fibroids, which might be causing excessive bleeding. These problems may be suspected as a result of examination, but they can only be detected actually during the D & C when the doctor can feel inside the uterus with a curette.

92. Normal post-operative course after D & C

There should be very little bleeding after a D & C; sometimes staining will last for a week; sometimes a woman will find that she passes small clots into the toilet. She may have cramps or backache for a day or two. Complications such as heavy bleeding are infrequent. Avoid douching and tampons until bleeding stops. Condoms should be used during intercourse, for the first ten to fourteen days, for the cervix does not close right away. Resume bathing immediately and anticipate returning to normal work a few days after the operation.

93. Complications are rare after a D & C

A D & C poses few complications relative to other operations on the uterus. Perforation of the uterus occurs occasionally. (See p. 199) Cervical stenosis (sten-OH-siss)—in which the cervix is scarred during the operation and fused shut by scar tissue—is a very rare complication which may occur a long time afterwards. In the case of cervical stenosis, menstrual blood, mucus or pus (if the woman is postmenopausal) may accumulate behind the barrier that is closing the cervix and cause pain or swelling of the uterus. Unusual reactions to general anaesthesia are a risk in any surgical procedure.

94. Irregular menstrual bleeding: the most common reason for D & C

A D & C is generally performed to diagnose the cause of irregular menstrual bleeding or postmenopausal bleeding, but sometimes it will cure the problem as well. If no obvious cause for the irregular bleeding is found and all the pelvic organs are normal then the diagnostic label will be dysfunctional uterine bleeding.

95. Some specific causes of irregular uterine bleeding

    a. Endometrial polyps—small growths on the lining of the uterus—thought to be related to excess oestrogen stimulation

    b. Simple hormone imbalance, often related to stress

    c. Fibroid polyps

    d. Chronic inflammation of the endometrium (*endometritis)*

    e. Cancerous or precancerous growths

96. Hormone therapy as an alternative treatment for irregular uterine bleeding in healthy women under thirty-five

When women under thirty-five are having irregular periods, with no reason to suspect serious disorder, hormone imbalance is a likely cause. If a cervical smear is normal and the doctor feels the pelvis is normal on examination, no treatment is needed. If the periods are still troublesome after six months or so, hormone treatment to correct it may be suggested before a D & C is tried. This usually involves *no more than a few months* of hormone therapy to give the body time to retrieve its own balance, and in most cases is less dangerous than D & C and general anaesthesia.

In women under thirty-five in whom hormone therapy fails, or in women over thirty-five, a D & C is the preferred treatment. For women bleeding after menopause, a D & C is the treatment of choice.

WARNING: In women over 35 a diagnostic curettage should be performed before starting hormone therapy to make sure that there is no cancer, further symptoms of which could be hidden by hormone treatment.

97. Recommendation: D & C is not for teenagers

Menstrual irregularity is common among teenagers and usually rights itself in time without treatment. If it is severe or disabling, it can be treated with hormones, and is more easily corrected than irregular bleeding in older women. (See p. 23) A D & C is more dangerous for a young woman who has had no pregnancies because the cervix is often very difficult to dilate, may tear, and the cervical lacerations affect future fertility. *Seek another opinion*, therefore, if your doctors recommend a D & C as the first line of treatment for a teenager. Don't forget that gonorrhoea and non-specific genital infection may first be detected because of irregular periods.

98. D & C is frequently suggested at time of tubal ligation

With the woman's permission, a D & C is frequently performed at time of tubal ligation (sterilization) to eliminate the chance of a pre-existing pregnancy or any polyps. However, women have remained pregnant after this operation.

99. Other reasons—and non-reasons—for a D & C

D & Cs are often done in the treatment of Asherman's Syndrome (scarring in the uterus) and during infertility work-ups associated with laparoscopy and tubal lavage (See p. 102)

WARNING: *It is a common fallacy that a D & C is "good" for a woman as a periodic "cleaning-out". This is nonsense.* If a woman exhibits no menstrual irregularity, then the inside of her uterus is probably in excellent shape and there is no reason in the world that she should undergo an operation to have it scraped off.

D & C is not in itself a treatment for infertility; it may serve as a necessary part of the diagnostic work-up for infertility but not before many other steps take place. In infertility investigations, an endometrial biopsy (usually taken at a formal D & C) can confirm that ovulation has occurred and that tuberculosis is not the cause of infertility. (See p. 354) WARNING: It is also *not* a treatment for cramps, no matter how severe these are (see Dysmenorrhoea, p. 311) unless there is a need to make a diagnosis that only a lab test on the endometrial tissue can prove.

100. Opinion: If a doctor wants to do a D & C and can't give one of the above good reasons for it, check with another doctor

One of the most important ways to evaluate a doctor is to judge whether he or she suggests unnecessary surgery. A great many doctors use the D & C as a diagnostic measure when less radical measures would suffice. *No surgery should ever be routine.* If you have the slightest doubt about the necessity for any operation, check with one or several other physicians and corroborate the first opinion before going ahead.

101. Laparoscopy as a diagnostic procedure

This is a method of looking directly at the pelvic organs and is discussed completely on p. 102.

102. Hysteroscopy (hiss-ter-OSS-copy): a new diagnostic procedure

In this procedure, the inside of the uterus is visualized by a tube attached to a viewer, similar to a laparoscope, inserted through the cervix. This procedure may be used to remove lost IUDs or to see if there are any abnormalities in the endometrium, for instance, fibroids, as part of an infertility work-up. Some methods of blocking the Fallopian tubes for sterilization are performed with a hysteroscope. (See p. 86) This procedure is not widely available in Britain.

HYSTERECTOMY

103. What is a hysterectomy?

There are several types of hysterectomy, and the distinctions between them are vitally important. Get your doctor to spell out exactly what is to be removed.

a. *Radical hysterectomy* is the removal of tubes, ovaries, uterus, cervix *and* pelvic lymph nodes. WARNING: It should only be done in women with advanced cancer.

b. *Total hysterectomy* or *hysterectomy and bilateral salpingo-oophorectomy* (sal-ping-go-oo-for-ECK-tomy) is the removal of the uterus and cervix and the tubes and ovaries. If the uterus and cervix but only one tube and one ovary are removed, it is called *hysterectomy and unilateral salpingo-oophorectomy.*

c. *Hysterectomy* or *simple (rarely known as a "partial") hysterectomy* is the removal of the uterus and cervix.

d. *Subtotal hysterectomy* is the removal of the uterus but not the cervix.

Radical and total hysterectomies cause symptoms of menopause and climacteric. The hormone supply diminishes; physical and emotional changes are severe in many cases. If a woman already past menopause has the operation, the changes will not affect her greatly. Younger women may suffer much more and should take hormone treatment to prevent the severe symptoms of the climacteric too early in life.

Simple hysterectomy does not change a woman's hormonal status: she still has her ovaries. She does not menstruate, however, and needs no contraception. A hysterectomy in which only one ovary is removed also leaves a woman's hormone supply at normal levels.

104. Opinion: Hysterectomy is often an unnecessary operation

A number of factors contribute to this:

a. Some doctors dealing with women who have already completed their families use hysterectomy as a preventive measure against cancer and other degenerative diseases which increase in incidence as women grow older.

b. Some doctors perform hysterectomies when a woman wants to be sterilized; a simple and much less dangerous tubal ligation would do as well.

c. Some physicians perform hysterectomies for disorders in which a simple and much less dangerous D & C would serve.

About 19 per cent of British women have this operation in one form or another. In the past, and especially in the United States, it was used too frequently as an easy answer to female problems. The attitude of the gynaecologist is an important factor, which you should assess when a hysterectomy is suggested. It is a good idea to have your partner or a friend with you to give support during the discussion.

105. Opinion: How to avoid having an unnecessary hysterectomy

A hysterectomy is a major operation, useful only to correct major disease, like cancer or fibroids. *Anything less than major disease or injury should be disqualified as a reason for having the operation.*

Never accept a hysterectomy to achieve simple sterilization.

Never accept hysterectomy for menstrual irregularity, unless a D & C or hormones have been tried previously, or unless you have large fibroid tumours.

Always get at least one other opinion from your GP or family planning doctor or alternatively from doctors associated with different hospitals, if hysterectomy is recommended.

Always know whether your doctor is recommending a simple or a total hysterectomy with removal of the ovaries. Know whether you are going to lose both ovaries or just one. These differences are *critical*—and they require a decision by the patient, not just her doctor. If there is not an *excellent* reason for the ovaries to be removed, opt for a simple hysterectomy, for this will leave you with an undisturbed hormonal cycle. If only one ovary is diseased, keep the other one, especially if you are under fifty; it will provide you with some if not all the hormones you need and make the change of life less troublesome. (See p. 279)

Talk to other women who have had hysterectomies. Their experience may be valuable when you make your own decision.

Never accept hysterectomy as preventive medicine. It may be your doctor's view that the reproductive organs are unnecessary baggage for a woman who has completed her family, and is on her way to climacteric and possibly the degenerative diseases that afflict older people. This is a useless line of thinking; the odds are excellent that you will *not* get cancer of the uterus so the risk of the operation is greater than the risk of cancer if disease is not already present.

106. Abdominal hysterectomy—the most common form of this surgery

Abdominal hysterectomy involves general anaesthesia. An incision is made in the lower abdomen either vertically or horizontally at the level of the top of the pubic hair (which is shaved before surgery). Some surgeons pride themselves on making this horizontal incision as close to the pubic hair as possible so that the resulting scar is all but invisible. It is called a Pfannenstiel incision, after the doctor who perfected it. *Request this incision.* Surgical values being equal, the Pfannenstiel incision is much more desirable cosmetically, and has better strength in healing. If large tumours are present, a Pfannenstiel incision may not be possible.

The uterus is removed, as well as the cervix; the top of the vagina is closed. This wound just heals over, allowing intercourse as before. The bladder has to be moved a bit during the surgery.

A woman may need to have her bladder emptied with a catheter if she can't pass urine after the operation. As the bladder relaxes into its natural position and the trauma to the surrounding muscles lessens, she can pass urine normally. The woman will probably receive intravenous fluids until her bowel starts working again and she can eat and drink normally. This should take two to four days.

In the few days immediately after the operation, a woman will experience considerable pain. Her specialist can prescribe painkillers to ease the discomfort. *She should get out of bed and walk around as soon as possible, preferably the first day after the operation.* This prevents lung congestion that could lead to pneumonia; it makes leg muscles contract, helping to prevent phlebitis (clots in the veins, see p. 47); it encourages the circulation that promotes healing and helps the bowel to function normally again. When the nurse suggests this first walk, you may with all your heart wish to resist. But the suggestion is a good one and should be followed, despite the pain.

The hospital stay for hysterectomy is usually eight to ten days, depending on how quickly the individual recovers. Full recovery will need another three to six weeks' rest at home, and some women will probably not feel at full energy until some months after the surgery. Every prior arrangement must be made to allow the recuperation she needs. Women in good physical condition or who have wanted to have a hysterectomy because of unpleasant symptoms usually recover quickly.

107. Vaginal hysterectomy

Vaginal hysterectomy involves the same removal of organs, except that the incision is made through the top of the vagina. Recovery time is generally less than for an abdominal hysterectomy; there is less pain, because it is the vagina, not the belly, which must heal. Vaginal hysterectomy has some limitations. First, the uterus must be small enough to be drawn out through the vagina—this excludes women who suffer from large fibroid tumours of the uterus. It is not usually used in total hysterectomy, where diseased tubes and/or ovaries are being removed, as the surgeon cannot assess the extent of the disease so well vaginally.

For stress incontinence and other forms of pelvic relaxation (see p. 308), vaginal hysterectomy may be combined with vaginal repair. Most surgeons leave a catheter in the bladder after these operations, which is removed three to five days later, as there may be bruising of the bladder and vaginal walls.

108. Sexual response is not affected by hysterectomy

The physical aspects of sex should not be affected by hysterectomy—except that sex must be avoided until the woman is fully healed. Most women say that sex after hysterectomy is just as good or better than before, but some attest that it does *feel* different—probably because there are contractions of the uterus during orgasm which a woman who has had her uterus removed no longer feels.

Sexual response of a woman should not be affected by partial hysterectomy. In the case of total hysterectomy, the removal of the ovaries and the interruption of the hormone supply may have an important effect in altering (not always lessening) physiological responses to sex (see p. 377). If vaginal dryness or severe hot flushes occur, discuss hormone therapy. (See p. 278)

109. Complications of hysterectomy

a. Urinary-tract infections sometimes occur because of the catheter in the bladder after surgery (see No. 61 above).

b. Pelvic infection is a possibility. Blood may collect in the area where the uterus was, and then become infected. This is more common after vaginal than abdominal hysterectomy, because the vagina contains more bacteria that could infect the area than does the skin of the abdomen. Antibiotics are the common treatment; sometimes if pus has collected in the area where the uterus was, a drain must be placed through the top of the vagina to let it out.

c. Wound infection in the abdomen is a possibility. This usually appears around the fourth or fifth day after surgery. The treatment is antibiotics and heat pads. The rate of wound infection is much higher in obese women.

d. The bladder is the principal organ that must be moved to allow removal of the uterus. Therefore, bladder damage is relatively more common than other complications; it can usually be repaired on the spot, with no after-effects. The greater difficulty comes when the damage to the bladder is not recognized during surgery and grows more severe after the surgery is over.

In less than one per cent of cases, and more frequently in complicated surgery, a *fistula* (FISS-tue-la) may form to complicate bladder function. A fistula is a small canal (the word comes from the Latin word meaning tube or pipe) which allows the contents of one hollow organ to drain into another. As a result of damage to the bladder or ureter during hysterectomy, a fistula forms and the urine may begin to leak out into the vagina. Treatment is usually to place a catheter in the bladder and allow it to drain for several weeks while the fistula seals itself. Further surgery is sometimes needed. A woman can be up and around during this waiting period, but the scope of her activity is limited.

110. Post-operative care for hysterectomy

After the six-weekly post-operative check-up, you may not need to attend hospital again. Annual checks of the breasts and a vaginal examination to check the size of your ovaries can be done by your doctor. Vaginal smears are not required unless the uterus was removed for cancer. The gynaecologist will want to see you until he or she is satisfied that all is well if the uterus has been removed for cancer, infection or endometriosis.

111. Long-term complications of hysterectomy

a. *Hernia:* In overweight women or women who have suffered a post-operative infection in the wound, a hernia through the abdominal scar is a possible long-term complication. In this case the stomach muscle and fibrous tissue give way and a bulge appears under the skin. Some hernias are small and give no discomfort, others must be repaired surgically.

After hysterectomy, the top of the vagina can also herniate. Again, the treatment depends on the seriousness of the discomfort.

b. *Prolapse of the ovary:* After both abdominal and vaginal hysterectomies, there is a new empty cavity where the uterus used to be. In some women the ovaries may fall into this area behind the vagina and cause pain during intercourse. Rarely, surgery may be needed to pull the ovaries back into place.

112. Psychological complications of hysterectomy

Hysterectomy can have profound psychological effects that few women can anticipate. These stem from a feeling of having been cut off from one source of womanhood, from feelings of mutilation, or from the feeling (common in major surgery) that one has actually seen death. If a woman has had a total hysterectomy and develops severe hot flushes the psychological problems may be aggravated by the physical. She should use oestrogen replacement for *short periods of time.* (See p. 279) Mild depression following hysterectomy is common: if it is severe or prolonged, seek professional help.

If you know you are about to have a hysterectomy, and you are scared, do not be surprised if husband, children, and doctors are no comfort. They cannot be expected to understand what you are about to go through. Seek the advice and comfort of other women who have been through it and know how bad it was and *how bad it was not.*

113. Fibroids of the uterus: the most common reason for hysterectomy

Fibroids of the uterus are benign tumours of the uterine muscle, which occur in 25–35 per cent of all women. Their cause is unknown, but they do seem to run in families. They tend to decrease in size after menopause (when oestrogen supplies are low) and increase in size during pregnancy (when oestrogen is high) and in women on high-dose birth control pills.

If the fibroids are small, they may give no symptoms—and surgery to remove them is unjustified. Indeed a woman may live comfortably and without any symptoms with small fibroids for years and years. (By "small", doctors usually mean that the tumour does not make the uterus bigger than it would be at three to four months of pregnancy.)

114. Symptoms of uterine fibroids

a. The most common symptom is increasingly heavy menstrual bleeding, sometimes to the extent of haemorrhage. If untreated, this can leave a woman severely anaemic. Bleeding is heaviest if the fibroid is on the *inside* of the uterus, right under the endometrial surface (submucous).

b. If the tumours are large, they can press on other pelvic organs, such as the bladder and rectum, causing constipation and sometimes kidney infections that only hysterectomy will assuage. For a few women, severe backache may be a symptom of fibroids.

Like all tissue, a tumour must have a blood supply to stay alive. If a fibroid loses its blood supply, dies, or twists on the uterus, severe pain will result.

Any or all of these symptoms—bleeding, severe abdominal pain, severe backache—should at once take you to a doctor.

115. If fibroids are discovered on examination

A doctor who discovers small fibroids may do nothing about them.

OPINION: If they make the uterus larger than it would be at 16 weeks' pregnancy, have them removed. Beyond that size, they begin to cause pressure on the other organs. Since these tumours become cancerous in fewer than 1 in 200 women, their presence alone should not alarm you. However, if you have fibroids, have yourself examined at least twice yearly to assure that the tumours are not changing or growing fast. If you have no symptoms and they are not growing, there is little point in having them removed.

116. Myomectomy: removal of the fibroids alone

In a myomectomy, fibroid tumours alone are removed; the uterus is left in place. It may only be a stop-gap measure—that is, it can be done if small fibroids are rendering a woman infertile or causing heavy periods as a way of allowing her to conceive a child or keep her uterus. In about 20 per cent of cases, a hysterectomy is needed later on. But the myomectomy may have given the woman those few years she needed to have the children she wanted. A woman who becomes pregnant after a myomectomy should be delivered in a fully equipped hospital as she needs careful monitoring and probably has a higher chance of needing a Caesarean section than a woman whose uterus has not been scarred.

OPINION: Some specialists don't like to do myomectomies. They feel the woman will just have to come back for a hysterectomy later on, so why not do the whole job in the first place? *This may make good sense to a doctor, but it is no answer for a woman who wants a child or who just does not want her uterus out.* While myomectomy is less radical than a hysterectomy, it may be more difficult technically, with greater blood loss. If the fibroids are unusually large, and the uterus very distorted, it is *not* the recommended treatment. However, if you really desire a myomectomy and your doctor refuses, get at least one additional opinion. A specialist in the treatment of infertility is a good choice.

117. Other reasons for hysterectomy

a. *Irregular bleeding* with no obvious cause that has not been stopped by D & Cs, or hormone treatments.

b. *Pelvic infection and pelvic inflammatory disease.* Women who have suffered from these disorders, often in the aftermath of gonorrhoea or infection (see pp. 298-308), may develop serious scarring of the tubes and ovaries. The scar tissue knits these organs together with the uterus, and may cause infertility, severe dysmenorrhoea and severe pain during sexual intercourse. A diagnosis of pelvic inflammatory disease should be confirmed by laparoscopy (see p. 102) and antibiotics should be tried to resolve the infection before surgery is attempted. Sometimes conservative surgery, such as lysis of adhesions, may work, and you should discuss this possibility. *However, in severe cases—and most heartbreakingly, among young women—the condition cannot be checked except by total hysterectomy.* So never imagine that venereal disease can always be cured quickly, without complications.

   c. *Pelvic relaxation* (See No. 63 above)

   d. *Cancer of the uterus, cervix, or ovary* (see below)

   e. *Endometriosis or adenomyosis* (see No. 131)

   f. *Postnatal haemorrhage.* On rare occasions, a woman will haemorrhage so extensively after delivering her child that the only way to stop the bleeding and save her life is by removing the uterus. This is an emergency operation, usually conducted soon after delivery.

118. Subtotal hysterectomy (supracervical)

This is a rare procedure, in which the uterus is removed *but not the cervix*. It is used for women who have widespread pelvic infection or severe endometriosis that make removal of the cervix impossible without damage to the ureters or bladder. A woman who has had a supracervical hysterectomy must still have cervical smears because she must continue to guard herself against cervical cancer.

OVARIAN CYSTS

119. Ovarian cysts

Ovarian cysts are very common, usually benign, swellings, filled with fluid, that appear and sometimes disappear spontaneously. Most ovarian cysts are *functional*—that is, something goes slightly wrong in the normal menstrual cycle and excess fluid collects around the follicle or corpus luteum, then disperses by itself.

Sometimes, the cysts retain their fluid and actually collect more fluid, creating a cystic mass filled with the normal secretions of the ovaries. If this grows large, it must be removed surgically.

120. How ovarian cysts are detected

Frequently, ovarian cysts have no symptoms and are only detected by the examining doctor. Sometimes they are indicated by pain on the affected side as well as by menstrual irregularity.

If the cyst is less than 5 cm in diameter, in a woman under forty, another examination in three to six weeks is indicated. If the cyst has grown, *then* surgery is indicated. (In many cases, it will have disappeared.) In older women, ovarian enlargement is more serious and requires immediate evaluation by laparoscopy or laparotomy.

121. Birth control pills may shrink functional cysts

When a woman takes birth control pills, her ovaries do not always go through the changes of complete follicle development and corpus luteum formation because she is not ovulating. *Thus, women on the pill almost never develop functional cysts of the ovary.* Sometimes the pill can be used to shrink functional cysts. This treatment should last for no more than two months: if the cyst has not disappeared, it is probably *not* a functional cyst. Further diagnosis is in order.

122. Other tumours of the ovary—benign or malignant
These include:
a. Dermoid cysts and other benign tumours
b. Polycystic ovaries
c. Cancer of the ovaries

123. Dermoid cysts (cystic teratomas)
These are common, benign tumours of the ovary in young women. They are fairly startling because they are believed to be embryological remnants—frequently containing teeth, hair, brain and thyroid tissue. Usually they are detected during a routine gynaecological examination and can be confirmed by X-ray of the lower abdomen, which may reveal calcium in the embryologic content. Dermoid cysts do not usually cause menstrual irregularity.

Preferred treatment is surgical removal of the cyst, which can often be performed without removing the entire ovary.

124. Polycystic ovaries (the Stein-Leventhal Syndrome)
Laparoscopy and ovarian biopsy is required for a diagnosis of polycystic ovarian syndrome. It has another name—the Stein-Leventhal Syndrome (after Irving Stein and Michael Leventhal, the American doctors who first described it in 1935). This rare syndrome describes a group of women suffering from hormone imbalance, with accompanying obesity, excess body hair, and chronic menstrual irregularities. In addition, they have enlarged ovaries with a great many follicle cysts. This part of the condition is called polycystic ovaries. These women frequently have difficulty conceiving. (See p. 93)

125. Cancer of the ovaries
Ovarian cancer often shows very few symptoms. It is more common in women who have not had children. Women over 35 should have a regular vaginal examination, combined with a cervical smear. Unexpected weight loss or swelling of the lower part of the abdomen should be investigated.

126. Polyps

Polyps are *benign* growths of glandular tissue which occasionally pop up in little lumps on the cervix or the endometrium. Cervical polyps are usually discovered during a regular pelvic examination or may cause bleeding after intercourse. Endometrial polyps almost always cause irregular vaginal bleeding, and if a D & C is done to relieve the symptom, the cause will be discovered at that time. A D & C is the best treatment for cervical or endometrial polyps and will usually get rid of them for good. Occasionally, a cervical polyp in a young woman can be removed on an outpatient basis. If bleeding continues, a D & C is needed. Polyps are more common around menopause and are probably related to endocrine imbalance.

127. Bartholin's abscess

The Bartholin's glands are located at the lower part of the entrance to the vagina. Sometimes a minor irritation can inflame the gland, sometimes they can be infected by gonorrhoea; in either case, the entrance to the gland is blocked and the gland fills with pus and fluid and swells up. If there is pus inside, an abscess is formed and a very painful, hot swelling can occur.

128. Treatment of Bartholin's abscess

If an abscess forms, and infection is clearly present, a woman should have herself checked for gonorrhoea. Antibiotics will usually clear the abscess. Warm baths that help bring the infection up to the surface so that it can drain will relieve swelling and pain. If antibiotics and heat do not make the abscess drain, a doctor can incise it with a needle or small knife for immediate drainage. For women who suffer repeatedly from these abscesses, a permanent solution—marsupialization (mar-SOUP-ee-ill-ization)—is suggested. In this process, the gland is literally turned inside out so that fluid or pus cannot accumulate.

129. Bartholin's cysts

A Bartholin's cyst is just like a Bartholin's abscess except that the cyst is filled with fluid, the abscess is filled with pus. If small, a Bartholin's cyst need not be treated. Small cysts sometimes occur after childbirth, if the episiotomy (see p. 141) cuts across the duct of the Bartholin's gland. If the cyst becomes annoyingly large, proper treatment is removal of the gland or marsupialization. This is a relatively simple operation. Compared with Bartholin's abscess, a Bartholin's cyst is not painful.

130. Cyst and abscess of Skene's glands

In exactly the same way as the Bartholin's glands, the Skene's glands—located just below the urethra—can become infected or cystic. Treatment is usually removal of the cyst or abscess by removal of the gland—again a simple procedure.

131. Endometriosis (en-doe-mee-tree-OH-siss)

Endometriosis is a little-understood condition in which cells lining the uterus somehow appear outside the uterus—for example, in the pelvic cavity, behind the uterus, on the ovary and the tubes, in the cervix and vagina, and even sometimes on the skin of the vulva and the abdomen. The disease usually strikes women in their late twenties.

Common symptoms may be

a. Severe menstrual cramping in women who previously had little or no discomfort

b. Chronic pelvic pain

c. Pain during sexual intercourse

d. Infertility (because endometrial tissue may adhere to the Fallopian tubes, altering tube motility, causing scarring and preventing conception)

e. Irregular periods

For endometriosis to be diagnosed, most or all of these symptoms must be present, and the diagnosis must be confirmed by laparoscopy.

Adenomyosis is a condition when the cells of the endometrium occur in the muscle of the uterus.

132. Treatment of endometriosis

a. For many years, the main treatment method was hormones, given in the form of very high-dose birth control pills. In many cases, this treatment made the patches of endometriosis shrink. Low-dose pills can often keep mild endometriosis under control. Obviously, pregnancy is impossible under these circumstances.

b. Some women have used progestogens (synthetic progesterone) such as medroxyprogesterone acetate (Provera) in high doses with great success.

c. *Good news—watch the papers:* A very promising new drug, Danol, seems to have had the best results yet. It may have other beneficial side effects, such as decreasing the severity of cystic disease of the breast. (Ref. 12)

d. Surgery can work as well. The surgeon removes all patches of endometriosis he or she can find, and may burn small areas with diathermy.

CANCER

133. Cancer is a malignant (invasive) distortion of cell development which can affect any part of the body. Probably a group of diseases, rather than a single disease, it is the subject of intense research today, of two types:

a. *Basic research* to determine what causes cells to undergo the changes that eventually become a malignancy, and thereafter to multiply rapidly and spread throughout the body.

b. *Applied research* on how to detect the disease early and treat it. Applied research may *seem* more important, because of its assault on the concrete problem. But most of our great scientific breakthroughs required, somewhere along the line, research into the *basic* nature of the problem in its most abstract dimensions. For example, it is probable that Watson and Crick (and their unheralded colleague, Rosalind Franklin), in their Nobel Prize-winning work on the basic make-up of DNA, the genetic material in every cell, contributed greatly to applied cancer research. But they weren't *thinking* of cancer necessarily; they were just trying to find out more about cells and the genetic package they carry. Basic research is slow and painstaking but essential if we are to learn more about cancer.

134. A carcinogen is a substance which starts the cancer process

A carcinogen (car-SIN-o-jen) alters a cell so that it becomes free of normal limitations on growth and can reproduce itself without control. It may be a virus (which causes breast tumours in mice) or a chemical (such as hydrocarbon, present in air pollution, which causes tumours in animals and is implicated in lung cancer in humans), a high dose of radiation, or a hormone (which is implicated in tumours of the breast and genital organs). Cancer may also be associated with failure of the body's immunological responses, and the resultant inability to eliminate abnormal cells.

135. A promoter is a substance which speeds the cancer along once it has started

After the carcinogen has prompted the cell to change, certain *promoter* substances can hasten the process and contribute to the growth of the tumour. Hydrocarbons and hormones act as promoters in animals, and may do so in humans as well.

136. The "latent period" is the time it takes for cancer to express itself

The time from initiation of the cancer by the carcinogen to the time that the cancer invades and is expressed and observable in the body is called the "latent period". For cervical cancer, it is about two to ten years; for breast cancer, as long as ten to thirty years. The latent period may be shortened by promoter agents. *Thus, even a tumour that has started may not appear without a promoter to encourage it.* Thus control of promoter substances is *vital* to cancer control, a fact which should make us all dedicated environmentalists. It is during the latent period that cancer, if the cancer can be detected, is most easily arrested and cured. (See No. 179 below)

137. The risk of breast cancer

Breast cancer is the largest single cause of death among women in Britain—though lung cancer caused by more smoking among women is catching up fast. Over 29,000 new cases of breast cancer are detected each year. The chance that a British woman will get breast cancer is 1 in 16 and 1 in 18 women die from breast cancer.

Some women run a *higher* statistical risk than others. These include women who:

a. Have a family history of breast cancer, especially at a young age

b. Have been exposed to high doses of radiation

c. Have early menarche and late menopause

d. Have their first child after age thirty or who have no children at all

e. Have previously had cancer of the colon, or endometrium

Some women have a *lower* statistical risk of developing breast cancer. These include women who:

a. Have a pregnancy before age eighteen, and have many pregnancies

b. Have late menarche and early menopause

c. Breast-fed several children over long periods of time (not such an important factor as was once thought)

d. Have their ovaries removed at a young age (not to be encouraged as a prophylactic method) (Refs. 13, 14, 15, 16)

138. What causes breast cancer?

The causes of breast cancer have not yet been established. Experimental work has been done in animals to test several theories of causation centred on

a. Viruses

b. Oestrogen (and other sex hormones)

c. Immunological breakdown

d. Excess radiation to the chest

e. Other factors such as prolactin levels, diet and environmental pollution.

139. Environmental pollution

The pollutants in the air, water and food supply are largely industrial wastes, the products of our advanced society. However, economic and industrial progress might be being made at the cost of human health. Some researchers now believe that perhaps 75 per cent of human cancers are caused by environmental factors, and breast cancer could be included here.

140. The viral theory of cancer causation

Certain viruses cause breast cancer in mice. Particles very similar to these viruses have been found in the breast milk and breast tumours of women. An enzyme has been isolated—reverse transcriptase—from human breast cancers which is known to occur only in viruses that cause cancer. (Refs. 17, 18)

In addition, some women with breast cancer have an antigen in their blood which causes the body to develop antibodies which in turn react *against* tumour tissue. This is the way the body normally reacts against a virus. The antigen seems to be identical in all breast cancers; sometimes blood serum from women who have the antigen and the antibodies it triggers can be given to women who aren't having the antigen-antibody reaction to help them fight their own cancers. This work is still highly experimental but very exciting. (Refs. 19, 20)

141. Oestrogen as a carcinogen and as a promoter substance for cancer

During the last fifteen years, because of birth control pills containing oestrogens, oestrogen-replacement therapy during menopause, and the addition of DES—diethylstilboestrol—into feed for fattening livestock, women have been receiving more than their normal share of oestrogen. Thus, the possible links of oestrogen with cancer—both as an initiating carcinogen and as a promoter substance—have caused great and continuing controversy.

WARNING: *There is strong evidence that DES is a carcinogen.* (See No. 194 below)

It is associated with a tumour of the vagina which is virtually unknown except in the daughters of women who received DES during early pregnancy. The DES causes some changes in the cells of the vagina and cervix, so that after puberty, when hormones appear in large quantities, the cancer appears. In this case, oestrogen may act as carcinogen *and* promoter. (Refs. 21, 22) Mothers who took DES may have a higher risk of breast cancer, although this data is debatable. (See No. 195 below)

Continuous oestrogen replacement in menopause and the high-oestrogen sequential birth control pills have been associated with endometrial cancer, and neither is recommended now. (Refs. 23, 24, 25. Also see p. 278)

Some "purists" will say that this is not enough to prove that oestrogenic compounds are carcinogenic. *However, this is one case where guilt by association is grounds for condemnation.* Oestrogens have caused cancers in test animals; the DES daughters are the tragic guinea pigs in an inadvertent "test" on people. That should be proof enough that low-oestrogen birth control pills should be used instead of high-oestrogen compounds; and that livestock should be fattened with something other than DES.

No matter what doubts many have about this theory of carcinogenesis, there is no doubt that oestrogen is a promoter substance for breast cancer. In test animals, cancers initiated by viruses are promoted to maturity by oestrogen. While studies show birth control pills *decrease* the incidence of benign breast disease, they may *increase* the speed with which pre-existing tumours grow. (Refs. 26, 27, 28) This is a hotly debated issue at present. Watch for further studies.

Obviously then, anyone who is at high risk for breast cancer (see No. 137 above) should not take oestrogen! Everyone else should proceed with utmost caution, always using combined oestrogen-progestogen therapy if it is absolutely necessary. (See p. 279)

142. The role of progesterone in cancer is debatable

In mice and dogs, progestogens (artificial progesterone compounds) can serve as promoters of breast tumours. However, in humans, evidence suggests that progesterone may have a protective effect and progestogens are currently being tried as treatment for breast and genital cancer.

143. The role of prolactin in causing or promoting breast cancer

Prolactin is the hormone which triggers lactation at the end of a pregnancy, allowing a woman to breast-feed her baby. (See p. 154) At all other times, it is blocked by the prolactin-inhibiting factor produced in the hypothalamus, responding to high levels of oestrogen and progesterone in pregnancy and during the normal menstrual cycle.

Sometimes the prolactin-inhibiting factor is stopped, and

prolactin released when it shouldn't be. High prolactin levels have been found in women who have breast cancer and many people believe prolactin works with oestrogen in causing breast cancer. But the association does not prove that high prolactin levels cause cancer. For example, a high prolactin level is produced by phenothiazines (tranquillizers such as Largactil used in high doses for mental disorders), but no higher rate of breast cancer has been found in women on long-term treatment.

Drugs which elevate prolactin levels include

a. *Phenothiazines* (feen-o-THIGH-a-zeens), a group of tranquillizers

b. *Tricyclic antidepressant drugs* (Aventyl, Norpramine, Pertofran, Tofranil, Sinequan and others)

c. *Methyldopa*, also prescribed for hypertension.

If you take these drugs, have yourself examined periodically for breast cancer and watch for further reports of the effects of these drugs.

Do not stop these drugs out of fear for cancer! If they do increase the risk, then this is only one of many factors involved in the disease (see No. 137 above). It is much more important to keep your hypertension under control, for example, than to avoid the slight possibility of increased breast cancer risk.

144. Immunological breakdown and the spread of cancer

One theory proposes that cancer is most common in childhood and in old age, when the immune system is not well developed or is deteriorating and cannot fight off invading cancer cells. That is why, it is believed, breast cancer occurs more frequently in older and post menopausal women. The strong, healthy body does not necessarily give in to the onslaught of cancer: for example an intense inflammatory reaction around a tumour means that the body's immune system is fighting it; the prognosis in these cases may be better, for the tumour so resisted may be less likely to metastasize (me-TASS-ta-size)—to spread. In addition, women who have the antigen/antibody reaction in their blood have good prospects for a cure. (See No. 140 above)

145. Excess radiation to the chest causes breast cancer

Women who were exposed to radiation in Japan during World War II, and women who have received multiple doses of radiation during treatment of tuberculosis have higher incidence of breast cancer. (Radiation therapy of various benign diseases such as acne is to be condemned.) This is the reason that the use of mammography for routine screening of all women (see No. 150) needs further research. The risk may be greater than the benefit in young women. (Refs. 29, 30)

146. The earlier breast cancer is detected, the better chance for a cure

If all breast tumours could be detected before they were one centimetre in diameter, the cure rate would be 80–90 per cent.

Like other cancers, breast cancer has a premalignant stage, a carcinoma-in-situ stage and an invasive stage. The earlier you find it, the better your chance of a cure *without* a radical mastectomy and the better your chance that mastectomy will not be followed by a recurrence.

An excellent series of articles on screening, treatment, management and chemotherapy for breast cancer can be found in the *British Journal of Hospital Medicine,* Vol. 23, No. 1, January 1980.

147. How breast cancer is detected

There are five major ways in which breast cancer is detected. No method is 100 per cent foolproof

    a. Self-examination;
    b. Examination by a doctor or nurse;
    c. Low-dose mammography;
    d. Thermography;
    e. Newer experimental methods.

148. Self-examination

Women should learn to examine their breasts as soon as they have passed puberty. Do the examination every month on the last day of menstrual bleeding or immediately after the menstrual period ends. This timing will eliminate some of the unnecessary alarm that women feel when they examine their breasts during the week before menstruation, when swelling, tenderness, and prominence of the glandular tissue of the breasts are quite normal. (After menopause any time will do.)

First. Look at your breasts in the mirror. Look for symmetry. Look to see if either breast has any bumps protruding or if there is any tightening of the skin, as though over a swelling or any puckering. If you press your hands on your hips, you will accentuate your breasts and be better able to observe them. Bend forward and look again.

Second. Still looking into the mirror, raise your hands over your head and watch to make sure that the nipples move upward with the rest of the breast. If either nipple seems stuck, if it doesn't move upward, and this is a change, see a doctor right away.

Third. Lie down on a firm surface. With your left hand, feel all areas of your right breast; keep your right arm behind your head. With the fingers flat, move round the breast, pressing the tissue against the chest wall. Then switch sides. Put your left hand behind your head, examine your left breast with your right hand. Remember to gently squeeze both nipples to see if there is any discharge. A small amount of crusty discharge is normal. A bloody discharge is not, nor is a heavy discharge that seems continuous, not drying.

What you are feeling for and looking for is any swelling, or lump or any change in the texture under the skin of the breast. Breast tumours start out very small—the lump might feel like a pea or a marble under the skin, perhaps like a group of tiny pebbles. Remember, you are looking for something *under the skin:* an eruption, a pimple or sore perhaps from the chafing of a bra is almost surely not cancer. Compare the same areas in each breast. In addition, try not to confuse the ribs, and the overlying muscles with a lump in the breast, or—and this is harder to differentiate— the breast glands that normally swell depending on what stage of the menstrual cycle you are in. *When in doubt, see a doctor.* It may be embarrassing to be told that the lump you thought you felt was really a rib—but it's also comforting.

A leaflet illustrating the technique of breast self-examination is available from the Health Education Council and can probably also be found at your local family planning clinic or at your local GP's surgery.

149. Examination by a physician

When you have your annual or six-monthly gynaecological examination, make sure your doctor includes an examination of the breasts.

The doctor will feel the breasts with both hands, prodding, pushing, to make sure that no lump or thickening is present. You must undress for this procedure. *Examination through the clothes or inside the bra is inadequate.*

No woman should depend entirely on examination by a doctor in guarding herself against breast cancer. *You must do self-examination every month!*

150. Low-dose mammography

Mammography is a kind of breast X-ray which is currently the most effective method of detecting incipient tumours *before they are large,* at a stage when they can be completely cured with surgery or other therapy.

The trouble is, X-ray itself is a known carcinogen. If straightforward breast X-ray of women on a regular basis had been used, it could have caused more cancer than it prevented. Low-dose mammography, so called because the radiation exposure is much less, could be a useful new development and is currently being tested in Britain to see how effectively it can be used in screening women.

151. Who should have routine mammography?

Some women run a relatively high risk of breast cancer and regular low-dose mammography may be useful for them. They are women

a. Over fifty;

b. Aged forty to forty-nine, with strong history of breast cancer in the family, or history of cancer in one breast;

c. Over thirty-five years old with a history of cancer in one breast.

Reports should be appearing in the next few years on the pros and cons of low-dose mammography, so *watch for them.*

In the meantime, younger women with an increased risk of breast cancer (See No. 137 above) should examine themselves routinely and have a doctor check them every four to six months.

152. Opinion: Thermography is not as reliable as mammography

Thermography tests for hot spots on the breast with the idea that they may indicate incipient cancer. The great advantage of this method is that it is apparently without side effects. The disadvantage is that the method produces false results in many cases. At the present time it cannot be relied upon as the sole screening method for women in the high-risk group. (See Nos. 137 and 151 above) It is now more or less discredited in Britain.

Some experimental methods of screening currently being tested include ultrasound, computerized tomography (CT scans) and other heat methods. *Watch for news!*

153. Benign breast lumps that disappear sometimes occur in young women

Malignant tumours of the breast are very rare in women under 25. Sometimes, as the breasts develop, lumps will appear that are no danger at all. These should be observed by a doctor over time. Only if they don't go away is further treatment in order.

154. Pain is not usually a symptom of cancer

Generally, cancer is not accompanied by pain until it is far advanced. Pain is, however, a frequent sign of fibrocystic disease of the breast, as is premenstrual tenderness. (See No. 156 below)

155. Nipple discharge is a possible symptom of cancer

A small amount of crusty discharge from the nipple is normal. Only if it is continuous or heavy and *doesn't dry* is there something to worry about.

A watery or milky discharge sometimes results from vigorous manipulation of the breasts during sexual relations. Some tranquillizers, by their effect on the hypothalamus, can cause milky nipple discharge. Similar discharge can occur when there is some malfunction of the hypothalamus after childbirth or after stopping the pill. (See p. 51) If the discharge persists or is heavy, consult a doctor. The problem is not cancer in some cases, but a hormone specialist will probably be needed.

If the nipple discharge is bloody, brownish or green, and occurs in one breast only, this may be an important sign of malignancy. In this case, or any case which disturbs you, a smear of the discharge can be sent for a smear to detect any malignant cells. In addition, mammography can be done if there is no palpable mass and the woman is over age thirty-five.

156. Fibrocystic disease of the breast

Fibrocystic disease of the breast usually occurs in women over twenty-five and probably results from a hormonal imbalance that can be triggered by a vast range of causes. It is believed that the imbalance allows oestrogen to predominate in the body and stimulate the growth of the glands and fibrous tissue of the breast, creating a number of small lumps and distentions, usually in the outer areas of the breast. Some women will experience the growth of cysts that seem to come and go; some will experience growths in the fibrous tissues.

The major symptom is both the visible swelling *and pain* (a pretty good indication that the condition is *not* cancer). Padded bras with very good support are essential treatment. If the cysts grow large, aspiration (see No. 159 below) may be a good treatment. Usually, fibrocystic disease comes in spurts and goes away. It is not dangerous in itself, but a woman who suffers from it is considered a higher than average risk for breast cancer and should have herself checked routinely. In severe cases, Danol (see p. 322) has been shown to have good results. (Ref. 31) An interesting recent report shows that cutting down on foods containing xanthines (coffee, tea, colas, chocolate) can reverse or reduce cystic disease. (Refs. 32, 33) Try this method, coupled with examinations by your doctor. The anti-prostaglandin drugs may help too. (See p. 313)

157. Fibroadenomas: benign tumours of the breast

These are the most common tumours in young women. Characteristically they are firm, round and movable, and feel like a marble under the skin of the breast. These can usually be removed simply under local anaesthesia.

158. Breast abscess

Some masses in the breast and discharges from the nipple occur because of infections in the glands and ducts of the breast. These are common after childbirth or during breast-feeding. They can be treated with antibiotics but occasionally have to be drained surgically.

159. What happens if a breast lump is detected?

If a breast lump is detected, or suspected, see a doctor *immediately.* Don't wait to see if the lump will go away; don't try not to think about it; have it checked. *Fewer than one-fifth of the breast lumps discovered by self-examination are cancerous.* A number of benign breast diseases can produce suspicious symptoms that are not cancer. *In 80 per cent of all cases,* lumps detected by any means will turn out to be benign.

The doctor may attempt to aspirate the lump with a syringe in the surgery. If there is any fluid in it, that will be drawn off and usually sent for a smear. Fluid generally indicates that the lump is a benign cyst. However, it is important that a woman who has had a cyst aspirated returns for a check-up within a few weeks. *If the cyst reappears, it must be biopsied,* i.e., removed for pathological examination (see No. 160).

Sometimes the lump is not a cyst but just a benign mass that has grown in the breast. It can be removed in hospital under local or general anaesthesia.

160. A biopsy is necessary to prove malignancy

The lump or part of the lump should be removed and sent to the pathologist to determine the exact nature of the problem. It is standard procedure in some hospitals to have a woman sign a consent form to do a biopsy, send the specimen for frozen section, and on the basis of the preliminary report, allow the surgeon to proceed with further surgery if cancer is reported. *This should be avoided.* Waiting for the permanent sections of tissue gives a better guarantee that there will be no error in the biopsy reading. A second opinion on the pathology slides may be requested by the woman and the slides may be posted or hand-delivered to a pathologist at a specialist cancer centre or university hospital. *Of great importance, this small delay gives a woman the chance to know what may be about to happen to her.* She can discuss with her doctor which surgery and combined therapy are best for her. She knows what to expect and has some chance to adjust, or if she has objection to surgery, she can stop it.

161. Outpatient biopsy
Some surgeons now perform biopsies on an outpatient basis. The woman waits a few days for preparation and reading of the permanent slides. This delay does not alter long-term survival or complication rate. (Ref. 34)

Procedures for biopsy include:

a. *Needle or drill biopsy*: most reliable for large and/or superficial lesions, but unreliable for small and deep lesions. These methods have the advantage of not leaving a scar.

b. Deep or small lesions picked up on mammography usually require *open biopsy under general anaesthesia.* Performing this procedure under general anaesthesia prevents patient discomfort and also better enables the surgeon to remove the lesion completely, control bleeding, and restore the shape of the breast. However, admission to the hospital is not always needed.

162. Treatment of breast cancer
The treatment of breast cancer must be aimed first at removing the local disease (the cancer in the breast and in the nearby lymph nodes) and secondly, at eradicating the cancer from the rest of the body if there is indication that it has spread. Surgery and radiation therapy are the two options for treating the local disease. Chemotherapy, hormonal therapy, immunotherapy, and radiation therapy are the methods of treating advanced disease.

163. Surgery for breast cancer—mastectomy
Mastectomy is surgical removal of the breast. A "partial" mastectomy removes part of the breast tissue; a "total" mastectomy removes all of the breast; a "radical" mastectomy removes the breast, lymph nodes, and chest muscles; a "modified radical" mastectomy leaves the muscles.

Until about ten years ago, *radical mastectomy* was the only kind. At the time, the operation created wonderful improvement in the survival statistics for women with breast cancer. About forty years ago, the death rate for breast cancer began levelling off—at 25 per 100,000 women per year. Twenty years ago, researchers began looking at those statistics and wondering why there had been no further improvement. Perhaps the radical procedure was not necessary for everybody; perhaps greater selectivity was in order. Some physicians began performing *total mastectomy*, in which the chest muscles were left intact and the lymph nodes removed only in cases of large tumours. *The mortality rates have remained about the same.* Today, we are at the point with another twenty years of hindsight, where a variety of treatments other than radical mastectomy are being used for breast cancer, with greater and greater demand from patients and doctors that individuals be treated with different therapies suitable for *them*.

Many experts now believe that the modified radical mastectomy is the treatment of choice for all breast cancers which are large (over 5 centimetres in diameter). This is also one of the options in the treatment of early breast cancer.

164. Normal care after mastectomy

The usual hospital stay after a total or modified radical mastectomy is seven to ten days. A woman can expect pain in the incisional area and under the arm if the lymph nodes have been removed, but this is not severe and is readily controlled. Small tubes are left beneath the skin and connected to a suction pump to drain blood and tissue fluid and help the skin adhere to the chest wall. They are removed within a few days.

Within the first five days, begin exercises to maintain the full range of motion in the shoulder and arm on the side where the surgery took place. This means that an already hurting area will hurt more—but it is absolutely imperative that the exercises be done. Not to do them is to risk having a frozen shoulder. (See No. 165d below) Most of the exercises involve just lifting the arm from the shoulder, strengthening the grip, reaching a little higher every day as recovery progresses.

After radical mastectomy, a woman may feel numb on the side of her chest which has been operated on or may find that the area is very sensitive to touch for up to a year afterwards. Avoid this sensitive area during intercourse. Find a position that is comfortable for you and your partner without placing weight against the chest.

165. Possible after-effects of mastectomy

a. *Lymphoedema (swelling of the arm)* is the most common long-term post-operative complication after radical or modified radical mastectomy—occurring in about one case in three. It can occur immediately, or years later, because of the blockage in the small lymph vessels that ordinarily drain from the arm into the lymph nodes of the armpit. Women who have had post-operative infections or who receive radiation treatment to the under-arm area are more likely to experience this complication.

Some methods of controlling lymphoedema are

1. Diuretics (medicines that cut down the amount of water the body retains),

2. Low-salt diets which do likewise, and

3. Elastic sleeves. Physical-therapy machines are available which massage the arm, starting at the hand and gradually pushing all the accumulated fluid toward the shoulder. This treatment may have to be repeated frequently; an elastic sleeve is a must in conjunction with a physical therapy machine. They are provided by the NHS where they are needed.

Exercise of the arm and shoulder is the very best way to prevent lymphoedema and to keep it under control after it occurs.

b. *Frozen shoulder, with pain whenever it is moved,* can be a problem if post-operative exercises are neglected. Heat treatments can help; some doctors suggest steroid injections into the shoulder joints, as though treating arthritis. Again, the best way to avoid this unnecessary complication is to do the suggested post-operative exercises, no matter how much they hurt at the time.

166. Emotional after-effects of mastectomy

Most women suffer depression and anxiety after this operation, partly because they have been sick with cancer and fear its recurrence, mostly because they feel mutilated, and anticipate rejection by friends and lovers. Some people say that every woman who undergoes mastectomy needs psychotherapy. That may be extreme; psychotherapy is best kept for counselling *abnormal* emotional responses. Crying and depression after mastectomy is, if it is any comfort, a normal response. Seek help first from the Mastectomy Association (1 Colworth Road, Croydon, Surrey; 01-654 8463). They will come and see you in the hospital, or at home; they've been through it too. Just meeting a woman who has recovered, who knows what the bad time is like, how important the exercises are, will be a source of strength for you.

Sexual partners adjust to mastectomy far more easily than many women expect them to. Discuss your feelings openly with both the men and the women in your life. Resume sexual activity as soon as possible. (Medically, sex is fine as soon as you come home from the hospital.) A woman may find it more difficult to adjust if she does not have a loving relationship in her life, but *talk* to the people around you—*don't retreat* —you need them now, and they will rise to the occasion. (Ref. 35)

And remember: the most important thing about the thousands of women who have had mastectomies in this country is not that they have come through harrowing and serious surgery but that they have, for the most part, stopped their cancer spreading.

167. Prostheses—artificial breasts—after mastectomy

a. An exterior silicone prosthesis can be fitted and matched to the other breast before the woman leaves the hospital. It looks fine when you are dressed. It is not a good idea to wear it with your bra when you are making love—because of the possible discomfort and also because your partner needs to make his or her own adjustment to your surgery.

b. Reconstruction of the breast through plastic surgery, right after mastectomy or later on, is a growing medical practice, and women should encourage research into its possibilities.

If the cancerous lesion has been small, and a total or modified radical mastectomy was performed, some surgeons now leave more skin than usual so that a silicone prosthesis can be placed under it. Initial reports show that when this is done in cases of cancer detected early, there is no additional risk of recurrence. (Ref. 36) But because recurrent growth can invade the implant it is not normally put in until three years after the mastectomy

Check on the possibility of such an implant *before* you have your surgery—especially if you are not having a radical mastectomy. (The possibility of prosthesis implanting is all the more reason to wake up between the biopsy and the surgery.) (See No. 160 above)

Many people believe that the worst psychological effect of mastectomy could be stopped if a fairly normal-looking prosthesis could be placed under the skin. (Ref. 37) This is one area of medical development in which women should be vitally concerned.

168. Radiation therapy for early breast cancer

Recent studies have shown that the survival rates for women with *early* breast cancer treated by high doses of radiation are the same as those treated with mastectomy. This is not appropriate therapy for far-advanced cancers. The radiation is given by radiotherapy machines and by implants with small needles containing radioactive material. The needles are left in the breast for a short period of time to allow a concentrated dose of radiation to be delivered to the area surrounding the tumour without burning the skin. (The bulk of the tumour must be removed by partial mastectomy before radiation.)

The advantages of radiation therapy are mainly in the great improvement in cosmetic result. A good radiotherapist can treat the tumour and leave very little or no change in the appearance of the breast afterwards. The crucial issue is to find a *good radiotherapist*. This is a relatively new mode of treatment, so not many doctors have great expertise. The ones available are usually at teaching hospitals which usually house the regional cancer centres where these exist.

169. The concept of hormonal dependence of tumours and its use in treatment of breast cancer

Approximately 40–60 per cent of breast cancers which occur in premenopausal women are dependent upon oestrogen for growth. This is known by the fact that the removal of the ovaries, which was previously routine in premenopausal women with breast cancer, caused regression of the tumour in 40–60 per cent of the women. If the tumours did not respond to removal of the ovaries, then removal of the adrenal glands and sometimes of the pituitary gland was helpful in some women.

It is now possible to predict which tumours will respond to the removal of these other endocrine glands. This is done by the analysis of the tumours for the presence of receptor proteins. If the breast tumour contains the receptor proteins for oestrogen, progesterone, or androgen, it means that the tumour probably needs that particular hormone for growth. Women who do not have these receptor proteins are found to have little chance of benefit from further surgery, so they are spared the unnecessary removal of the organs.

Most tumours in postmenopausal women are found not to contain oestrogen receptors, but some contain androgen receptors and respond well to the removal of the adrenal, glands the major source of androgen.

The converse use of receptor protein information is that, if the receptor proteins are absent, the tumour may respond well to administration of that hormone as a therapy. Make sure this test is done when you receive treatment for breast cancer.

170. Chemotherapy

Chemotherapy involves the administration of powerful anti-tumour drugs to women in whom there is indication that the tumour has spread from the breast to other parts of the body. In the initial treatment of breast cancer, women should have at least some of the lymph nodes removed from under the arm. (This is usually done at the time of the original biopsy if there is a high suspicion of cancer.) If tumour is found in the lymph nodes (some experts say in 4 or more nodes) then chemotherapy is recommended in addition to the surgery or radiation. This is especially important therapy in premenopausal women. If no tumour is found in the nodes, then usually no chemotherapy is given.

If, at a later time, the tumour recurs, then chemotherapy and sometimes radiation are used to treat the patient.

The best results are likely to be obtained in hospitals dealing with a large number of cancer cases, which is why some women may be referred out of their district.

171. Immunotherapy

WATCH FOR FURTHER NEWS: Some researchers working with the *immunological response theory* (see No. 144 above) are experimenting with ways to transfer immunity from women who have developed high levels of antibody to tumours to women who have not. The goal is to eliminate the tumour cells from the blood stream of the second woman. Other similar projects involve attempts to determine ways in which to stimulate a woman's own immune system to react more violently against the tumour cells. (Ref. 20) Substances such as BCG (a vaccine against tuberculosis) are being used as stimulants to the entire immune system, hopefully to filter out the abnormal cells that are present. These treatments have been used in conjunction with chemotherapy, but have not proved very useful to date.

Interferon is a protein substance which appears naturally in the blood of a person with a viral infection. It is very expensive to produce. Early studies have shown optimistic results in treating several cancers, including breast cancer.

172. When do you know the cancer will not return?

It is certainly wise for women who have had a tumour removed from one breast to suspect that cancer might recur in the other breast, and to follow to the letter her instructions for post-operative care, to check herself frequently, and to have low-dose mammography (see No. 151 above) once a year.

Some cases recur as late as ten to fifteen years, but most doctors estimate that after five years, a woman has a good chance of non-recurrence.

178. Breast abscess
Some masses in the breast and discharges from the nipple occur because of infections in the glands and ducts of the breast. These are common after childbirth or during breast-feeding. They can be treated with antibiotics but occasionally have to be drained surgically.

CERVICAL CANCER AND OTHER TUMOURS OF THE REPRODUCTIVE TRACT

Cancer of the cervix is unique in that an easy smear test (see No. 177 below) makes early detection sure and simple, allowing complete cure in over 90 per cent of cases.

Other tumours and cysts, both cancerous and non-cancerous, are common in the reproductive tract: almost all are curable through drugs and/or surgery. In general, the two major ways that a woman can guard herself against these diseases is to have regular examinations with a smear, and to be alerted by any change in her normal menstrual cycle.

174. Cervical cancer
Approximately 4,000 new cases of cervical cancer are detected and about 2,000 women die of the disease each year in England and Wales, almost always because they did not have the routine examinations that could have led to early detection and treatment.

175. Cervical cancer is related to sexual activity
Cervical cancer almost never occurs in sexually *inactive* women.
It seems to occur more frequently in women who
a. Started sexual activity at an early age;
b. Had an early first pregnancy;
c. Have multiple sexual partners.
Only 10 per cent of the women who contract the disease have never been pregnant. Jewish women show lower rates of cervical cancer than women from other cultural backgrounds. At one time, this was attributed to the fact that Jewish men were always circumcised. It is still thought it may be linked to levels of sexual hygiene.

176. Herpes II virus may cause cervical cancer

The herpes II virus (see No. 25 above) is now widely held to be a factor in developing cervical cancer. The exact cause and effect is not clear, except that women with positive blood tests for herpes II show a higher incidence of cervical cancer. (Ref. 4) A woman who has had herpes is by no means a sure victim of cervical cancer; any more than a woman who has had a cystic mastitis will surely get breast cancer.

177. Smear tests to detect cervical cancer early

Tiny scrapings are taken with a speculum from the external part of the woman's cervix, as high up in the canal as possible. (This causes a small cramp at most and is usually completely painless.) Then the cervical cells are analysed in a laboratory, if cancer is present, the cell changes on the slide will show it. The test detects cancer in its earliest and most frequently curable stage. Cytologists suggest that two tests should be done in one year if a woman has not had regular smears taken. After that, they should be done every five years up to age 35 and every two or three years after that. More frequent screening is preferable, but at present the NHS cannot afford it.

ACTION: See how well your community is provided with this service and use your community health council to press for improvements.

If abnormalities have been noted in the past, the test should be performed more frequently. The test is not 100 per cent accurate, with a small number of false negatives and positives. (Smears can also be done on cells from the breasts, lungs, and other organs to look for malignancy.)

178. Where to obtain a smear test

Women attending family planning clinics will automatically be offered smear tests at regular intervals. Or you can ask your general practitioner to do one for you. There is also a screening programme with built-in recall for women over 35 and younger women who have had three or more pregnancies. Free smear tests are also available at local well woman clinics and in the mobile units run by the Women's National Cancer Control Campaign.

179. The several stages of cervical cancer

The disease passes through several stages before it becomes invasive and begins to metastasize. In the earlier stages, there are no symptoms at all. The smear test is used to detect the disease prior to invasive cancer and can be supplemented by colposcopy. (See No. 183 below)

a. The earliest stage is *dysplasia* (dis-PLAYS-ya). The most superficial cells have begun to change and are mildly abnormal. Some women with dysplasia will develop more severe changes, others will return to normal. No one can predict who will fall into which group, *so all cases of dysplasia are treated or watched closely with repeat smears.*

b. The second stage is called *carcinoma-in-situ:* a cancer is present, but limited to the outside layers of the cervix. (This is the latent stage, see No. 136 above) This stage is not reversible, but is completely curable. Treatment is cone biopsy in a young woman (see No. 181 below) or hysterectomy in a woman whose family is complete.

c. The third stage of cervical cancer is called *invasive*. The disease has spread beyond the outer layers of the cervix and later invaded the pelvis. Treatment is either radiation and/or surgery, depending on the extent of the tumour.

180. Steps after an abnormal smear

The first thing to do after a smear test shows abnormal cells is to repeat it, just to make sure the laboratory has not made an error. Lab results are classified as follows:

A class 1 result—test is normal; no cancer.

A class 2 result—test indicates either infection of the cervix or mild dysplasia. Most of these cases will revert back to normal so a repeat smear is done. If the class 2 reading persists, then colposcopy is frequently done to localize and remove the abnormal areas.

A class 3 smear signifies moderate to severe dysplasia.

Class 4 and 5 smears indicate carcinoma-in-situ, or invasive cancer.

Women with class 3 tests or worse *must* have colposcopy (see No. 183) or cervical biopsy.

181. Cone biopsy of the cervix

In order to determine the full extent of the abnormality, a cone-shaped wedge of tissue is removed from the cervix and sent to the lab to be examined by the pathologist. This will be final proof that invasive cancer is not present. The biopsy is done in the hospital under anaesthesia.

Cone biopsy of the cervix is a relatively safe procedure, but has a degree of complications, such as bleeding, stenosis (narrowing) of the cervix, infertility and incompetent cervix (see p. 163). RECOM-MENDATION: *Colposcopy is preferable* for diagnosis. Cone biopsy should be reserved for proven carcinoma-in-situ.

182. Other types of cervical biopsy

More limited biopsies can be taken using Lugol's iodine to stain the cervix and show up the abnormal skin and then using a special instrument like a paper puncher to punch out the abnormal cells. These are called punch biopsies and do not affect the internal cervical opening and future reproductive capacity. The surgeon can also take a ring of tissue from the squamo-columnar junction of the cervix, which is where the two types of cells which make up the cervix join. This is where abnormal cells usually start.

183. Colposcopy: a new method of diagnosis and biopsy for cervical cancer

Colposcopy was developed on the Continent fifty years ago. Doctors in Britain and the USA are now becoming skilled in it. The cervix is cleansed and observed directly through a microscope. Any abnormal areas are biopsied and sent for pathological report. In 75 per cent of the cases, colposcopy bypasses the need for hospital admission and cone biopsy. However, if the entire suspicious area of the cervix is not visualized, a biopsy will be recommended. Make sure you have a skilled colposcopist. If you doubt his or her technique, get a second opinion before having surgery.

184. Steps to be taken if dysplasia is noted on biopsy

If dysplasia is noted on the smear and colposcopy is adequate for evaluation and treatment, then follow-up smears should be taken every three months for the first year and every six months thereafter. Some doctors are treating dysplasia with cryosurgery (see p. 297) that freeze-cauterizes the lining of the cervix and allows removal of affected tissues. Women who undergo this procedure should have themselves checked thereafter to make sure that dysplasia does not recur.

WARNING: *Cryosurgery to treat dysplasia must always be perfor-med by a specialist in cancer therapy who will use the colposcope to identify the correct area. It is a risky procedure if used improperly to treat more advanced stages than dysplasia.* Even in the treatment of dysplasia by cryosurgery, long-term studies are not yet available to show whether this is a safe treatment.

In cases of severe dysplasia, where carcinoma-in-situ seems a

351

very likely next stage, hysterectomy may be suggested. This removes the risk of cervical cancer entirely, but it is a major abdominal operation that involves risks of its own. Think it over carefully, and seek an additional opinion.

Diathermy cauterization has also been used for treatment of dysplasia, but follow-up is mandatory because the tissue treated is destroyed (as in cryocautery) and therefore histological evidence that the area of abnormal cells has been destroyed is lacking. Regular smears must be done annually or more frequently if advised by the cytologist.

185. What to do if carcinoma-in-situ is discovered

If the disease has progressed to the stage of carcinoma-in-situ, have a cone biopsy to rule out invasive cancer. If all the tumour seems to have been removed, and if the woman desires more children, she can go ahead and have them *if she is very closely watched by her doctors.*

If she has completed her family, hysterectomy is usually suggested. However, if a woman wants to avoid hysterectomy and the doctor thinks that all the tumour was removed with cone biopsy, then it is quite safe to have frequent smear tests (every three months). If the carcinoma-in-situ returns, the woman should proceed with hysterectomy.

Some doctors are using therapy with laser beams in the treatment of carcinoma-in-situ. Again this is an experimental method with no long-term studies available.

186. Opinion: Simple hysterectomy is recommended treatment for cervical cancer in-situ if hysterectomy is needed at all

Simple hysterectomy (see No. 103 above), vaginal or abdominal, is the proper treatment for cervical in-situ cancer. *The ovaries need not be removed.* Afterwards, a woman will still experience normal hormone cycles, with all that these mean to general well-being. Smear tests are a vital part of postoperative care, for a small number of women who will also develop carcinoma-in-situ of the upper vagina, also detectable by the smear.

187. Steps to be taken if invasive cancer is discovered

A woman with invasive cancer should be referred to a hospital with special experience of treating the disease. Treatment usually involves radiation and/or surgery. Chemotherapy is not as well developed as radiotherapy and surgery. Women should remember that even at this more advanced stage, cervical cancer can be controlled sometimes for years and in many cases, cured completely.

188. Cancer of the body of the uterus or endometrial carcinoma
Cancer of the endometrium, the lining of the uterus, accounts for 3,500 new cases and 1,500 deaths yearly. It occurs mostly in postmenopausal women and is more common in women who have never been pregnant. This cancer seems to be associated with

a. excess oestrogen production, for instance in women who are not ovulating regularly, and with

b. general metabolic and endocrine imbalance, as in diabetes, hypertension and obesity. Women who do not ovulate for long periods of time, should receive progestogen for several days every three to six months, to prevent the constant effect of oestrogen on the endometrium.

Recently, a possible increase of this type of cancer has been reported in women who have been receiving solely oestrogen during menopause (Refs. 24, 25). Women using oestrogen for menopausal symptoms should also take progestogen periodically to counter the effects of oestrogen on the endometrium. (See p. 283)

189. Bleeding is a major symptom of endometrial cancer
In the earliest stages of this tumour, a woman will frequently experience heavy menstrual bleeding, bleeding between periods, or bleeding after menopause. In this phase, it is impossible to determine whether cancer, polyps or just hormonal imbalance causes the bleeding, so a D & C should be performed for diagnosis.

190. Stages of endometrial cancer and the treatment for each
a. The earliest stage is *hyperplasia*. In young women, in women who have been taking oestrogen, or in women who are not good risks for surgery, high doses of progestogens may be used for three to six months in an effort to reverse the hyperplasia. Oestrogens should be stopped. After this time, have a repeat D & C to make sure that the hyperplasia has disappeared, followed by yearly endometrial biopsies or washings (see No. 191 below). If the hyperplasia is severe or does not respond to progesterone therapy, a total hysterectomy is the usual treatment.

b. The next stage is carcinoma-in-situ, when the tumour is in the uppermost layers of the endometrium. Treatment is hysterectomy and removal of the ovaries.

c. *If the tumour is invasive,* the woman should be treated with surgery alone or with radiation (radiotherapy) depending on the extent of the spread.

Chemotherapy with progestogens, is frequently used and tumour masses may shrink, even in advanced cases.

191. Endometrial biopsy and washing

Endometrial cancer is not always detected by the routine smear test. However, several types of mini-suction or lavaging (washing) devices can obtain cells from the lining of the uterus for pathological reading. Some doctors prefer using endometrial biopsy (mini-curettage) to obtain these samples. (see p. 101) These tests can performed in the clinic with minimal discomfort. *Certain women should have these routinely:*

a. Those in high-risk groups (See No. 188 above) starting oestrogen therapy

b. Those already on oestrogen therapy more than one year

c. Those who have had hyperplasia

d. Those with mildly irregular bleeding at menopause

192. Good news: Cure rates for cancer of the cervix and uterus are excellent

Even when the disease becomes invasive, the chances of its being controlled and reversed through surgery and/or radiation and possible chemotherapy are excellent, in the early stages, especially for endometrial cancer. No woman with either disease should feel hopeless. She should welcome the treatment and prepare to live on for a long time.

193. Ovarian cancer should be checked for after menopause

Women who are postmenopausal should continue to have routine gynaecological examinations, for at the present time this is the only way to detect early cancer of the ovary. Most tumours of the ovary are benign, not malignant, but any abnormal enlargement should be evaluated. Childless women have an especially high risk of ovarian cancer. Some families also have a high incidence.

194. Cancer of the vagina

a. *Squamous cell cancer of the vagina* is a rare tumour found mainly in older women.

b. *Clear-cell adenocarcinoma* is a cancer of the glandular tissue of the vagina that has been found in the daughters of women who took DES (diethylstilboestrol—die-ethyl-still-BES-troll) and related compounds during early pregnancy.

DIETHYLSTILBOESTROL (DES)

195. Warning: Girls whose mothers took DES in early pregnancy should be checked for vaginal cell changes

DES is an artificial oestrogen, which in the United Kingdom was given to an estimated 7,500 women early in pregnancy in an effort to prevent miscarriage. It was mainly used between 1948 and 1960, with peak use in the early 1950s.

a. In 1971, American doctors reported a startling new rise in the incidence of *clear-cell adenocarcinoma* of the vagina among girls whose mothers had received the drug. (Ref. 21) Although only a few cases have been reported in Britain it is suspected that there are several latent cases.

b. The other abnormality of the cervix and vagina occurring in DES-exposed girls is *adenosis,* a proliferation of the glandular tissue of the cervix, extending into the vagina. The adenosis does not appear to progress to the clear-cell cancer in most cases. However, all young women whose mothers were exposed to DES should have regular colposcopic checks from puberty.

c. Disturbing American reports have shown that as many as 75–85 per cent of young women with DES exposure may have abnormalities of the uterus as well. (Ref. 38) In addition, women exposed to DES in utero, appear to have a higher incidence of incompetent cervix (see p. 163) when they get pregnant. (Ref. 39) Recent studies have also shown an increased incidence of tubal pregnancy miscarriage and premature deliveries.

d. There are also worries that DES-exposed women may be at higher risk of cervical dysplasia. (Refs. 40, 41) So smear tests every six months are essential. These reports await confirmation.

196. Evaluation of women exposed to DES

Any woman who took DES or related drugs during pregnancy should make sure her daughter has at least one examination by colposcopy. (See No. 183 above) The test can usually be done at a clinic; if this is not possible, then under general anaesthesia. Biopsies of the cervix of any abnormal areas in the vagina are done at this time. A girl should be examined first at about age fourteen or whenever she starts having any vaginal bleeding or sexual activity.

If adenosis or any other abnormalities are noted to confirm the DES exposure, smears are recommended every six months. If any abnormalities are noted on the smears, then the colposcopy will be repeated. If any malignancy, or premalignant condition is detected, make sure this is treated at a cancer centre. Surgery is not the proper treatment of adenosis.

The proper way of evaluating DES daughters for abnormalities of the uterus has not been established. Within a year or so, if the reports of uterine abnormalities are corroborated, it may well be that certain women with DES exposure will be evaluated with hysterosalpingograms as well. (See p. 102)

Other American reports suggest that the mothers who took DES may be at higher risk of the development of breast cancer. (Ref. 42) These women should be very careful to do routine self-breast examinations and to have routine screening examinations. (See No. 148 above)

197. Boys may be affected by DES too

Some studies show that males exposed to DES in the uterus may have a significant increase in genital abnormalities such as cysts, small testicles, and low sperm counts. (Refs. 43, 44) They should be examined by a urologist.

ANAEMIA

Anaemia refers to a shortage of pigment (haemoglobin) which allows the cells to carry oxygen. The strength of the body depends on the reliability and quality of its blood supply, and when the blood is deficient, the body is not getting the oxygen and other nutrients it needs to function well. Because healthy women bleed every month, anaemia is always a threat; it can result from something as simple as one over-heavy menstrual flow. Sometimes anaemia is the *principal* disease process, sometimes, the secondary result of another disease or injury.

198. Blood count: the principal test for anaemia

There are two ways to perform a blood count.

a. A blood sample is taken and measured for haematocrit or packed cell volume (PVC)—the percentage of red blood cells in the total volume of blood taken. For healthy women who are not anaemic, the red blood cell count is between 36 and 50 per cent.

b. *Haemoglobin* is a protein in the red blood cells that carries oxygen. Another kind of blood test shows the haemoglobin value in the sample of blood taken—a woman is not anaemic if the haemoglobin value is over 12.0 grams per 100 millilitres (ml) of blood.

One of these tests should be part of a routine medical examination of any kind, including a gynaecological examination. Many other types of tests can be performed on blood samples, so *always ask for which tests the blood is being taken.*

199. Bone marrow: the source of red blood cells
Red blood cells are manufactured in the bone marrow. For this process to occur, many elements must be present. The bone marrow must have adequate supplies of iron and certain vitamins such as folic acid (which can be found in green leafy vegetables and liver) and Vitamin B-12. In addition, the genes which govern the formation of the protein haemoglobin must be normal.

200. General symptoms of anaemia
Symptoms characteristic of anaemia, no matter what the cause, include: fatigue, light-headedness, headaches, and, occasionally, numbness and tingling in fingers and toes. You may notice that your nail beds or palms are pale.

201. Types of anaemia relevant to women
a. Hereditary anaemias
b. Vitamin-deficiency anaemias
c. Iron-deficiency anaemia

202. Hereditary anaemias
The four most common types of hereditary anaemia found here (mainly in immigrants) are:

a. *Thalassaemia*, in which the production of the haemoglobin molecule is not totally synchronized. Parts of the molecule are underproduced, leaving an excess of other parts. This excess (alpha-chains) clutter up the red blood cells, making them abnormal and causing them to get stuck in the spleen and bone marrow as they pass through the circulation. Here the cells are destroyed, causing an enlarged spleen and other effects such as jaundice.

b. *Spherocytosis*, in which the red cells are perfectly round, a shape which makes them get stuck in the spleen. As in thalassaemia the spleen enlarges and the person becomes anaemic because of the loss of red cells;

c. *Glucose-6-phosphate-dehydrogenase deficiency (G-6-P-D deficiency)* in which an enzyme is missing from the red cells so that they are destroyed if certain drugs are taken; and

d. *Sickle-cell anaemia,* the most common hereditary anaemia in Britain today.

203. Sickle-cell anaemia, a hereditary anaemia affecting black people

A recessive gene (see p. 212) is inherited from ancestors and carried by some of their descendants. Along with the other anaemias mentioned above (No. 202), sickle-cell anaemia is a recessive-gene disease and approximately 5–10 per cent of black people carry the trait for it.

A person with sickle-cell trait has one normal and one abnormal gene for producing haemoglobin. Such a person may not be anaemic—but can pass the trait on to children. If both father and mother have sickle-cell trait, the odds are one to four that their child will have sickle-cell anaemia.

Sickle-cell *trait* is not, therefore, dangerous in itself.

In *sickle-cell anaemia,* the haemoglobin molecule in the red cells is abnormal. When enough of the haemoglobin molecules have a low-oxygen content, the red cells tend to form into a sickle shape in the blood stream. The abnormal cells get stuck in the small blood vessels, the liver, and the spleen, and break down there, causing anaemia. Unfortunately, treatment and control of this disease is limited and people with sickle-cell anaemia have a chronic debilitating disease which may cause an early death.

204. How to prevent sickle-cell anaemia

Because of the severe nature of the disease, and the current lack of good treatment methods for sickle-cell anaemia, black men and women may want to consider being tested for sickle-cell trait. A simple blood test will determine whether you carry the trait. If both partners have sickle trait, there is a one in four chance that this couple would have a child with sickle-cell anaemia.

It is sometimes possible to detect sickle-cell anaemia antenatally by placental puncture or blood sampling using fetoscopy (see p. 218) so that abortion will be an option if it is determined that the fetus is affected by the disease. These techniques carry a high risk of miscarriage (20–25 per cent) at the present time. Couples who both have sickle trait may also want to consider artificial insemination as a preventive method. (See p. 110)

205. Vitamin-deficiency anaemias

In women, these anaemias are most commonly caused by a lack of folic acid or, in older women, a lack of vitamin B-12. They are called megaloblastic anaemias (*megalo* meaning big; *blast* for cell) because on a blood smear, the cells are larger than normal.

206. Folic-acid-deficiency anaemia

Folic acid comes from green leafy vegetables and meat, especially liver.

A lot of people hate liver and some don't like salad either. If you won't eat lettuce, try to eat spinach, cabbage or broccoli. If you eat neither greens nor liver, take supplements of folic acid.

Folic-acid deficiency is quite common during pregnancy (see p. 174) when the fetus is drawing on the total supply in a woman's body. In addition, there are reports of folic-acid deficiency among women on the pill.

Certain drugs such as phenytoin used for fits cause folic-acid-deficiency anaemia if a supplement is not taken. Alcoholic women suffer from this anaemia as well.

207. Vitamin B-12 deficiency anaemia

More common in older women, this disease occurs when a substance in the stomach (intrinsic factor), which normally allows B-12 to be absorbed, runs into short supply. This is "pernicious anaemia". Other diseases such as regional ileitis may cause poor absorption of B-12 from the digestive tract. Treatment requires monthly B-12 injections; pills of B-12 are not absorbed by these women.

In very rare cases, vegetarians who eat no eggs or milk (in addition to no meat) also become deficient in B-12. These women need supplemental B-12, and for them pills are fine.

208. Remember: good nutrition can prevent and cure most vitamin-deficiency anaemias

Somehow, good nutrition often stops after childhood. This silly mistake can take a severe toll on a woman's health. *A woman must feed herself as well as she feeds anyone in her family.*

209. Iron-deficiency anaemia

This type of anaemia is the most common among women.

Bone marrow contains more than enough iron to supply a normally menstruating woman who eats properly. Menstrual flow normally carries iron out of the body, but the iron is usually replenished during the weeks of the cycle when the woman is not bleeding.

However, a number of other factors can interrupt this course of events.

a. During pregnancy, iron-deficiency anaemia is common as the fetus makes inroads into the woman's iron supply.

b. If for any reason menstrual flow is very heavy, too much iron can be lost and the manufacture of red blood cells slowed down so that anaemia results.

c. Surgery or serious injury, with accompanying severe loss of blood, can cause this anaemia.

Iron-deficiency anaemia differs from vitamin-deficiency anaemia in that the red blood cells become abnormally small instead of abnormally large.

210. Who runs a high risk of iron-deficiency anaemia?

Women with poor diets, heavy periods, pregnant women, women using IUDs, women who have had major surgery or sustained a severe injury are all at a high risk for iron-deficiency anaemia. These women should ask their doctors to check for anaemia, and, if present, iron supplements should be used.

ARTHRITIS

Arthritis refers generally to a whole group of diseases which cause painful swelling, redness, and sometimes damage to joints. Aches and pains in the joints do not signify arthritis unless there is swelling, heat, redness, or changes which show up on the X-ray of the joint. In the public mind, arthritis is more associated with age than sex. However, some forms affect women particularly.

211. Types of joint disease common in women
   a. Rheumatoid arthritis
   b. Degenerative joint disease or osteoarthritis
   c. Lupus erythematosus
   d. Tendonitis—"tennis elbow", "housemaid's knee"
   e. Infectious disease—e.g., gonorrhoea, rubella

212. Rheumatoid arthritis

Rheumatoid arthritis occurs three times more often in women than in men, more often in northern climates, and increases in incidence with age. It is thought to be passed on genetically. It is estimated that one million people in Britain have some form of this disease.

213. Rheumatoid arthritis is an autoimmune disease

In this disease as well as in other autoimmune diseases such as lupus and rheumatic fever, the body manufactures antibodies that work against its own normal functioning. The antibodies of this autoimmune disease can attack the membranes covering the joints (called synovia—sin-OH-via), the membrane covering the heart—the pericardium (perr-ih-CARD-ium)—the lungs and their coverings (pleura), and the abdominal cavity (peritoneum—per-ih-toe-NEE-um), and can cause inflammation of parts of the eyeballs.

Rheumatoid arthritis affects the joints specifically; in severe cases, it can affect the heart and/or liver and spleen. *It is an inflammation, not an infection; it cannot be cured,* but it can be controlled.

214. Course of rheumatoid arthritis

The synovia, membranes that cover and lubricate the joints so that they move easily and painlessly, become inflamed, usually in the fingers, knees, hips, spine. When the inflammation becomes severe, the cartilage, ligaments, and tendons (joint supports) around the joint also become inflamed and begin to degenerate. The course of the disease varies with the individual: it can affect one joint, it can affect many; it can be very painful for a time; then for no apparent reason, the discomfort will stop until the next attack, which likewise may occur for no apparent reason. Rheumatoid arthritis can get worse or can remain about the same for years. It all depends on the individual. Most people have the mild form of rheumatoid arthritis, where the joint supports are not involved.

215. How rheumatoid arthritis is diagnosed

Any swelling, redness, and pain in the joints should be investigated. Rheumatoid arthritis is typically indicated by swelling in the finger joints closest to the palm and by the presence in the blood of a protein called "rheumatoid factor".

216. Treatment of rheumatoid arthritis

The principle of treatment is to prevent the inflammation from spreading to the cartilage, tendons, and ligaments that support the joints, and to relieve the pain and swelling so the arthritis sufferer can live more or less comfortably with the disease.

There are several elements to treatment:

a. Aspirin and aspirin compounds and several new anti-inflammatory drugs;

b. Regular periods of rest during the day; coupled with regular activity;

c. Application of heat to the affected areas.

For severe cases, treatment may be:

d. Injections of gold salts;

e. Anti-malarial drugs;

f. Penicillamine;
g. Corticosteroids;
h. Phenylbutazone, indomethacin, and other drugs;
i. Surgery.

217. Aspirin as a treatment for rheumatoid arthritis

Aspirin is the most widely used treatment for mild rheumatoid arthritis, for it fights inflammation while dulling pain. Depending on the individual's needs, a doctor may allow a dosage of up to sixteen pills a day. (Never decide yourself how many aspirin per day is your limit; consult with a doctor, for even this most common remedy can be overindulged with bad side effects.)

The cheapest soluble aspirin is as good as any aspirin on the market. Forget advertising. The *essential* ingredients in aspirin are always the same, by law. Other ingredients may be added but these deal with other disorders besides arthritis—for example, ingredients may be added to aspirin to prevent stomach discomfort.

Rheumatoid arthritis sufferers take a lot of aspirin and may have difficulty tolerating it in such large amounts. It may produce stomach upset or at the worst, actual stomach bleeding.

Try taking the aspirin with some antacid liquid or on a full stomach. If that doesn't work, try coated aspirin, which is easier on the stomach, or an aspirin with antacid in it. Most arthritis sufferers find a way to live with large amounts of aspirin; if they don't, they must resort to stronger, combination anti-inflammatory drugs that have their own side effects. (See No. 218 below)

Other signs of aspirin overdose are ringing in the ears or temporary hearing loss. This condition reverses itself as soon as the dosage is cut back. The side effects of aspirin mean essentially that there is a limit on how much you can take. That in turn means there is a limit on how much pain you can alleviate.

Other pain-killers, such as paracetamol or codeine, may be used along with the aspirin, *but these drugs do not relieve the inflammation*, only the pain.

218. New drugs that can be used instead of aspirin

There are several new drugs which are now used widely with great success in treating arthritis. The most widely used of these is ibuprofen (Brufen). which, like aspirin, is an anti-inflammatory as well as anti-pain agent. In fact, some people find it works better than aspirin. The side effects are similar to aspirin and apparently no more severe. Another new drug with much potential is naproxen (Naprosyn). All these drugs await long-term usage data, but at present seem very useful, especially for rheumatoid arthritis and osteoarthritis. They are the anti-prostaglandin drugs, which usually work for dysmenorrhoea as well. (See No. 80 above). Another drug, Sulindac, is being widely promoted, but has no great advantages at present.

219. Periods of rest each day are essential for arthritis sufferers

The more motion, the more inflammation. If the joints get a rest, the inflammation is controlled. Rest may not be a simple matter to arrange, especially if your arthritis affects the joints you need to work with: a typist with arthritic fingers, for example, has a problem that wouldn't be so bad if she were a sales executive. In such a case, more aspirin will probably not help; you may just have to change your job.

220. Local heat as relief for arthritis

A warm bath or an infra-red lamp may ease the pain. After applying heat, try gently exercising the joint.

221. Muscle weakness. the role of physical therapy

Arthritis sufferers tend to sit still, to rest their aching joints. *Too much* rest may lead to a loss of tone in the muscles around the joints. When a woman returns to the activity she had given up because of arthritis, she may find she can't do it any more—this time because she isn't strong enough. This is why a programme of physical therapy should be set up for all arthritis sufferers. This will include range-of-motion exercises, isometrics, and heat treatments. Ask for a referral to a physiotherapist if you have moderate or severe arthritis.

222. Gold-salts injections: a treatment for severe rheumatoid arthritis

It is unclear why injections of gold salts reduce the pain and spread of severe arthritis, but they do, and if careful attention is paid to possible side effects, they may be very helpful. Before regular therapy begins, a small test dose should be given to test for possible allergy. If there is no allergy, then the shots are usually given once a week. It takes six to eight weeks, generally, to get a response. If the spread of the arthritis is stopped, then a monthly shot may suffice as maintenance. Oral gold salts are currently being tested.

Gold salts cause some *rare* side effects, including kidney damage and bone marrow damage. Therefore, have blood counts and urinalysis before each injection. Other side effects, also rare but not so dangerous, are skin rash and the appearance of small ulcers in the mouth. If any side effect appears, notify your doctor, who will probably stop the medication.

Penicillamine is a drug with similar effects and side effects as gold salts. It seems to work for some women who do not respond to gold. (Ref. 45)

223. Antimalarial drugs as a treatment for severe rheumatoid arthritis

Certain drugs commonly used to treat malaria also seem to have good anti-inflammatory effect when used against rheumatoid arthritis. These include chloroquine and hydroxychloroquine (Plaquenil). Like gold salts, they need some time to begin working: four to six weeks. Some individuals experience side effects—nausea, vomiting, and skin rashes, loss of hair colour. More serious is dimness of vision or photophobia, an abnormal sensitivity to light, or the sensation of seeing halos around lights. Women who are using these drugs to treat arthritis should have eye examinations every three to six months, so that any accumulation of the drug in the eye can be discovered, and the dosage cut down or out.

224. Corticosteroids: useful as treatment only for severe rheumatoid arthritis

The corticosteroids are a group of drugs which can be highly effective in relieving pain and stopping the spread of arthritic in-flammation through the joint supports. *However, they should only be used in very severe cases: they have dangerous known side effects.* Low-maintenance doses can usually be taken safely, but in higher doses, steroids can cause unhealthy weight gain, stomach ulcers, and bone degeneration. *A patient using steroids must be under constant observation.* Any sign of incipient side effects should be reason enough to try something else.

OPINION: In fact, unless you are being *crippled* by arthritis, this treatment is probably excessive. If your doctor prescribes corticosteroids as the first or only course of therapy, get another opinion before consenting.

225. Phenylbutazone, indomethacin, and tolmetin sodium as treatment for severe arthritis

These strong anti-inflammatory drugs should be used only in very severe cases and only for a very short time, because prolonged use can lead to rash, stomach ulcer, and deterioration of the bone marrow leading to anaemia. Tolmetin sodium seems to have fewer side effects and so is probably the best of these. Again, before accepting these drugs as a first therapy, get another opinion and if you are on them for even a brief time, get frequent blood counts.

226. Opinion: Surgery is sometimes the safest treatment for severe arthritis

Although surgery is usually the treatment of last resort, in the case of severe arthritis, it is sometimes less dangerous and more sure of success than some of the stronger drugs. Because of enormous recent advances in orthopaedic (bone and joint) surgery, damaged joints can be fixed mechanically; total replacement of hip and knee joints is now quite frequently carried out. If you are so crippled by arthritis that it has put you on the inactive list for the foreseeable future, and you are being advised to try powerful drugs, consider surgery as a possibly safer alternative. But make sure you consult with orthopaedic surgeons who have performed the particular operation you may need many times: orthopaedic surgery is as highly specialized as open-heart surgery, perhaps even more so.

Some specific surgical corrections of crippling arthritis include replacement of the hip joint, replacement of the knee joint and elbow, repair of the kneecap and microsurgery on the tiny joints of the fingers and toes. The simplest form of surgery for arthritis is a synovectomy—removal of the inflamed membranes that cover the joint. This certainly gives temporary relief and, some doctors feel, may prevent the spread of the arthritis to the tendons, ligaments, and cartilage surrounding the joint. (This alleged prophylactic effect has not yet been proved.)

227. Experimental drugs as treatment for severe arthritis

Experiments are now being conducted with drugs which attack the autoimmune response that permitted the arthritis in the first place. They are called immunosuppressive drugs. Obviously, any therapy that affects the body's *autoimmune* reactions may also threaten its *immune* reactions and the risk of infection is high. However, this line of research does hold out much hope.

228. Degenerative joint disease—osteoarthritis

About 5 million people in Britain have some form of osteo-arthritis, degenerative joint disease. Unlike rheumatoid arthritis, it is not an autoimmune reaction, but comes from the normal wear and tear of life.

365

Swelling and pain in the joints are similar to that of rheumatoid arthritis, but there is no rheumatoid factor in the blood, no inflammation that may spread to other organs. Osteoarthritis originates in the joint and stays there and is more common in the lower extremities and spine.

The single most important predisposing factor in osteoarthritis is overweight. Other orthopaedic problems may cause the condition: for example, a crippled hip may force the body's weight on to the knee, creating an imbalance in the distribution of weight and overloading the knee joints. Trauma or injury to a specific joint may also lead to osteoarthritis. For example, a sports injury that permanently hurts the knee may make the knee weaker and less capable of carrying the weight which cannot be shifted on to another joint.

229. Treatment of osteoarthritis

Treatment should be to lose weight, if you are heavy, and to *keep* yourself light. Rest frequently; use a firm mattress and a bed board to give your body extra support. Sometimes, crutches or a cane can help take the pressure off the joint. Aspirin is the first order of treatment for pain. In severe cases, surgery may be needed. Some doctors inject steroids into the joint to relieve the pain and swelling, but this is of limited use and the side effects (See No. 241 below) may make it counterproductive.

230. Lupus erythematosus (generally called lupus or L.E.)

Lupus (in Latin, it means wolf) occurs mainly in women in their twenties and thirties, and particularly in black women. The cause is still unknown. It is on the increase in Britain.

It is an immune complex disease, affecting the primary vascular and haemological systems in which the body builds antibodies against the ribonucleic acids which are important in cell metabolism and chromosomes. (See p. 210) Antibodies against the nucleic acids are found circulating in the blood of lupus patients and serve as the basis for the tests which diagnose the disease (called antinuclear factor tests). The damage to the body occurs when the antibodies join with their antigens (the nuclear materials) and form deposits in the lining of the blood vessels.

As with the other autoimmune diseases, there is virtually no way at present to see lupus coming or to prevent it. WARNING: Some drugs cause a reaction indistinguishable from lupus; this is called "drug-induced lupus". The drug which most commonly causes this side effect is *procainamide (Pronestyl)*, used for severe irregularities of the heartbeat. Other drugs such as phenothiazines (a group of tranquillizers) and several antihypertensive drugs such as hydralazine can cause this reaction. If you develop any lupus-like symptoms after starting a new drug, notify your doctor.

231. Symptoms of lupus

These include:

a. Fever

b. Weakness and fatigue

c. Arthritis (in 90 per cent) which is usually not as severe as rheumatoid arthritis

d. Rash on face, neck, and arms

e. Anaemia

Except for the rash, these are rather non-specific symptoms, so that the disease must be verified by tests. (See No. 230 above) In most cases of lupus, the disease is very mild, limited to rash, arthritis and intermittent fever. In the more severe cases, circulating antibody-antigen complexes interact with certain cell parts, usually in the lining of blood vessels. In the most acute cases there is damage to the kidneys, heart, and brain. There is also a high incidence of spontaneous abortion in lupus patients. However, even in the most severe cases there is a good chance, with drug therapy, for the sufferer to live a normal and quite comfortable life.

232. Treatment of lupus

Treatment with aspirin is now generally avoided. Patients with skin and joint problems are often given anti-malarial drugs which keep the disease manageable. In severe cases, steroids may be used to control the initial flare-up. This should be quickly followed by controlling treatment with non-steroidal anti-inflammatory drugs or steroids on alternate days. Experimental treatment involves plasma exchange.

233. Rheumatic fever

This disease begins as an infection and seems to *develop* into an autoimmune disease. It does not primarily affect women but is included because it may be confused with rheumatoid arthritis. Rheumatic fever usually begins with an infected throat that goes untreated. The highest-risk age group is ages five to fifteen: about 25–35 per cent of all sore throats and fevers in this age group are due to the streptococcus bacteria ("strep").

If a streptococcal infection goes untreated, a small number of people will develop rheumatic fever. Why only a small number, no one knows. In most people, the infection is cleared by the body itself. In those who develop rheumatic fever, the strep infection leads to the autoimmune reaction because the antibodies which the body forms to fight the streptococcal infection also react against other body organs—especially the valves of the heart and the joints. Antibodies which react with the heart muscle can be detected in the blood stream of most victims of rheumatic fever. Once the autoimmune reaction sets in, rheumatic fever has started.

234. Symptoms of rheumatic fever
These include:
a. Aches and pains moving from joint to joint
b. Fever
c. Chorea (Sydenham's) which is characterized by sudden involuntary movements in parts of the body, occurring most frequently in children (see p. 50)
d. Skin rash and nodules under the skin
e. A history of a recent cold and sore throat

The disease is confirmed by the presence of a heart murmur or other evidence of heart disease, and by blood tests detecting a recent streptococcal infection and the presence of continuing autoimmune reaction. Don't allow the diagnosis to be made without proof, because many viral illnesses can give aches and pains in the joints and fever.

235. Treatment of rheumatic fever
The infectious part of the disease can be treated with antibiotics. The autoimmune part of the disease is treated like rheumatoid arthritis, depending on severity. The attack may last six to twelve weeks. Restricted activity is required for all sufferers and total rest for those with severe heart involvement. Aspirin is used to control the symptoms of arthritis. In the most severe cases, steroids are needed to keep the inflammatory response under control. The final outcome of the disease is variable. Usually, the disease resolves without remaining heart disease. Sometimes, there is severe damage to the valves of the heart, which may show up at a later time and is a major but declining cause of heart trouble for women during pregnancy. People who have had rheumatic fever are more prone to develop it again, so that everyone who has had the disease should take prophylactic penicillin or sulphonamides until at least age 18.

236. Tendonitis ("tennis elbow")
Tennis elbow is an old term that has come into use again because

of the recent popularity of tennis. It is actually *tendonitis*, a form of bursitis, involving inflammation of the tendon of the lateral portion of the elbow. It comes from repeated strain on the tendons of the elbow, which is often caused more by poor tennis form than by the rigours of competition. There is a debate over treatment—some say "Rest", others say "Continue to play". The symptoms seem to go away within six months, no matter what the treatment.

237. Infections that can cause arthritis

Some infectious diseases which invade the body generally can also invade the joints, causing the pain, swelling, and heat symptomatic of arthritis.

a. Gonorrhoea, when not discovered early, may cause a very painful arthritis. The treatment for gonorrhoea at this stage is usually hospitalization and antibiotics by intravenous drip.

b. Bacterial endocarditis is an infection of the lining of the heart which may also be accompanied by arthritis.

c. Hepatitis, a viral infection of the liver, is often preceded by arthritic symptoms.

238. Rubella can cause arthritic symptoms

Rubella, so dangerous to the fetus in early pregnancy (see p. 219), can cause arthritis symptons during its acute stages in adults. The joint pain usually disappears when the disease has run its course. Many adults who are vaccinated against rubella experience pain and occasionally swelling in their joints afterwards.

239. Other diseases sometimes accompanied by arthritis

Psoriasis (sore-EYE-a-sis) is a common skin disease in both men and women. About 7 per cent of those who have it also have arthritis. The joints involved and the treatment is very similar to rheumatoid arthritis. Ulcerative colitis and regional ileitis are bowel disorders which may be accompanied by arthritis.

240. Joint tap: a diagnostic test for type of arthritis

In a joint tap, a doctor removes some fluid from a joint to see which type of arthritis is present. The fluid can be cultured to discover an infection and otherwise analysed. This is a very safe procedure when done under sterile conditions and is very essential for diagnosis. The skin over the joint must be cleansed carefully and then a small needle is placed into the joint and fluid withdrawn. The same procedure should be used for injecting steroids into the joints.

241. Use of steroid injections into the joints to treat arthritis.

Some doctors recommend injections of steroids directly into the joints to relieve arthritis inflammation and pain. This treatment usually affords only temporary relief. It should be used *only* when the pain is crippling and all less powerful treatments have failed to relieve it. Steroid injections should never be used if infection is present and should only be administered under the most sterile conditions. The recipient must be checked frequently for undesirable reactions.

VARICOSE VEINS

242. What are varicose veins?

There are two types of blood vessels in the body—*arteries*, which carry the blood from the heart, and *veins*, which carry the blood back to it. Veins generally have much thinner walls than arteries, and are somewhat more easily damaged.

The further away the veins are from the heart, the greater the force of gravity against the flow of blood—imagine what an uphill fight it is for the leg veins with the help of the leg muscles, for example, to push the blood back to the heart. Sometimes the force of gravity, along with extraneous pressure, can cause the veins in the legs and the anogenital area to swell. The valves that help the blood along are not strong enough to do their job. This means that the blood does not move along on its upward course but rather rolls back, like the backup in a flooded pipe, and the veins bulge outward. These bulges are called varicosities—varicose veins (the word comes from the Latin *varix* which means a dilated vein).

Varicose veins are actual weaknesses in the walls of the vein, and not related to blood pressure or the temporary distention of the veins as during athletic activity.

243. Varicosities occur in the outer veins close to the skin surface

The body has two vein systems—the *superficial veins*, which are close to the surface of the skin, and the *deep veins*. Varicosities develop in the superficial veins, usually in the legs.

244. Causes of varicose veins

a. Heredity may be a major factor. If your mother or father had them, you may have inherited thin-walled veins and should take care not to aggravate pressure on your legs.

b. If a woman suffers from phlebitis (clots in the deep veins of the legs that are, in themselves, a much more serious disorder than

370

varicose veins), this can add pressure on the superficial veins and cause varicosities. (See p. 47)

c. Prolonged standing over many years can put too great pressure on the veins of the legs and cause varicosities.

d. Prolonged pressure on the veins through many years of wearing tight corsets and garters that cut into the upper leg can contribute to varicosities.

e. Pregnancy or abdominal tumours can block the return of blood through the pelvic area to the heart, causing pelvic varicosities.

f. High levels of progesterone produced during pregnancy may dilate the veins and cause varicosities. Often the varicosity will disappear after childbirth; sometimes it is there to stay.

g. Some women react to the birth control pill by developing varicosities. Consider changing to a lower-hormone combination. (See p. 47)

245. Varicose veins of the vulva during pregnancy

The sheer weight of carrying a child, coupled with the high hormone levels, may cause painful varicosities in the vulva during pregnancy. Wear tights or elastic pants to support the veins, which will probably go down after delivery.

246. Haemorrhoids (piles) are varicose veins of the anus

Many women suffer a bout of piles or haemorrhoids, particularly during pregnancy. These are varicosities in the veins of the anus caused by pressure and constipation, and complicated in some women by heredity. Most of the veins go down after the birth, but may enlarge in subsequent pregnancies. Treatment for severe piles is not recommended until several months after delivery.

247. Symptoms of varicose veins in the legs

Varicosities in the legs become more frequent as a woman grows older and the accumulated wear and tear on her body begins to have its effect. Varicosity symptoms are

a. A feeling of heaviness in the legs (literally the pressure of blood unable to resist the downward pull of gravity);

b. Swelling (oedema);

c. Sometimes by dryness of the skin over the area of the veins. The severity of the varicosities can range from little spidery marks to severely disfiguring, tortuous veins covering the entire leg.

248. Prevention and treatment of varicose veins

a. Although it is hard to avoid the predestination of heredity, women can do a lot to avoid varicose veins. If either of your parents suffers from varicosities, start wearing support stockings or tights early in life; put your feet up when you are sitting; try not to choose a career which will keep you on your feet all day. Wear good solid shoes that exercise your calf muscles properly. Avoid excessive weight gain, and include plenty of fibre in your diet.

b. The injection of irritating materials directly into the vein (sclerosing agents) is one method of treatment. Injections are usually made into areas where the veins bulge significantly. A reaction is set up inside the vein and a clot forms which closes off that area of the vein and decreases the bulging. These injections generally give only temporary relief, for at times the vein can open again and the problem recur. About 15 years ago the injections were combined with bandaging the leg. This method seems to give fairly good results in moderately severe cases and is not followed by recurrence as was the isolated injection method. One complication is the severe irritation which occurs if some of the sclerosing agent gets outside the vein into the leg tissues. Make sure you are treated by a doctor who has performed this procedure often.

c. Stripping of the veins: this is performed under general anaesthesia and involves making several incisions at various places along the veins of the leg. A wire is threaded throughout the entire length of the vein (or as far as possible) and a knob is placed over the end. The thick wire is then pulled and the entire vein comes out with the device. Elastic bandages are immediately placed to prevent bleeding. The woman will have to wear elastic stockings for several weeks after surgery, to allow for healing. The postoperative period involves little discomfort and there are few complications, the main one being bleeding from the torn ends of the veins. This procedure helps cosmetically, but the varicosities may recur as other vessels dilate from the same factors which caused the problem in the first place.

12

SEXUAL HEALTH

The notion of what is "normal" in sex changes from age to age, from culture to culture, from generation to generation. Mothers and daughters may differ radically on the subject; private citizens may be astounded at the views on sex held by the law. The line between public acceptance of a sexual practice and private consent is always unclear. What *is* clear, however, is that a satisfactory sex life is important in the overall physical and mental health of a woman. This aspect of health has long been overlooked by medical and lay people alike.

It is far beyond the scope of this book to discuss the infinite variety of normal sexual practices. We have suggested several readings in the reference section. We will discuss the normal sexual response of women and a few of the major sexual problems. Also, when certain sexual activities may have associated medical problems we will discuss these.

In general, the normal range of sexual expression includes abstinence, masturbation, heterosexuality and homosexuality. There is nothing inherently dangerous, either physically or psychologically, in any of these practices. What is *not* normal or healthy in sex is a situation in which a woman is forcing herself or being forced by others to assume a role for which she has no respect, which makes her feel uncomfortable or anxious, or which makes her dislike herself. Sex should be enjoyable and contribute to a woman's feeling of well-being. Sex is not normal if it becomes compulsive or ritualistic. And violence in sex, whether between consenting parties, or rapist and victim, is not normal at all.

NORMAL SEXUAL RESPONSE
1. Female sexual arousal and orgasm
Although sexual arousal may start with an emotional-psycho-

logical impulse—for example, a fantasy—it involves specific physical responses in all parts of the body, particularly the nervous system, the endocrine system and the genital organs. We all owe a great debt to the researchers Masters and Johnson for finally recording the physiological parameters of female orgasm. They coined the term 'sexual response cycle'. The various stages of this are:

a. *The first stage: excitement*

In the early stages of sexual excitement, the blood vessels of the genital and pelvic area begin to enlarge and lubrication of genital area begins. The vagina expands, enough to accept a penis virtually regardless of size. The lower third becomes congested with blood, so that the woman who has had children still has a pleasurably tight vagina, even though in the unstimulated state the entrance may feel lax. The walls of the uterus become engorged with blood and the uterus enlarges, pushing slightly out of the pelvic cavity. (This movement of the uterus places the cervix in a position that generally heightens the chances of fertilization.)

b. *Second stage: the plateau phase*

As sexual arousal builds to what Masters and Johnson call "the plateau stage", vascular tissue of the pelvis grows congested along with the tissues and muscles surrounding the entrance to the vagina. Vaginal lubrication occurs. Heart rate and breathing speed up.

Unless these changes take place, a woman will not find intercourse especially pleasurable. Thus, it is essential to allow sufficient time for sexual arousal before attempting intercourse.

c. *Third stage: orgasmic phase*

A series of rapid contractions occur in the muscles around the vagina and pelvic floor. Throughout the body muscles tense then relax, producing a sensation of intense pleasure.

d. *Last stage: resolution*

After orgasm, body tissues gradually return to normal. Heart rate and breathing slow to their usual rate. The couple feel (psychologically) close and relaxed together.

2. The clitoris—the most sensitive of all female genital structures

The clitoris is a small hump of erectile tissue near the upper rim of the vagina and over the pubic bone, which is the most sensitive of all the female genital organs. Both the first stage of sexual arousal and the orgasm itself are triggered by sensations which are most intense in the clitoris. *Thus, there is no physiological difference between "vaginal orgasm" and "clitoral orgasm".*

Women who have felt sexually deficient because they cannot achieve orgasm simply through the friction of penile thrusting should know that they are normal. At least 30–50 per cent of women need additional clitoral stimulation, usually manual, in addition to intercourse to achieve orgasm. Penile thrusting causes *indirect* stimulation to the clitoris which may not be enough for some women. (See No. 15 below)

3. Lubrication of the vagina during sexual arousal

The amount of vaginal lubrication during sexual arousal varies from woman to woman, and an individual woman can experience more or less at various times of the menstrual cycle or at different times of her life. If there is no lubrication at all, intercourse can be very painful and not pleasurable. If this is an occasional problem, additional lubricants available without prescription may be used. If this is a chronic problem, and you suspect a psychosexual basis, consider therapy.

During or after menopause, severe vaginal dryness may stem from oestrogen deficiency. Try lubricants such as KY Jelly (*not* Vaseline; if you are using a cap or sheaths it damages the rubber). If these fail, consider a low-dose oestrogen cream. (See p. 274)

4. All orgasms are not the same

Although all orgasms are physiologically the same, the intensity of contractions may vary considerably, depending on the stimulus, the time of the cycle or the woman's mood.

5. Multiple orgasm

Some women at certain stages of their lives are capable of having multiple orgasms. (Physiologically, all women are capable, but many women simply do not experience this reaction.) A woman who can have multiple orgasms is in no way more mature or more healthy than a woman who has only one orgasm.

6. Sexual arousal without orgasm

If a woman is sexually aroused but does not reach her climax, she does not experience "resolution" and her blood vessels may be engorged, her body tense for hours afterwards.

Many women find that intercourse is pleasurable even if they do not have an orgasm. However, prolonged and repeated sex without the relief of orgasm may produce pelvic congestion with persistent backache and abdominal and genital pain. (See pp. 314-15)

7. Fantasies during sex are normal

Fantasies often heighten sexual arousal. Many people fantasize about other people besides their partners during sex; many people fantasize about violence. Remember, as peculiar as a fantasy may seem to you, it endangers no one as long as it is only in your mind. A woman who finds she is *acting out* her more dangerous fantasies—e.g., engaging in actual violence during sex—should seek counselling. And any woman who finds that her partner is acting out violent fantasies should send him for therapy or end the relationship.

8. Oral-genital and anal sex

These are both normal and widely practised sexual activities. There are some cautions, however. If one partner has a herpes infection (cold sores) of the mouth, oral-genital sex should be avoided because the virus can be spread to the genital area. (See p. 295) Vaginal intercourse immediately following anal sex can result in vaginal infections if the penis has not been washed very carefully before insertion into the vagina. Lubricants should be used during anal sex to avoid tearing of the anus resulting in fissures.

Don't feel you ought to practise either oral-genital or anal sex unless you want to. The only reason for either is if they are mutually enjoyable.

9. Group sex

These practices of sex for physical pleasure only are on the rise and for short periods of time may well suit a woman's needs and be considered normal. There are definite risks to sex with a large number of partners, mainly the many types of sexually transmitted diseases. (See p. 298) If this is your sexual pattern, make sure to get regular checks at a VD clinic.

10. Vibrators

These are battery or electrically operated devices used by many women during masturbation and in lovemaking between partners. They produce intense, rapid orgasms which individual women may or may not enjoy. There are some reports of vaginal bruising or lacerations mainly caused by inserting the device into the vagina before turning on the power—turn it on before insertion. The vibrators which strap on to the hand or are handheld and used for general body massage and clitoral stimulation are very safe.

SEXUAL DYSFUNCTION

11. What is sexual dysfunction?

Sexual dysfunction (diss-function), the inability to have satisfying sexual relations, can be caused by a number of emotional or physical problems, many of which can be improved or cured by recently developed therapy techniques.

The word "frigidity" has been used to describe sexual dysfunction in women. Like calling menstruation "the curse", calling an unsatisfied woman "frigid" is pejorative; it blames a woman for something which may not be anyone's "fault". *It is time to stop using this word.*

12. What causes sexual dysfunction?

a. Ignorance—about one's own or one's partner's sexual physiology and anatomy.

b. Miseducation—for example, childhood taboos about sex that linger, consciously or subconsciously, into adulthood.

c. Specific, unresolved emotional conflicts—such as inordinate attachment to one parent

d. Current tensions between partners

e. Fear of losing control

f. Lack of confidence or anxiety about one's own sexual performance

g. Fatigue

h. Physical illness

i. Depression

FEMALE SEXUAL PROBLEMS

13. Lack of sexual desire

Most women find that at one time or another in their lives, they do not feel the need for sexual activity. They lose interest in having sex with anyone; in masturbating; even erotic fantasies stop. How long this lack of interest has to last for it to be labelled abnormal is hard to say. If it persists for months in a previously good relationship, some new conflict between the partners may be the cause. Illness must always be suspected. Fatigue is a common cause; the harassed mother raising small children may just be too tired for sex; likewise the overworked businesswoman. Disinterest in sex may also occur after severe trauma such as rape (see No. 34 below) or emergency hysterectomy.

If a woman has never had any interest in sex, this probably indicates a basic emotional conflict about sexuality—and if she is unhappy about her state, she should see a doctor.

Only when the lack of interest is prolonged over many months should it be considered unhealthy.

14. Inhibited sexual excitement

Some women, though mentally interested in sex, find that they sometimes cannot become physically aroused; others, though highly aroused during sexual activity, cannot achieve orgasm. Very few women are orgasmic 100 per cent of the time, and this is normal. Lack of orgasm should only be considered a "problem" if it persists. A woman can try masturbation or seek additional clitoral stimulation from her partner. If this does not work, consider sex therapy.

15. Many women need additional clitorial stimulation to achieve orgasm

Thirty to fifty per cent of all women have this entirely normal sexual need. Some women have orgasms only when the partner is stimulating the clitoris (with mouth or hands). If the couple finds this pattern upsetting or boring, they can alter it by longer foreplay and manual stimulation of the clitoris during intercourse by either the woman herself or her partner.

16. Vaginismus (involuntary muscle spasm at the entrance to the vagina)

Vaginismus (vadge-in-IS-mus) occurs when the muscles of the vagina contract so forcefully that a woman is unable to have intercourse. Some women with this problem also find that they cannot insert a tampon or a diaphragm. A gynaecological examination can make the diagnosis, for the muscles will be able to be observed and palpated in spasm. Treatment is usually begun by teaching the woman to dilate her own vaginal muscles with her fingers or dilators. The object is to make the woman relax and gain control over her pelvic muscles. OPINION: Surgery is not recommended for this problem! Many women who actually have vaginismus are operated upon to "open a rigid hymen". Of course, the surgery does not work for vaginismus. Make sure the diagnosis and treatment are begun by reliable physicians. Always get a second opinion if surgery is recommended.

17. Dyspareunia: pain during intercourse

Dyspareunia (dis-par-YOON-e-ah) can be caused by several physical problems such as endometriosis (see p. 331), pelvic infection (see p. 287), and occasionally be a retroverted (tipped backward) uterus. A woman experiencing pain repeatedly during intercourse, should have a gynaecological examination. If the doctor finds no abnormality, the pain can frequently be traced to one of the above causes of sexual dysfunction. (See No.12 above). Occasionally, ovaries are bumped during intercourse, which can cause a severe, sharp pain. A change of position during sex will help this problem.

SEXUAL PROBLEMS OF MEN
18. Common sexual problems of men

a. *Premature ejaculation* occurs when a man does not have voluntary control over the timing of ejaculation, usually causing ejaculation before he desires. This becomes a problem if he ejaculates within the first few minutes of sex play and before the woman has had time to become sexually aroused. If this happens regularly, it can lead to mutual recrimination between partners and real misery. This problem can be caused by anxiety or by a man's early sexual experience, which may have created in him a desperate need to hurry. Therapy for this disorder has been highly successful and should be sought. (See No. 20 below)

b. *Impotence* (IM-po-tense), the inability to have an erection, afflicts virtually every man at some time or another, and if it happens occasionally, it is nothing to worry about. If men are tired, worried, drunk, "not in the mood", they may become impotent as a result. Unfortunately, however, men tend to be terribly frightened by impotence. Victimized by a notion of machismo that dictates they must always be able to perform, they can feel so defeated by an occasional bout of impotence that they worry themselves into a permanent siege. The answer is to discuss the cause of the impotence (to rule out fatigue and anxiety) and take steps to alleviate it; one of these may be marital or sex therapy.

c. *Retarded ejaculation.* Some men cannot ejaculate inside the vagina. They are able to maintain an erection but must masturbate to achieve ejaculation. Most of the time, the problem is psychological in origin, and for couples seeking to have a child, it can be most distressing. First, the man should see a doctor for an examination. Then, *the couple* should seek sexual counselling.

TREATMENT OF SEXUAL PROBLEMS
19. How to deal with sexual dysfunction

a. Read. This is the best cure for ignorance, the source of much sexual difficulty in couples, and today, there are innumerable books on the market which give explicit advice. Men particularly tend to be ignorant of the geography of a woman's genitals; in fact, an awful lot of men and women manage to reach sexual maturity without knowing that the clitoris exists, much less where it is.

b. Talk. People have to tell each other their needs. If a relationship is warm, this should be possible without undue embarrassment. However, sometimes loving partners do not wish to hassle each other with sexual demands, and just let a growing problem lie silent between them. Say what you need; that is probably the best way of getting it.

c. If a woman doesn't understand her own sexual needs, masturbation may be a good way to find out about them—so that later she can communicate her feelings to her partner. She should also use a mirror to examine her genital area and locate the various parts.

d. Rule out physical illness. Consult your doctor. Your problem may have a simply physiological cause which can be discovered by examination and cured quickly.

e. If your partner has a sexual problem, don't automatically blame yourself. A frightened man may blame his partner for his impotence, for example, but he is not necessarily right. Don't assume that he is having trouble because you are a bad lover or because you have thin thighs.

f. Try to change the outward circumstances of sexual relations. Maybe you're both too tired to make love at night; try having sex after a good night's sleep. Try sleeping somewhere else. Try changing the atmosphere. There is much truth to the reports that people who stopped having sex altogether in their own homes, with the children softly snoring down the hall and the bathroom tap dripping, rediscovered their passion for each other on holiday, or for that matter, in the hotel down the road.

g. Sex therapy—a relatively new counselling speciality—should be considered.

20. How to find help

If you are reluctant to discuss your sexual life with your family doctor, you can seek help at a clinic specializing in sexual difficulties. The Family Planning Association or the National Marriage Guidance Council will tell you where to find your nearest clinic. Occasionally a referral note from your doctor is needed.

The British Association for Counselling publishes a directory of agencies offering therapy, counselling and support on psycho-sexual problems. They are at 1a Little Church Street, Rugby, Warwickshire. The Association of Sexual and Mental Therapists, at 79 Harley Street, London W1, also publishes a list.

21. What to expect at the clinic

The counsellor should:

a. take a long detailed history of your relationship, if you seek treatment as a couple (which is preferable), or of your individual sex life;

b. make sure you and your partner have both had a thorough physical examination recently; if the counsellor is a doctor she may do this herself;

c. discuss anatomy and physiology;

d. seek to discover emotional problems which may be contributing to the dysfunction;

e. possibly suggest exercises which can be done at home, in private.

A good counsellor will not suggest

a. that he or she observe you while you are making love;

b. that he or she have sex with you or your partner.

22. Exercises to treat sexual problems

Most treatment for sexual dysfunction is a modification of the Masters and Johnson "sensate focus exercises". The partners will be instructed to take the focus off the need to achieve successful intercourse and place it on more relaxed ways of giving each other pleasure. Privacy and relaxation are absolutely prerequisite. These exercises are used most often to treat persistently non-orgasmic women and men who suffer from impotence, or premature ejaculation. (See References and Further Reading for completely descriptive material.)

23. Avoid surgical treatment for sexual dysfunction unless it is recommended by a very reputable sex therapist, and verified by other medical opinions

In most cases, sexual dysfunction is *not* caused by anatomical problems in the genital area—so that surgery to somehow alter the genitals is a very unusual suggestion.

One suggestion is that the skin over the clitoris be surgically loosened so that the clitoris will be more stimulated during intercourse. Another is surgery to "open the hymen". A rigid hymen is very rare; when it is diagnosed, the woman can usually dilate it herself; and very often, the diagnosis is mistaken—the woman really has vaginismus (see No 16 above). Never accept this surgery, unless yours is one of the very rare cases which can be corroborated by several doctors.

24. Warning: Never consider transsexual surgery until you have had a careful trial of psychotherapy

Transsexuals are different from homosexual women in that they are not happy with their identity as women (which homosexuals are) but actually think of themselves as men.

Any woman who believes she is a transsexual could seek initial help from the National Marriage Guidance Council or from the Beaumont Society, Box 3084, London W. 1.

The general practice is to require intensive counselling for several years, and then to suggest that the woman live as a man for at least a year before surgery is contemplated. *No reputable surgeon would perform the transsexual operation without assurance that the patient had spent a very long time in therapy, and without the recommendation of a qualified psychiatrist.*

25. How physical illness and its treatment can cause sexual dysfunction

a. Almost any severe or prolonged illness can cause sexual problems. Kidney disease or diabetes, for example, which affect the endocrine system, are almost sure to decrease sexual interest.

b. Pain, even from an illness which is not otherwise serious except for its discomforts, may decrease sexual appetite; and the pain-killers needed to alleviate the discomfort may decrease it even more.

c. A person who is recovering from a serious illness may be afraid that sex will cause a recurrence, and therefore avoid sex altogether, sometimes quite needlessly. Heart-attack victims are a classic example. Although capable of sexual arousal, they fear the exertion of sex will lead to another heart attack. *Check with your doctor for assurance of exactly when sexual exertion is not dangerous after major illness or surgery.*

d. Medicines used to treat a disease may cause orgasm problems or impotence. Antidepressants, tranquillizers, sedatives, and drugs used to treat hypertension sometimes have this effect. If you note a sudden change in sexual function after starting a certain drug, check with your doctor. *A doctor should always tell you before-hand if a drug can be expected to cause sexual problems.*

e. Illness may touch off emotional/relational problems between partners which can lead to sexual dysfunction. Women who are having severe emotional reactions to breast surgery or hysterectomy, for example, may feel so bad about their bodies that they cannot resume sex. (See p. 344) Very often, the woman's fears of rejection are unfounded; she feels worse about her appearance than does her partner. Talking, plain communication, may alleviate the problem. Time as well as love and understanding often solve it. Seek outside help first from the self-help organizations; go to therapy as a final resort.

RAPE

The crime of rape (along with other sexual assaults) is on the increase. It is clearly a violent crime of male aggression against women. It is a means of humiliation and injuring women, made yet worse by the fact that those involved with the rape victim after the assault (doctors, lawyers, and police) may be caught up in sexist attitudes too and often contribute to the humiliating and misogynous aspects of the crime. Things are changing, but not quickly enough.

26. Rape fantasies: male and female

The prevalent belief about rape in this and other countries is that women cannot be raped unless they want to be. This is a nonsensical male fantasy. Many men have fantasized about raping women, about overcoming the resistance of an unwilling woman who finally gives in to the overwhelming power of the male. It is a power fantasy. The vast majority of men never act on it—but just because they have had the fantasy, they may lack sympathy with the rape victim.

It is no easier for a woman to resist an armed rapist than for a bank clerk to resist an armed robber. Because the robber gets away with the money, the clerk is not accused of collusion; why then should the woman be accused of collusion if the attacker gets away with the rape?

Women have fantasies about rape too, usually because they have somehow accepted the notion that men must be overpowering to be excitingly virile, or because responsibility for their sexual response is taken from them. This has no bearing on the reality of rape, for it is a romantic fantasy and rape is not a romantic crime: it is a violent crime.

27. Who is a rapist?

There are many kinds of mental and emotional problems that cause a man to rape a woman. This means that there is no clear formula or sign to warn the potential victim. A rapist might be immature, violent, insane or just drunk; he might be a relative, deliveryman or a passerby. And so unfortunately, a lone woman will often have to be on guard to avoid unwarranted attack.

383

28. How to help yourself

Try not to be alone or dawdle in risky areas, like dark streets or lonely parks. Don't stop in such places to give directions or the time. Avoid spots where gangs congregate.

If someone is following you, go into a public place, like a pub, and tell the landlord or phone a friend or the police. In a deserted street, walk into the middle of the road and shout for help. If the attack is imminent, run.

If driving alone, always check the back seat of the car before getting in. Drive with your windows and doors locked and never give lifts to a lone man. If you think you are being followed, drive on until you spot a police patrol or station. On public transport, never enter an empty compartment or one with a lone man. Try to sit near another woman, the emergency signal or the guard.

Over half of all rape incidents take place in the victim's home. Don't put your full name on the doorbell or in the phone book: use your initials. Install a safety chain or peephole and never open the door to a stranger without checking his identity first. Don't leave easily accessible windows open; good locks will also keep out burglars. If you think there is someone in the house, get out if you can or break a window to attract attention.

If your attacker is unarmed, you might be able to put up a fight and a well aimed blow could give you the chance to get away. The noise might also attract assistance. If he is armed, your life might be in danger and resisting could only make things worse.

29. What to do if you have been raped

1. First of all, report the crime to the police.

2. Contact a friend or a rape crisis centre or women's group. You will need someone to comfort and advise you and stay with you at the police station.

3. Do not wash or change your clothes: you may be destroying evidence.

4. Don't take alcohol or drugs.

5. Take a change of clothes to the police station.

6. Try to make a note about the attack and your attacker; this may help you when making your statement.

7. Get someone to spend the night with you or go to a friend's house, if you are nervous about staying home alone.

8. If you decide not to inform the police, talk to *someone* about the rape.

9. See a doctor to check for pregnancy, VD or injury. (See No. 32 below)

30. Official procedure after rape

You will be taken to the police station and may be kept there for several hours, whilst the following steps are undertaken:

1. You will be asked to make a statement. This will be taken down by a police officer, and you can ask for it to be a woman. Read the statement carefully and ask for any changes before signing it.

2. The officer dealing with your case will ask numerous detailed intimate questions.

3. A police surgeon will be called to give you an internal and external medical examination. You can ask for your own GP or a woman doctor to do this, if you prefer. These examinations are only to collect forensic evidence (Make sure that you see your own doctor afterwards to check for pregnancy, VD or internal injuries. See No. 32 below.)

4. You may be asked to look at identity pictures, show the police where the rape took place or view an identity parade.

If the case does eventually come to trial, you may be kept waiting several months before going to court. This can be a very nerve-wracking experience and many women feel that they are on trial, rather than their attacker. Your name cannot legally appear in the media when they report the trial, and during the court case, unless the judge directs otherwise, you can ask to remain anonymous and not have your name and address read out in court.

31. Legal aspects of rape

Rape is defined by the law as: The unlawful carnal knowledge of a female by force or fraud against her will. (Carnal knowledge means the penetration of the labia by the penis to any degree—full penetration and ejaculation need not take place in order to prove rape.)

This is too simple a definition. A rapist may inflict many kinds of sexual assault on an unwilling woman. These include beating, humiliation, urination or defaecation on the victim, oral or anal sex and the use of knives, bottles or sticks.

32. Medical procedure after rape

1. You should make a general examination (inspection) of your entire body. Make sure that the doctor writes down descriptions of any bruises, lacerations, redness, or pain anywhere on your body. If any evidence of trauma appears after you have left the hospital, make sure that you return and have the doctor note these and enter them into the medical record.

2. A pelvic examination should be performed, again to look for any evidence of trauma. This may be very upsetting: the last thing most women want after being raped is a vaginal examination. However, most are also happy to be reassured that there has been no damage done, or if there has, to have it repaired. Approximately 25–50 per cent of women have some physical trauma from the rape incident, so the general examination and the pelvic examination are *very* important.

3. During the pelvic examination, samples of the vaginal secretions should be taken for sperm and acid phosphatase (FOSS-fatase), a component of seminal fluid which would be present even if a man had no sperm (e.g. if he had had a vasectomy). *It is a very important corroborating piece of evidence in many cases and must be tested for.*

4. Tests for gonorrhoea should be done if the assault was more than twenty-four hours before the examination. Some examiners do these tests routinely, more as a public health measure than for their actual relevance to the case.

5. The anus and mouth must be examined if the attack involved these areas.

6. Most rape victims would like to receive preventive treatment for VD and pregnancy. If the woman desires it, she can receive two shots of procaine pencillin and probenecid (a drug to make the blood level of penicillin higher). Or she can wait and have the tests for gonorrhoea and syphilis repeated at three and six weeks (and again, in twelve weeks, for syphilis). If she is allergic to penicillin, this should be reported to the examiner and tetracycline or spectinomycin requested. (See p. 302)

7. Pregnancy prevention may be obtained in the form of the 'morning-after pill' (see p. 70), unless you were taking birth control pills or were otherwise protected against pregnancy at the time of the attack. Menstrual aspiration is another option if the period is delayed, and does not involve the side effects of the "morning-after pill". (See p. 189)

33. Physical after-effects of rape

a. Vaginal discharge and itching may occur. This can be due to candidal infection (see p. 288) if a woman received penicillin or tetracycline. (If you have a tendency toward candidiasis ask for a prescription to prevent this.) Some women will contract trichomoniasis (see p. 291) from the rapist, or any of the other vaginal infections that are spread by sexual contact. If a discharge develops, seek medical help. It is very unlikely to be syphilis or gonorrhoea if you received prophylactic antibiotics.

b. Bruises, swelling, pain not apparent immediately after the rape may show up later on. Go back to the same doctor you saw after the rape and make sure these are noted on his or her report.

c. Lacerations of the rectum may accompany rape cases which involve anal sodomy. Sometimes they do not bleed until you move your bowels. Report these to the police surgeon and to your doctor. If there is anal pain but no bleeding, report this as well. For treatment sometimes Vaseline will be helpful.

d. A follow-up medical examination should be scheduled for three to four weeks after the assault. At this time tests for venereal disease and pregnancy should be taken, if indicated. It will also be a reassurance that all things are medically well.

34. Psychological after-effects of rape

Initially, many women are stunned and appear calm, as though they cannot believe this assault has happened to them. Most women suffer tension, anxiety, even hysteria eventually. It is normal to be afraid to be alone, even for a few minutes; normal to be sleepless; normal to want to run away and disappear off the face of the earth. In time, these psychological reactions should pass—and if friends, family, and police are sympathetic, they will pass much more quickly.

The trouble is that people are so confused about rape victims that they often fail a woman when she needs them the most. Police and doctors are not reliably sympathetic; you may not want to tell your family because they would be too upset. If it's a choice between your mother and your brother, try to think which of them will care most about you and least about the rape.

The women's groups and rape crisis centres are enormously helpful to the rape victim—because they are understanding strangers. After calling the police, the doctor, and a close friend, call them—they can counsel you, comfort you, give legal advice, and help guide you past serious psychological trauma. It is probable that most adult women can come out of a rape without serious psychological therapy, provided they have early supportive help.

The most helpful emotion to have after a rape is rage. Too many women are afraid to get as angry as they would like.

The least helpful emotion after a rape is guilt. Too many women feel that they were somehow to blame for the incident.

The rage is justified; the guilt is groundless. Counsellors at the rape crisis centres and in the women's groups can help you cope with both emotions.

35. Sex crimes against children

The younger the woman, the more severe the psychological trauma in general after a rape. Children who are raped or otherwise sexually molested suffer the most—especially because the attacker is frequently a relative. If your child, boy or girl, has been assaulted in this way, seek referral to an expert through the rape crisis centre or family doctor. In such a case, the mother may be the last person able to get the child to speak frankly and master the nightmare.

13

ROUTINE HEALTH CARE
FOR WELL WOMEN

Throughout this book we have suggested that every woman should have a personal way of coping with the health events in her life—with pregnancy, change of life and illness. The suggestions below will help women stay in good health and help them to cope more easily with ill health, but above all to acquire the habit of preventive medicine.

1. Take the main responsibility for your own health care

You must assume responsibility for obtaining the best treatment and care available. Never just accept treatment or medicine without knowing first exactly what it is and what it is for. Use your friends, newspaper and magazine articles, the authorities, this book and your doctor as advisers to help you make the right choice on issues regarding your health.

2. Preventive medicine is a lifelong habit

The best preventive medicine protects your body from potentially harmful factors—eat properly and do not become overweight, get enough exercise and sleep, do not smoke or drink excessively. Only use medicines that are essential for treatment. Become a watchdog on environmental and health matters and try to interest your friends, neighbours and family in caring about these issues too.

3. Become well informed about health issues

Find a regular source of medical and health news that you enjoy reading and make sure that you keep abreast of the news. This will help you stay aware of the major health issues that might affect you or your family now or in the future.

4. Keep a health record

Try to find out about the health history of your family, e.g. whether any of your relatives have had diseases such as diabetes or hypertension. Keep a record of any serious illnesses, operations and what these entailed, for yourself and every member of your family. If you have a condition that might cause an emergency, such as allergy to penicillin or bad reaction to insect stings, carry this information with you on a card, locket or bracelet. You can also keep a note of your blood group. (For advice contact the Medicalert Foundation, 9 Hanover Street, London W1; 01-499 2261.)

5. Second opinions

If you are told that you have a serious condition and that drastic (but not emergency) treatment or surgery is needed, find out all you can about it. Read about it, question your doctor and ask about possible alternatives. If you do not feel completely satisfied, get a second opinion.

6. Know your medicines

If you are prescribed a drug, take the trouble to find out about it. How quickly should it help, how long should you take it, are there any side effects, does it interact with any other drug, food or alcohol? This information can be obtained from your doctor or chemist and applies to over-the-counter drugs as well as those on prescription.

7. If you are using more than one medicine, tell your doctor

If you have been prescribed medicines from different sources, for example from your GP, dentist and the hospital, make sure that you mention this to each one. You must be careful to avoid the potential side effects of different drugs reacting with each other.

8. Use the professionals as advisers, but take the main responsibility yourself

You may spend a great deal of time and consideration shopping for clothes, buying a household appliance or finding a school for your children. Apply the same philosophy to your health care and search hard for the best doctors, the best treatment and the best hospital available to you.

9. Routine examinations and screening tests will help keep you in good health

Well-woman clinics are run in some health authorities and will do cervical smears, test blood pressure and urine and examine your breasts. *You* must make sure that you have a cervical smear every five years until you are thirty-five and every two to three years after that. Your GP may be reluctant to do one (she or he is not paid for this service if you are under thirty-five or have not had two children).

Family planning clinics will give you regular cervical smears, check your weight and blood pressure and give you breast and pelvic examinations. During pregnancy, your urine should be tested for protein and sugar and your blood for anaemia. On your first visit you will also have a blood test for VD. You should check your weight regularly and any sudden gain or loss should be checked with your doctor. Women who smoke should consider having regular chest X-rays, and think seriously about giving up the habit.

The National Health Service pays for you to have your sight tested by an optician and subsidizes the cost of having your teeth checked by a dentist.

Consider the differences between the sparse services available on the National Health Service and the checks suggested in the table below, which appeared in the American edition of this book. Although there is an element of unnecessary medicine in this, it does show what standard of care women should aim to win for themselves and how far we still have to go.

SUGGESTED PROGRAMME OF HEALTH MAINTENANCE FOR WELL WOMEN: INTERVAL IN MONTHS BETWEEN CHECKS

	Age 16—40	Age 40—60	Age 60 +
General physical examination	36	24	24
Blood pressure check	12	6	6
Urine test for protein and sugar	12	12	12
Self breast examination	1	1	1
Breast examination	12	6	6
Mammography (over age 50)	—	12-24	12-24
Pelvic examination	12	6	6
Cervical smear	12	12	12

	Age 16—40	Age 40—60	Age 60+
VD testing, when appropriate	6-12	6-12	6-12
Rectal examination and test for blood in stool	12-24	12	12
Proctosigmoido-scopy (examination and biopsy of the colon)	—	—	12
Blood test for anaemia	12	12	12
Cholesterol and other blood fats (over age 50)	—	12	12
Eye examination	24	12	12
Dental examination	6	12	12
Tuberculosis testing (if appropriate)	12-24	12-24	12-24

References

CHAPTER 1: WELL-WOMAN CARE

General references

Black, Sir D. (chmn.). *Inequalities in Health: The Report of a Research Working Group.* London: Department of Health and Social Security, 1980.

Boston Women's Health Collective (UK eds. A. Phillips and J. Rakusen). *Our Bodies Ourselves: A Health Book By and For Women.* London: Penguin Books, 1978.

Concise Medical Dictionary. Oxford: Oxford University Press, 1980.

"Doing Better and Feeling Worse: Health in the United States". Cambridge, Massachusetts: *Daedalus: journal of the American Academy of Arts and Sciences* 106:1, 1977.

Garner, L. *The NHS: Your Money or Your Life.* London: Penguin Books, 1980.

Honigsbaum, F. *The Division in British Medicine.* London: Kogan Page, 1979.

The Report of the Royal Commission on the National Health Service CMD 7615. London: Her Majesty's Stationery Office, July 1979.

CHAPTER 2: PUBERTY, MENSTRUATION AND ADOLESCENCE

1. Frisch, R. E. and Renelee, R. "Height and weight at menarche and a hypothesis of critical body weight and adolescent events". *Science* 169: 397, 1970.
2. Hafez, E. S. E. "Reproductive life cycle". In Hafez, E. S. E. and Evans, T. N. (eds.). *Human Reproduction: Conception and Contraception.* London: Harper & Row, 1973.

393

General references

Birke, L. and Gardner, K. *Why Suffer? Periods and Their Problems.* London: Virago, 1979.

Brandenburger, B. and Curry, J. *Girl!.* London: Hamlyn Paperbacks, 1981.

Cooper, W. *The Fertile Years.* London: Hutchinson, 1980.

Diagram Group. *Woman's Body: An Owner's Manual.* London: Corgi. 1978.

Gordon, L. *Woman's Body, Woman's Right.* London: Penguin Books, 1976.

Novak, E. R., Jones, G. S. and Jones, H. W. *Novak's Textbook of Gynaecology,* 8th edition. Baltimore: Williams and Wilkins, 1970.

Romney, S. L., *et al. Gynaecology and Obstetrics: The Health Care of Women.* Maidenhead, Berkshire: McGraw-Hill, 1975.

Rose, G. *The Chemistry of Life.* London: Penguin Books, 1970.

Weideger, P. *Female Cycles.* London: Women's Press, 1978.

Wilson, D. *Skin Troubles.* London: Hamlyn Paperbacks, 1980.

Zackler, J. and Brandstadt, W. *The Teenage Pregnant Girl.* Springfield, Illinois: Charles Thomas, 1975.

CHAPTER 3: BIRTH CONTROL

1. Miale, J. B. and Kent, J. W. "The effects of oral contraceptives on the results of laboratory tests". *American Journal of Obstetrics and Gynaecology* 120: 264, 1974.
2. Royal College of General Practitioners' Oral Contraceptive Study. "Mortality among oral-contraceptive users", *The Lancet,* 8 October 1977, p. 727.
3. Potts, M., van der Vlug, T. T., *et al.* "Advantages of orals outweigh disadvantages". *Population Reports* Series A, No. 2, 1975.
4. Kane, F. J. "Evaluation of emotional reactions to oral contraceptive use". *American Journal of Obstetrics and Gynaecology* 126: 968, 1976.
5. Rinehart, W. and Piotrow, P. T. "OCs—Update on usage, safety and side effects". *Population Reports* Series A, No. 6, 1979.
6. Jain, A. K. "Cigarette smoking, use of oral contraceptives, and myocardial infarction". *American Journal of Obstetrics and Gynaecology* 126: 301, 1976.
7. Vana, J., Murphy, G. P., Aronoff, B. L. and Baker, H. W. "Primary liver tumours and contraceptives: results of a survey". *Journal of the American Medical Association* 238: 2154, 1977.
8. Greenblatt, D. J. and Koch-Weser, J. "Oral contraceptives and hypertension". *Obstetrics and Gynaecology* 44: 412, 1974.
9. Laraugh, J. H. "Oral contraceptive-induced hypertension—nine years later". *American Journal of Obstetrics and Gynaecology* 126: 141, 1976.

10. Brenner, P. F. and Mishell, D. R. "Contraception for the woman with significant heart disease". *Clinical Obstetrics and Gynaecology* 18: 155, 1975.

11. Robboy, S. J. and Welch, W. R. "Microglandular hyperplasia in vaginal adenosis associated with oral contraceptives and prenatal diethylstilboestrol exposure". *Obstetrics and Gynaecology* 49: 430, 1977.

12. Rifkin, I., Nachtigall, L. E. and Beckman, E. M. "Amenorrhoea following use of oral contraceptives". *American Journal of Obstetrics and Gynaecology* 113: 420, 1972.

13. Van Campenhout, J., Blanchet, P., Beauregard, H. and Papas, S. "Amenorrhoea following the use of oral contraceptives". *Fertility and Sterility* 28: 728, 1977.

14. Sandmire, H. F., Austin, S. B. and Bechtel, R. C. "Carcinoma of the cervix in oral contraceptive, steroid and IUD users and nonusers". *American Journal of Obstetrics and Gynaecology* 125: 339, 1976.

15. Kennedy, B. J. "Appearance and spread of human breast cancer". In Griem, M. L. *et al.* "Breast cancer: a challenging problem". *Recent Results in Cancer Research* 42: 31, 1973.

16. Kastrup, E. K. and Boyd, J. R. (eds.). *Facts and Comparisons.* St Louis, Missouri: Facts and Comparisons Inc., 1978, p. 107g.

17. Rosenfeld, A. G. "Injectable long-acting progestogen contraception: a neglected modality". *American Journal of Obstetrics and Gynaecology* 120: 537, 1974.

18. Joshin, S. "Local effects of pharmacologically inert IUDs in rats, baboons and humans". In Hefnaur, F. and Segal, S. J. (eds.) *Analysis of Intrauterine Contraception.* Amsterdam and Oxford: North Holland Publishing Company, 1975, pp. 339-48.

19. Zipper, J., Edelman, D. A. and Goldsmith, A. "An overview of IUD research and implications for the future". *International Journal of Gynaecology and Obstetrics* 15: 73, 1977.

20. Snowden, R. "Copper IUCDs and the pregnancy rate". *British Journal of Family Planning* 6, No. 4: January 1981, pp. 104-107.

21. Wortman, J. "The diaphragm annd other intravaginal barriers—a review". *Population Reports* Series H., No. 4, 1976.

22. Ryder, N. B. "Contraceptive failure in the United States". *Family Planning Perspectives* 5: 133, 1973.

23. Stopes, M. C. *Contraception, Birth Control, Its Theory, History and Practice,* 3rd edition. London: Putnam, 1931.

24. Belsky, R. "Vaginal contraceptives, a time for reappraisal?" *Population Reports* Series H, No. 3, 1975.

25. Rowlands, S. and Guillebaud, J. "Post-coital contraception". *British Journal of Family Planning* 7: 3, 1981.

26. Lippes, J., Malik, T. and Tatum, H. J. "The postcoital copper-T". *Advances in Planned Parenthood* 11: 24, 1976.

27. Bremner, W. J. and De Kretser, D. M. "The prospects for new, reversible male contraceptives". *New England Journal of Medicine* 295: 1117, 1976.

28. Rock, J. and Robinson, D. "Effect of induced intrascrotal hyperthermia on testicular function in man". *American Journal of Obstetrics and Gynaecology* 93: 793, 1965.

29. Fahim, M. S., *et al.* "Ultrasound as a new method of male contraception". *Fertility and Sterility* 28: 823, 1977.

30. Ross, C. and Piotrow, P. T. "Birth control without contraceptives". *Population Reports* Series 1, No. 1. 1974.

31. Billings, J. J. *Natural Family Planning: The Ovulation Method.* Collegeville, Maryland: Liturgical Press, 1973.

32. Evans, T. N. "Sterilization in women". In Hafez, E. S. E. and Evans, T. N. (eds.). *Human Reproduction: Conception and Contraception.* London: Harper & Row, 1973.

33. Wortman, J. "Tubal sterilization—review of methods". *Population Reports* Series C, No. 7, 1976.

34. Wortman, J. and Piotrow, P. T. "Colpotomy—the vaginal approach". *Population Reports* Series C, No. 3, 1973.

35. Darabi, K. F. and Richard, R. M. "Collaborative study on hysteroscopic sterilization procedures". *Obstetrics and Gynaecology* 49: 48, 1977.

36. Wortman, J. and Piotrow, P. T. "Vasectomy—old and new techniques". *Population Reports* Series D, No. 1, 1973.

37. Wortman, J. "Vasectomy—what are the problems?" *Population Reports* Series D, No. 2, 1975.

Suggested reading

Guillebaud, J. *The Pill.* Oxford: Oxford University Press, 1980.

CHAPTER 4: INFERTILITY

Further reading

Behrman, S. J. and Menge, A. C. "Immunologic Aspects of Infertility". In Hafez, E. S. E. and Evans, T. N. (eds.). *Human Reproduction: Conception and Contraception.* London: Harper & Row, 1973.

Eliasson, R. "Parameters of male fertility". In Hafez, E. S. E. and Evans, T. N. (eds.). *Human Reproduction: Conception and Contraception.* London: Harper & Row, 1973.

Newill, R. *Infertile Marriage.* London: Penguin Books, 1974.

Philipp, E. *Childlessness: Its Causes and What To Do About Them.* London: Arrow Books, 1975.

CHAPTER 5: HAVING CHILDREN

1. Gabbe, S. G., Ettinger, B. B., Freeman, R. K. and Martin, C. B. "Umbilical cord compression associated with amniotomy: laboratory

observations". *American Journal of Obstetrics and Gynaecology* 126: 353, 1976.

2. Leboyer, F. *Birth Without Violence*. London: Fontana, new edition 1977.

3. MacMahon, B., Cole, P. and Brown, P. "Etiology of human breast cancer: a review". *Journal of the National Cancer Institute* 50: 21, 1973.

4. Collea, J. V., Rabin, S. C., Weghorst, G. R. and Quilligan, E. J. "The randomized management of term frank breech presentation: vaginal delivery v. Caesarean section". *American Journal of Obstetrics and Gynaecology* 131: 186, 1978.

5. U.S. Food and Drug Administration. "Fetal alcohol syndrome". *FDA Drug Bulletin* 7: 18, 1977.

6. Clarren, S. K. and Smith, D. W. "The fetal alcohol syndrome". *New England Journal of Medicine* 298: 1063, 1978.

7. Meyer, M. B. and Tonascia, J. A. "Maternal smoking, pregnancy complications and perinatal mortality". *American Journal of Obstetrics and Gynaecology* 128: 494, 1977.

8. Pirani, B. B. K. "Smoking during pregnancy". *Obstetrical and Gynaecological Survey* 33: 1, 1978.

General references and suggested reading

Bing, E. *Six Practical Lessons for Easier Childbirth*. New York: Bantam Books, 1969.

Cartwright, A. *The Dignity of Labour? A Study of Childbearing and Induction*. London: Tavistock, 1979.

Dowrick, S. and Grundberg, S. *Why Children?* London: The Women's Press, 1980.

Greenhill, J. P. and Friedman, E. A. *The Biological Principles and Modern Practice of Obstetrics*. Eastbourne: Holt-Saunders, 1974.

Karmel, M. *Thank YOU, Dr Lamaze*. Garden City, New York: Dolphin Books, 1959.

Kitzinger, S. *The Experience of Childbirth*. London: Victor Gollancz, revised edition 1972.

Klaus, M. H. and Kennell, J. H. *Impact of Early Separation or Loss on Family Development: Maternal-Infant Bonding*. St Louis, Missouri: C. V. Mosby, 1977.

Olds, S. W. and Eiger, M. S. *The Complete Book of Breast Feeding*. New York: Workman Publishing Company 1972.

Phillip, E. *Childbirth: A Complete Guide to Every Problem*. London: Fontana, 1978.

Pryor, K. *Nursing Your Baby*. New York: Pocket Books, 1972.

Rakowitz, E. and Rubin, G. S. *Living With Your New Baby*. London: Hamlyn Paperbacks, 1981.

Romney, S. L., *et al. Gynaecology and Obstetrics: The Health Care of Women*. Maidenhead, Berkshire: McGraw-Hill, 1975.

1. Tietze, C. "The effect of legalization of abortion on population growth and public health". *Family Planning Perspectives* 7: 123, 1975.
2. Rudel, H. W., Kincl, F. A. and Henzl, M. R. *Birth Control, Contraception and Abortion.* New York: Macmillan, 1973, chapter 6.
3. U.S. Department of Health, Education and Welfare, Centre for Disease Control. "Comparative risks of three methods of mid-trimester abortion". *Mortality and Morbidity Weekly Report*, 26 November 1976, p. 370.
4. Grimes, D. A., Schulz, K. F., Cates, W. and Tyler, C. W. "Mid-trimester abortion by dilation and evacuation". *New England Journal of Medicine* 296: 1141, 1977.
5. Office of Population Statistics. *Abortion Statistics.* London: Her Majesty's Stationery Office, 1974, 1975, 1976, 1977.
6. Registrar-General, *Statistical Review of England and Wales 1968–73.* London: Her Majesty's Stationery Office.
7. Department of Health and Social Security. *Report on Confidential Enquiries into Maternal Deaths in England and Wales, 1970–72* and *1973–75.*
8. Office of Population Censuses and Surveys. *Abortion Statistics 1979.* London: Her Majesty's Stationery Office.
9. Savage, W. D. "Abortion and Sterilization". *British Journal of Family Planning*, April 1981, pp.8-12.
10. Grimes, D. A. and Cates, W. "Complications from legally induced abortions: a review". *Obstetrical and Gynaecological Survey* 34: 177, 1979.
11. U.S. Department of Health, Education and Welfare, Centre for Disease Control. "Abortion Surveillance 1976". August 1978.
12. Harlap, S., Shiono, P., Ramcharan, S., Berendes, H. and Pellegrin, F. "A prospective study of spontaneous fetal losses after induced abortions". *New England Journal of Medicine* 301: 677–81, 1979.
13. Daling, J. R. and Emanuel, I. "Induced abortion and subsequent outcome of pregnancy: a matched cohort study". *The Lancet* 2: 170–72, 1975.
14. Daling, J. R. and Emanuel, I. "Induced abortion and subsequent outcome of pregnancy in a series of American women". *New England Journal of Medicine* 297: 1241–45, 1977.
15. Richardson, J. A. and Dixon, G. "Effects of legal termination on subsequent pregnancy". *British Medical Journal* 1: 1303, 1976.
16. Brewer, C. "Induced abortion after feeling fetal movements: its causes and emotional consequences". *Journal of Biosocial Science* 10: 203, 1980.
17. Simms, M. *Report on Non-Medical Abortion Counselling.* Birth Control Trust, 1973, revised 1977.

General references and suggested reading

Ashton, J. R. "Characteristics of special groups of abortion patients from one health district". *Journal of Biosocial Science* 13: 63–9, 1980.

Ashton, J. R. "Components of delay amongst women obtaining termination of pregnancy". *Journal of Biosocial Science* 12: 261–73, 1980.

Ashton, J. R. "Experiences of women refused National Health Service abortion". *Journal of Biosocial Science* 12: 201–210, 1980.

Ashton, J. R. "Patterns of discussion and decision-making amongst abortion patients". *Journal of Biosocial Science* 12, 247–59, 1980.

Ashton, J. R. "Provision of induced abortion in Wessex Health Region: unmet need and feasibility of compensatory day care". *Journal of the Royal Society of Medicine* 73: March 1980.

Ashton, J. R. "The psychosocial outcome of induced abortion". *British Journal of Obstetrics and Gynaecology* 87: 1115–22, December 1980.

Ashton, J. R. "Sex education and contraceptive practice amongst abortion patients". *Journal of Biosocial Science* 12: 211–217, 1980.

Ashton, J. R., Chamberlain, A., Dennis, K. J., Rowe, R. G., Waters, W. E. and Wheeler, M. J. "The Wessex Abortion Studies: II. Attitudes of consultant gynaecologists to provision of abortion services". *The Lancet,* 19 January 1980.

Ashton, J. R., Dennis, K. J., Rowe, R. G., Waters, W. E. and Wheeler, M. J. "The Wessex Abortion Studies: I. Interdistrict variation in provision of abortion services". *The Lancet,* 12 January 1980.

Callahan, D. *Abortion: Law, Choice and Morality.* New York: Macmillan, 1970.

Denes, M. *In Necessity and Sorrow.* New York: Basic Books, 1976.

Family Planning Perspectives, a bimonthly publication of the Planned Parenthood Federation of America.

Francke, L. B. *The Ambivalence of Abortion.* London: Penguin Books, 1980.

Group for the Advancement of Psychiatry. *The Right to Abortion: A Psychiatric View.* New York: Charles Scribner's Sons, 1969.

Potts, M., Diggory, P. and Peel, J. *Abortion.* Cambridge: Cambridge University Press, 1977.

The Report of the Royal Commission of Inquiry: Contraception, Sterilisation and Abortion in New Zealand. Wellington: March 1977.

For information

The two main abortion charities in Britain are the British Pregnancy Advisory Service, which has branches in most large cities and whose headquarters are at Austy Manor, Wootton Warren, Solihull, West

399

Midlands (Henley-in-Arden 3225); and the Pregnancy Advisory Service at 40 Margaret Street, London W1 (01-409 0281).

CHAPTER 7: GENETICS AND ANTENATAL DIAGNOSIS

1. Cavalieri, L. "New strains of life-or-death". The New York *Times Magazine*, 22 August 1976, p. 8.
2. Saxen, L. "Embryonic induction". *Clinical Obstetrics and Gynaecology* 18: 149, 1975.
3. Smith, A. *The Human Pedigree: Inheritance and the Genetics of Mankind*. London: Allen & Unwin, 1975, p. 126.
4. NICHD National Registry for Amniocentesis Study Group. "Mid-trimester amniocentesis for prenatal diagnosis: safety and accuracy". *Journal of the American Medical Association* 236: 1471, 1976.
5. Simpson, N. E., *et al.* "Prenatal diagnosis of genetic disease in Canada: report of a collaborative study". *Canadian Medical Association Journal* 115: 739, 1976.
6. Mennuti, M. "Prenatal genetic diagnosis: current status". *New England Journal of Medicine* 297: 1004, 1977.
7. Golbus, M. S., *et al.* "Prenatal genetic diagnosis in 3000 amniocenteses". *New England Journal of Medicine* 300: 157. 1979.
8. Rorvik, D. M. and Shettles, L. B. *Your Baby's Sex: Now You Can Choose*. New York: Bantam Books, 1970.

CHAPTER 8: EVERYDAY GOOD HEALTH

1. Chase, D. *The Medically Based No-nonsense Beauty Book*. New York: Alfred A. Knopf, 1975, chapters 11–15.
2. Garfinkel, J., Selvin, S. and Brown, S. M. "Possible increased risk of lung cancer among beauticians". *Journal of the National Cancer Institute* 58: 141, 1977.
3. Menck, H. R., *et al.* "Lung cancer risk among beauticians and other female workers". *Journal of the National Cancer Institute* 59: 1423, 1977.
4. Farah, A. P. "Be armed against perspiration". *Family Health/Today's Health* 8: 58, 1976.
5. Wilson, L. A., Julian, A. J. and Ahern, D. G. "The survival and growth of micro-organisms in mascara during use". *American Journal of Ophthalmology* 79: 596, 1975.
6. U.S. Food and Drug Administration. "Proposal to establish monographs for OTC laxative, antidiarrhoeal, emetic and anti-emetic products". *Federal Register* 40, No. 56: 12902, 21 March 1975.
7. Finn, R. and Wainscoat, J. S. "Laxan nephropathy". *The Lancet*. 25 May 1975, p. 1202.
8. Chase, D., op. cit., p. 89.

9. Hughes, L. E. and Webster, D. J. T. "The treatment of early breast cancer". *British Journal of Hospital Medicine* 23: 22–31, 1980.

10. "Saccharin and chemical carcinogenesis". *Medical Letter on Drugs and Therapeutics* 19: 75, 1977.

11. Leff, D. N. "Megavitamin therapy: does it work?" *McCall's*. September 1974, p. 47.

12. "Myths of vitamins". *FDA Consumer*. U.S. Department of Health, Education and Welfare Publication No. (FDA) 74-2053, March 1974.

13. Committee on Nutrition of the Mother and Pre-school Child. "Oral contraceptives and nutrition". *National Academy of Sciences*. Washington, D.C., 1975.

14. Orbach, S. *Fat is a Feminist Issue*. London: Hamlyn Paperbacks, new edition 1979.

15. "Bypass operation for obesity". *Medical Letter on Drugs and Therapeutics* 20: 33, 1978.

16. "Stapling creates mini-stomach for obese patients". *Medical World News,* 16 October 1978, p. 17.

17. Cohen, S. and Booth, G. H. "Gastric acid secretion and lower-oesophageal-sphincter pressure in response to coffee and caffeine". *New England Journal of Medicine* 293: 897, 1975.

18. "Coffee and cardiovascular disease". *Medical Letter on Drugs and Therapeutics* 19: 65, 1977.

19. "Another look at coffee". *Harvard Medical School Health Letter* 3, No. 6: 5, 1978.

20. "High density lipoproteins (HDL)". *Medical Letter on Drugs and Therapeutics* 21: 1, 1979.

21. "Update on coronary artery disease". *Harvard Medical School Health Letter* 3, No. 4: 1, 1978.

22. Mendeloff, A. K. "Dietary fibre and human health". *New England Journal of Medicine* 297: 811, 1977.

23. "A holiday check list". *Harvard Medical School Health Letter* 3, No. 2: 1, 1977.

24. Slone, D., *et al.* "Relation of cigarette smoking to myocardial infarction in young women". *New England Journal of Medicine* 298: 1273, 1978.

25. Stolley, P. D. "Lung cancer: an unwanted equality for women". *New England Journal of Medicine* 297: 886, 1977.

26. "Heavy smokers reach menopause earlier than nonsmokers". *The Female Patient*, November 1977, p. 53.

27. Califano, J. A., Jr. National Cancer Programme Special Communication on Smoking, 28 March 1978.

28. Everson, R. B. "Individuals transplacentally exposed to maternal smoking may be at increased cancer risk in adult life". *The Lancet*, 19 July 1980, pp. 123–6.

29. Harlap, S. and Shiono, P. H. "Alcohol, smoking and the incidence of spontaneous abortions in the first and second trimester", pp. 173–6; and Kline, J., *et al.* "Drinking during pregnancy and spontaneous abortion", pp. 176–80: both in *The Lancet*, 26 July 1980.

30. "Marijuana". *Medical Letter on Drugs and Therapeutics* 18: 69, 1976.
31. U.S. Secretary of Health, Education and Welfare, 8th Annual Report to the U.S. Congress. "Marijuana and Health". 1980, p. 15.
32. Graham, J. G. P. *Cannabis and Health*. London: Academic Press, 1976, p. 297.

General references and suggested reading

Branca, P. (ed.). *The Medicine Show: Patients, Physicians and the Perplexities of the Health Revolution in Modern Society*. New York: N. Watson Academic Publications, 1978.

Camberwell Council on Alcoholism. *Women and Alcohol*. London: Tavistock, 1980.

Chase, D. *The Medically Based No-nonsense Beauty Book*. New York: Alfred A. Knopf, 1975.

Jacobson, B. *The Ladykillers*. London: Pluto Press, 1981.

Mayer, J. *A Diet for Living*. New York: Pocket Books, 1977.

Royal College of Psychiatrists. *Alcohol and Alcoholism: The Report of a Special Committee*. London: Tavistock, 1979.

For information on stopping smoking

Health Education Council, 78 New Oxford Street, London WC1A 1AH. Tel. 01-637 1881.

Produces leaflets and other publications on various health matters, including "The Smoker's Guide to Non-Smoking" (catalogue no. AS23) and "Why I Stopped Smoking" (catalogue no. AS3).

Action on Smoking and Health (ASH), Margaret Pyke House, 27-35 Mortimer Street, London W1A 4QW. Tel. 01-637 9843.

National Society of Non-Smokers, Latimer House, Hanson Street, London W1. Tel. 01-636 9103.

CHAPTER 10: CHANGE OF LIFE

1. Friederich, M. A. "Psychophysiology of menstruation and the menopause". In Romney. S. L., *et al*, *Gynaecology and Obstetrics: The Health Care of Women*. Maidenhead, Berkshire: McGraw-Hill, 1975, p. 603.
2. Rybo, B. and Westerberg, H. "Symptoms in the postmenopause: a population study. A preliminary report". *Acta Obstetrica Gynaecologica Scandinavia* 50: 25, 1971.
3. Ballinger, C. B. "Psychiatric morbidity and the menopause: screening of general population sample". *British Medical Journal* 3: 344, 1975.
4. Morrison, J. C., Givens, J. R., Wiser, W. L. and Fish, S. A. "Mumps oophoritis: a cause of premature menopause". *Fertility and Sterility* 6: 655, 1975.

5. Coulam, C. B. and Ryan, R. J. "Premature menopause. I. Etiology". *American Journal of Obstetrics and Gynaecology* 133: 639, 1979.
6. Meema, S., Bunker, M. L. and Meema, H. E. "Preventive effect of oestrogen on postmenopausal bone loss". *Archives of Internal Medicine* 135: 1436, 1975.
7. Nachtigall, L. E., Nachtigall, R. H., Nachtigall, R. D. and Beckman, E. M. "Oestrogen replacement therapy I: a 10-year prospective study in the relationship to osteoporosis". *Obstetrics and Gynaecology* 53: 277, 1979.
8. Avioli, L. V. "Senile and postmenopausal osteoporosis". *Advances in Internal Medicine* 21: 391, 1976.
9. National Institutes of Health. "Over-the-counter antacid preparations can have adverse effects on bone". *Journal of the American Medical Association* 238: 1018, 1977.

Suggested reading

Sheehy, G. *Passages: Predictable Crises in Adult Life.* London: Corgi Books, new edition 1977.
Studd, J. and Thom, M. *The Menopause.* London: Hamlyn Paperbacks, 1981.

CHAPTER II: DISEASES OF WOMEN

1. Fleury, F. J., *et al.* "Single dose of two grams of metronidazole for *Trichomonas vaginalis* infection". *American Journal of Obstetrics and Gynaecology* 128: 320, 1977.
2. Thelin, I., Wennström, A.-M. and Mardh, P.-A. "Contact-tracing in patients with genital chlamydial infection". *British Journal of Venereal Diseases* 56: 259–62, 1980.
3. "Herpes simplex viruses and cervical cancer". *Journal of the American Medical Association* 238: 1614, 1977.
4. Rawls, W. E., Gardner, H. L. and Kaufman, R. L. "Antibodies to genital herpes virus in patients with carcinoma of the cervix". *American Journal of Obstetrics and Gynaecology* 107: 710, 1970.
5. Handsfield, H. H., *et al.* "Asymptomatic gonorrhoea in men: diagnosis, natural course, prevalence and significance". *New England Journal of Medicine* 290: 177, 1974.
6. Singh, B., Cutler, J. C. and Utidijian, H. M. D. "Studies on the development of a vaginal preparation providing both prophylaxis against venereal disease and other genital infections and contraception". *British Journal of Venereal Diseases* 48: 57, 1972.
7. Smith, P. J. B. "The management of urethral syndrome". *British Journal of Hospital Medicine* 22 (6): 578, 1979.
8. Anderson, A., *et al.* "Trial of prostaglandin synthetase inhibitors in primary dysmenorrhoea". *The Lancet*, 18 February 1978, p. 345.
9. Henzl, M. L., Buttram, V., Segre, E. J. and Bressler, S. "The

treatment of dysmenorrhoea with naproxen sodium". *American Journal of Obstetrics and Gynaecology* 127: 818, 1977.

10. Corson, S. L. and Bolognese, R. J. "Ibuprofen therapy for dysmenorrhoea". *Journal of Reproductive Medicine* 20: 246, 1978.

11. Masters, W. H. and Johnson, V. E. *Human Sexual Response*. Boston: Little, Brown, 1966, pp. 119–22.

12. "Danazol [Danol]—a new drug for endometriosis". *Medical Letter on Drugs and Therapeutics* 19: 62, 1977.

13. MacMahon, B., Cole, P. and Brown P. "Etiology of human breast cancer: a review". *Journal of the National Cancer Institute* 50: 21, 1973.

14. Hoover, R., Gray, L. A., Cole, P. and MacMahon, B. "Menopausal oestrogens and breast cancer". *New England Journal of Medicine* 295: 401, 1976.

15. Vorherr, H. and Messer, R. H. "Breast cancer: potentially predisposing and protecting factors". *American Journal of Obstetrics and Gynaecology* 130: 335, 1978.

16. U.S. Department of Health, Education and Welfare. "Multiple fluoroscopies and breast cancer". *FDA Drug Bulletin* 6: 38, 1976.

17. Shimkin, M. B. "Epidemiology of breast cancer". In Griem, M. L., *et al.* "Breast cancer: a challenging problem". *Recent Results in Cancer Research* 42: 6, 1973.

18. Sarkar, N. H. and Moore, D. H. "Viral transmission in breast cancer". In Griem, *et al.*, op. cit., p. 15.

19. Mavligit, G. M., Gutterman, J. U. and Hersh, E. M. "Immunologic aspects of human cancer". In Castro, J. R., Meyler, T. S. and Baker, D. C. (eds.). *Current Concepts in Breast Cancer and Tumour Immunology*. New York: Medical Examination Publishing Company, 1974, p. 237.

20. Oettgen, H. F. "Immunotherapy of cancer". *New England Journal of Medicine* 297: 484, 1977.

21. Herbst, A.L. , Ulfelder, H. and Poskanzer, D. C. "Adenocarcinoma of the vagina. Association of maternal stilboestrol therapy with tumour appearance in young women". *New England Journal of Medicine* 284: 878, 1971.

22. Herbst, A. L., *et al.* "Age-incidence and risk of diethylstilboestrol-related clear cell carcinoma of the vagina and cervix". *American Journal of Obstetrics and Gynaecology* 128: 43, 1977.

23. Lyon, F. A. and Frisch, M. J. "Endometrial abnormalities occurring in young women on long-term sequential oral contraception". *Obstetrics and Gynaecology* 47: 639, 1976.

24. Ziel, H. K. and Finkle, W. D. "Increased risk of endometrial carcinoma among users of conjugated oestrogens". *New England Journal of Medicine* 293: 1167, 1975.

25. Smith, D. C., Prentice, R., Thompson, D. J. and Herrman, W. L. "Association of exogenous oestrogen and endometrial cancer". *New England Journal of Medicine* 293: 1164, 1975.

26. Lipsett, M. B. "Hormonal induction of breast cancer". In Griem, *et al.*, op. cit., p. 28.
27. Kennedy, B. J. "Appearance and spread of human breast cancer". In Griem, *et al.*, op. cit., p. 31.
28. Fasal, E. and Paffenbarger, R. S. "Oral contraceptives as related to cancer and benign lesions of the breast". *Journal of the National Cancer Institute* 55: 767, 1975.
29. McGregor, D. H., *et al.* "Breast cancer incidence among atomic bomb survivors, Hiroshima and Nagasaki, 1950–1969". *Journal of the National Cancer Institute* 59: 799, 1977.
30. Simon, N. "Breast cancer induced by radiation: relation to mammography and treatment of acne". *Journal of the American Medical Association* 237: 789, 1977.
31. Aksu, M. F. Tzingonnis, V. A. and Greenblatt, R. B. "Treatment of benign breast disease with Danazol [Danol]: a follow-up report". *Journal of Reproductive Medicine* 21: 181, 1978.
32. "Benign breast disease tied to coffee, tea, cocoa, cola". *Medical World News* 20: 11, 1979.
33. Minton, J. P., Foecking, M. K., Webster, D. J. T. and Matthews, R. H. "Response of fibro-cystic disease to caffeine withdrawal and correlation of cyclic nucleotides with breast disease". *American Journal of Obstetrics and Gynaecology* 135: 157, 1979.
34. Lou. M. A., Mandel, A. K. and Alexander, J. L. "The pros and cons of out-patient breast biopsy". *Archives of Surgery* 111: 668, 1976.
35. Witkin, M. H. "Sex therapy and mastectomy". *Journal of Sexual and Marital Therapy* 1: 290. 1975.
36. Watts, G. T. "Restorative prosthetic mammaplasty in mastectomy for carcinoma and benign lesions". *Clinics in Plastic Surgery* 3: 177, 1976.
37. Asken, M. J. "Psychoemotional aspects of mastectomy: a review of recent literature". *American Journal of Psychiatry* 132: 56, 1975.
38. Kaufman, R. H., Binder, G. L., Gray, P. M. M. and Adam, E. "Upper genital tract changes associated with exposure in utero to diethylstilboestrol". *American Journal of Obstetrics and Gynaecology* 128: 51, 1977.
39. Goldstein, D. P. "Incompetent cervix in offspring exposed to diethylstilboestrol in utero". *Obstetrics and Gynaecology* 52: 73s, 1978.
40. Fowler, W. C. and Edelman, D. A. "In utero exposure to DES". *Obstetrics and Gynaecology* 51: 459, 1978.
41. Robboy, S. J., *et al.* "Squamous cell dysplasia and carcinoma in situ of the cervix and vagina after prenatal exposure to diethylstilboestrol". *Obstetrics and Gynaecology* 51: 528, 1978.
42. Bibbo, M., *et al.* "A twenty-five-year follow-up study of women exposed to diethylstilboestrol during pregnancy". *New England Journal of Medicine* 298: 763, 1978.
43. Gill, W. B., Schumacher, G. F. B. and Bibbo, M. "Structural and functional abnormalities in the sex organs of male offspring of

mothers treated with diethylstilboestrol (DES)". *Journal of Reproductive Medicine* 16: 147, 1976.

44. Bibbo, M., *et al.* "Follow-up study of male and female offspring of DES-exposed mothers". *Obstetrics and Gynaecology* 49: 1, 1977.
45. "Penicillamine for rheumatoid arthritis". *Medical Letter on Drugs and Therapeutics* 20: 73, 1978.

General references and suggested reading

Cancer and the Worker. New York: New York Academy of Sciences, 1977.

Clark, J. *Pre-menstrual Tension*. London: Hamlyn Paperbacks, 1980.

Committee of the American Rheumatism Association of the Arthritis Foundation. *Primer on the Rheumatic Diseases*, 7th edition. New York: The Arthritis Foundation, 1973.

Conn, H. F. (ed.). *Current Therapy, 1979*. Philadelphia: W. B. Saunders, 1979.

Dalton, K. *Once a Month*. London: Fontana, 1978.

Dalton, K. *Premenstrual Syndrome and Progesterone Therapy*. London: Heinemann Medical, 1977.

Evans, P. *Cystitis and How to Cope With It*. London: Granada, 1979.

Fernandes, L. *Arthritis and Rheumatism*. London: Hamlyn Paperbacks, 1980.

Gardner, H. L. and Kaufman, R. H. *Benign Diseases of the Vulva and Vagina*. St Louis, Missouri: Mosby, 1969.

Joseph, S. *Heart Trouble*. London: Hamlyn Paperbacks, 1981.

Kilmartin, Angela. *Cystitis: A Complete Self-Help Guide*. London: Hamlyn Paperbacks, 1980.

Lever, J., Brush, M. and Haynes, B. *PMT: The Unrecognized Illness*. London: Melbourne House, 1979.

Thorne, G. W., *et al.* (eds.). *Harrison's Principles of Internal Medicine*. New York: McGraw-Hill, 1977.

CHAPTER 12: SEXUAL HEALTH

Information on sex

Brecher, R. and Brecher E. (eds.). *An Analysis of Human Sexual Response*. New York: Signet, 1966.

Friday, N. *My Secret Garden*. New York: Pocket Books, 1974.

Gadpaille, W. J. *The Cycles of Sex*. New York: Charles Scribner's Sons, 1975.

Masters, W. H. and Johnson, V. E. *Human Sexual Response*. Boston: Little, Brown, 1966.

Sexual dysfunction

Barbach, L. G. *For Yourself*. Garden City, New York: Doubleday,

1975, Anchor, 1976.

Belliveau, F. and Richter, L. *Understanding Human Sexual Inadequacy*. London: Coronet Books, 1971.

Kaplan, H. S. *The Illustrated Manual of Sex Therapy*. London: Souvenir Press, 1976.

Kline-Graber, G. and Graber, B. *Women's Orgasm*. New York: Popular Library, 1976.

Masters, W. H. and Johnson, V. E. *Human Sexual Inadequacy*. Boston: Little, Brown, 1970.

Marriage

Gottner, J., Notarus, C., Gonso, T. and Markman, H. *A Couple's Guide to Communication*. Champaign, Illinois: Research Press, 1976.

Divorce

Weiss, R. *Marital Separation*. New York: Basic Books, 1977.

Women in Transition. Brighton: Harvester Press, 1980.

Mental Health

Brown, G. W. and Harris, T. *Social Origins of Depression: A Study of Psychiatric Disorder in Women*. London: Tavistock, 1978.

Ernst, S. and Goodison, L. *In Our Own Hands: A Book of Self-Help Therapy*. London: The Women's Press, 1981.

Miller, J. B. (ed.). *Psychoanalysis and Women*. London: Penguin Books, 1974.

Park, C. C. and Shapiro, L. *You Are Not Alone*. Boston: Atlantic/ Little, Brown, 1976.

Stanway, A. *Overcoming Depression*. London: Hamlyn Paperbacks, 1981.

Rape

Amir, M. *Patterns in Forcible Rape*. London: University of Chicago Press, 1971.

Brownmiller, S. *Against Our Will: Men, Women and Rape*. London: Penguin Books, new edition 1977.

Index

Body temperature: infertility and sperm production and, 97, 101, 106; rhythm birth control and, 78

Boils, 295; cloxacillin for, 295

Bone marrow, anaemia and, 357, 359

Bone thinning and loss. See Osteoporosis

Bottle-feeding, nursing and, 157; supplemental, 157; weaning and, 157

Bowel habits (bowel hygiene), 234; constipation and (see Constipation); cystitis and, 304; laxatives, 234-5; regulating, 234; routine stool exams, 392; vaginal hygiene, 225; vulvovaginitis and, 266, 267, 268; wind pains, 235-6

Brain damage: birth defects, 158, 217; breech birth and, 158; Caesarean section and, 172; cerebral palsy, 158, Down's Syndrome, 213-14; prematurity and, 166; tumours, infertility and, 96

Brandt-Andrews method of delivery of placenta, 141

Brassieres, use of, 13

Braxton Hicks, contractions, 136, 138

Bread, 246; high-fibre, 252

Breakthrough bleeding, the pill and, 42

Breast cancer, 180, 281, 286, 333-48; benign breast diseases and, 339; biopsies, 341-2; breast-feeding and, 157; causes, 333-6; chemotherapy, 347; Depo-Provera and, 55; DES and, 355-6; early detection, 337-40; examination by a doctor, 338, 390-1; high-risk categories, 334-5; hormonal dependence of tumours and treatment of, 346-7; latent period, 332-3; mammography and (see Mammography); mastectomy and (see Mastectomy); oestrogen and prolactin and, 334-5; the pill and, 45, 46, 51, 334-5; pregnancy risks and, 182; radiation therapy, 336-7, 345-6; risk statistics, 333, 337, 348; self-examination, 337-8, 391; varieties of treatment, 342-7

Breast-feeding, 123, 153-7; as best nutrition for newborn, 153-5; as contraception, 153, 156; food substances—recommended daily allowances, 260-2; groups and information on, 157; how milk is produced, 154-5; how to start, 156; the pill and, 52; premature infants and, 157; preparing breasts for, 156; weaning to bottle, 157

Breasts (breast changes): abscess, 341; benign tumours, 341; brassieres and, 13; and breast-feeding (see Breast-feeding); cancer (see Breast cancer); cosmetic surgery, 241; enlargement in newborn, 264; examining, 337-8, 391; fibroadenomas, 341; fibrocystic disease, 340-1; oestrogen and progesterone effect on, 23; oestrogen-replacement therapy and, 281; the pill and, 43, 45, 46, 51, 334-5; in pregnancy, 117, 130; puberty and premature development of, 12-13; soreness, 12-13; tenderness, abortions and, 196; tenderness, menopause and, 275, 276, 280, tenderness, normal before menstruation, 23

Breast surgery, cosmetic, 241-2 (see also Mastectomy); avoiding silicone injections, 241, reduction and enlargement, 241-2; silicone implants, 241

Breath, shortness in pregnancy, 128

Breathing exercise, in labour and delivery, 140

Breath odour, 226

Breech birth, 158, 160, 171, 172

Bridgework, dental care and, 244

Bromocriptine (Parlodel), 105, 106

Brown, Lesley, 110-11

Bulk stool softeners, 234

Butenandt, Adolf, 36

B vitamins. See under Vitamins

Caesarean section, 146, 158, 169-72, 176; anaesthesia, 172; incisions, 170; procedure, 170-1; repetitions, 172; when necessary, 171-2

Caffeine, use of 251, 258

Calcium: breast-feeding and, 155; need in pregnancy, 120; osteoporosis and, 282-3; recommended daily allowance, 260

Calculus (tooth decay), 242-3, 244

Calendar method of rhythm birth control, 77; and temperature method combined, 78

Calories, 245, 246

Cancer, 332-56 (see also specific kinds): breast (see Breast cancer); carcinogens, 332, 334, 353; causes, 333-6; cervical (see Cervical cancer); chemotherapy, 347; DES and, 355-6; endometrial (see Endometrial cancer); herpes and, 296, 349; IUD and, 61; latent period, 332-3; oestrogen-replacement therapy, 281; the pill and, 45, 51-2, 334-5; promoters, 332, 335; research, 332; statistics, 333; uterus/endometrial carcinoma, 353-4; vaginal, 354-6

Candidiasis (thrush or moniliasis), 288-91, 293, 386, chronic, 290-1; diagnosis, 291; in little girls, 266, 267; side effects of medications, 43-4, 291; symptoms and treatment, 32, 288-91

Cannula, 189

Capacitation, sperm, and, 92; and infertility, 99

Carbohydrates, 243, 245 (see also Sugar); recommended daily allowances, 260

Carcinogens, 332, 334-5, 353; DES and, 335-6; oestrogen and, 333, 334-5, 346, 353, 355-6

Carcinoma-in-situ: cervical, 350, 352; endometrial, 353

Cardiovascular disease, 281-2 (see also Arteriosclerosis; Heart disease; Hypertension; Stroke); oestrogen-replacement therapy and, 281-2

"Carrier state" genes, 211

Catheterization, as cause of cystitis, 304, 306

Cattle (livestock), DES and, 334

Caudal anaesthesia, 143

Cauterization sterilization, 83-6

Cell differentiation and division (see also Differentiation, cellular and organic): birth defects and, 210; chromosomes and, 207-8, 209; induction and, 209

Cephalopelvic disproportion, Caesarean section for, 171, 172

Cerclage, 163

Cerebral palsy, 158, 167

Cervical cancer, 51, 55, 277, 348-54; biopsy, 350; causes, 348; Depo-Provera and, 54-5; DES and, 355; herpes and, 295, 296, 349; hysterectomy for, 352; latent period, 332-3, 350; the pill and, 51; pregnancy and, 180; sexual activity and, 348; smear tests, 296, 342, 349, 352; stages and treatment, 349-54

Cervical cap, 63-6

Cervical mucus, 21, 38, 137, infertility and, 92, 95, 102, 108; and rhythm birth-control method, 78-9

Cervical rings, 56

Cervical smear, 100, 277, 296, 342, 349, 352

Cervicitis, 176, 297, 306; advanced, 297; cystitis and, 306

Cervix (cervical glands), 21-2; abortions and, 190-1, 199; adenosis, 355; cancer (*see* Cervical cancer); cervicitis (*see* Cervicitis); effect of oestrogen and progesterone on, 20-21; eversion (ectropion), 297; incompetent and immature delivery, 163-4, 355; infertility and, 92, 95, 101; laminaria to dilate, 199; mucus (*see* Cervical mucus); polyps, 330; pregnancy, labour and delivery and, 118, 136, 138-40, 159, 163-4; subtotal hysterectomy (supracervical), 328

"Chadwick's Sign," 118

Chancroid, 302

Change of life, *See* Menopause

Charcoal, for wind pains, 235

Chastity belts, 81

Chemical contraceptives, *See* Vaginal chemical contraceptives

Chemicals, industrial (*see also* Environmental pollution): infertility and, 97; and pregnancy dangers, 181-2

Chemotherapy, 347, 352, 354

Childbirth. *See* Delivery (childbirth)

Childlessness: abortions and (*see* Abortions): adoption and, 111; infertility and, 91-111; pregnancy and child-bearing and, 112-85

Children (little girls), 264-9 (*see also* Adolescence; Babies); abortions (*see* Abortions); assaults and rape of, 388; breast enlargement in, 264; confusion as to sex of, 265; dental care, 242-4; developmental problems, 265-6; foreign objects in vagina, 267; genital swelling and discharge, 264; imperforate hymen, 265; labial agglutination, 267-8; masturbation, 269; premature development of breasts and pubic hair, 265-6, urinary infections, 268; vaginal discharge and related problems, 266-8 (*see also* Vaginal problems in little girls); virginity and, 269; vulvovaginitis, 266-8

Chlamydia, 293

Chloasma (mask of pregnancy), 45, 129

Chloroform, toothpastes with, 243

Cholesterol, 36, 48-9, 246, 251-2; lipoproteins and, 252; stress and, 259; test for, 392

Chorea, Huntington's, 212

Chorea, Sydenham's 46, 50, 368

Chromosomes, 207-9; anomalies and birth defects and, 210, 212-14; and drug use and pregnancy risks, 182; functions of, 207-8; genes and, 207-8, 211; mutations and, 208, 210; non-disjunction, 213; role in normal development, 207-9; and sex determination, 209

Cigarettes (nicotine). *See* Smoking

Cilia, 21

Circadian Phase Shift ("jet lag"), 234

Cirrhosis of the liver, alcohol and, 256

"Clap," *See* Gonorrhea

Cleanliness. *See* Hygiene

Clear cell adenocarcinoma, 355

Clergy, and abortions, 204

Clinics, abortion, choosing, 202

Clitoris, 374-5; in female arousal and orgasm, 374-5, 376, 378, 381

Clomid (clomiphene citrate), 105-6, 107, 109

Cloning, 111

Clothing: body odour and, 226; pregnancy and, 121

Clotting disorders. *See* Blood-clotting disorders

Cloxacillin, for boils, 295

Coffee, 251, 258; decaffeinated, 251

Coitus interruptus, 103

Colic (wind pains), diet and breast-feeding and, 155

Collagen, 239; and wrinkles, 239

Collagen sponge diaphragm, 66

Colon cancer, high-fibre foods and, 252

Colostrum, 155

Colour blindness, 210

Colouring hair, *See* Dyes, hair

Colposcopy, 351

Colpotomy, 82, 86

Committee on the Safety of Medicines, 232

Conception and development of pregnancy, 113-18 (*see also* Conceptus; Fertility; Infertility; Pregnancy); immunology of conception, 95, 98-9; 109; moment of conception, 113

Conceptus, 114, 165; cell division and, 209; miscarriage and, 162

Condoms, use of, 72-3; after childbirth, 152; for birth control, 72-3; effectiveness, 73; to prevent VD, 30, 72, 300.

Condyloma lata, 301

Condylomata acuminata (venereal warts), 294

Cone biopsy, 350-1

Congenital birth defects, 210-11 (*see also* Birth defects; specific kinds)

Constipation, 234 (*see also* Bowel habits); avoiding, 131; and menstrual cramps, 313; in pregnancy, 125, 131

Contact dermatitis, perfumes and, 230

Contact-lens wearers, the pill and, 50

Contraceptives (contraception), 35-90 (*see also* Birth control; specific kinds); abstinence, 89; antifertility vaccines, 80; breast-feeding and, 153-4, 156; condoms and other male methods, 72-75; creams, foams, jellies, 66-70; diaphragm, 63-6; hormonal long acting, 53-5, IUD, 55-63, 71; oral, 35-55, 89-90; pessaries, 67-8; the pill and, 35-55 (*see also* Pill, the); post-abortion, 196; postcoital (morning-after pills), 70-1; rhythm method, 75-9; vaginal chemicals, 66-70; voluntary sterilization, 80-89

Cooking and shopping, healthful, 246-7

Copper-containing IUDs, 56-7, 61, 71

Copper 7 (Cu7), 56-7, 61, 71

Copper T, 56-7, 61, 71

Corpus luteum (yellow body), 18, 20, 22 in pregnancy, 114, 116-17; problems infertility and, 92, 93-4, 95, 101, 106-7

Corticosteroids (*see also* Steroids): for acne, 33-4; for arthritis, 364, 370; and infertility, 95-6

Cortisone, 36

Cosmetics, 228-31; allergies, 228, 230; deodorants and antiperspirants, 230; mascara and eye infections, 230-1; nail polish, 231; perfumes and contact dermatitis, 230; preferred hair care, 228-9; reading labels, 228, 232

Cosmetic surgery (plastic surgery) 238-42; after mastectomy, 242, 345; breasts, 241-2, 345; eyelid repair, 241; face lift, 240; nose, 239; qualified surgeons for, 238; wrinkles, 239

Cotton underpants, use of, 225, 288

Counselling: abortions and, 203-4; and genetic testing, 218-19; sex therapy, 380, 382, 383; and Tay-Sachs disease, 216; The British Association for, 380

Cramps: abdominal, in pregnancy, 131; abortions and, 196; IUD and, 59-60; in labour and delivery, 136, 138-9; legs, in pregnancy, 133 menstrual (dysmenorrhea), 23, 43, 311; miscarriage and, 162

Ejaculation: premature, 379, 381; retarded, 379

Elastic sleeves, 344

Elderly, the: health care and, 6; menopause and, 270-85

Elective induction of labour, 147

Electrolysis, hair removal by, 227

Embolus; the pill and, 45, 46-7; pulmonary, 47

Embryo (see also Fetus): differentiation and formation of organs in, 114 (see also Differentiation, cellular and organic)

Emergency births, 149-50

Emotional changes (psychological problems), 25, 44, (see also Anxiety; Depression; Mood changes; Stress; Tension); abortion and, 201-2; dieting and, 25, 30-1; dysmenorrhea and, 311, 312-13; false pregnancy and, 161; hysterectomy and, 325-6; identical twins and, 161; mastectomy and, 344-5; menopause and, 270, 276, 284-5; miscarriage and fetal death and, 165-6; overeating and, 248; the pill and, 44, 46; pregnancy and, 135-6, 161; rape and, 387-8; and sexual dysfunction, 377, 378; tranquillizers and, 257

Employment, stress and fatigue and, 259

Endocrine glands (endocrine function), 92 (see also Hormones; specific aspects, kinds, problems); infertility and, 92, 93, 95, 98, 99

Endocrinologists (endocrinology), 226

Endometrial cancer, 51, 277, 279, 281; biopsy and washing, 100-1, 354; bleeding as major symptom, 353; cure rates, 354; stages and treatment, 353-4

Endometriosis, 331; infertility and, 94, 107; symptoms and treatment of, 107, 331

Endometritis, in abortions, 199

Endometrium, 15, 16, 20, 21, 199, 331; biopsy, 21, 100, 101, 354; cancer (see Endometrial cancer); D & C and, 317; effect of oestrogen and progesterone on glands of, 20; implantation and pregnancy and, 113, 115, 116; infertility and, 94, 100, 101; menopause and, 277, 278, 279, 281; oestrogen-replacement therapy and, 281; the pill and, 42, 44, 51; polyps, 330; in puberty and menstruation, 15, 16, 20, 21

Energy, stress and fatigue and, 259

Enterocele, 309

Environmental factors: and health, 223-4 (see also Environmental pollution; specific aspects, kinds); and inherited characteristics, 210

Environmental medicine, 206

Environmental pollution, 206, 208, 334; breast-feeding and, 154; cancer and 332, 334; and changes in pregnancy, 181-2; infertility and, 95-6

Epididymis, 98

Epidural anaesthesia, 142-3, 147

Epilepsy, the pill and, 46, 51

Episiotomies, 123, 141, 143, 152, 309-10

Ergometrine, 192

Ethinyl oestradiol, 37-8, 89-90

Ethnic groups, birth defects and, 211, 214 (see also specific aspects, groups, kinds)

Ethynodiol diacetate, 38, 89-90

Eugenics, 206

Examinations and screening tests, routine physical, 390-2 (see also specific aspects, kinds, problems)

Exercise (athletics, physical therapy, sports), 253; acne and, 34; adolescent girls and, 27, 34; arthritis and, 363; avoiding now-and-

then strenuous kind, 253; backache in pregnancy and, 132, constipation and, 234; dysmenorrhea and, 314; energy, stress, and fatigue and, 259; essential for good health, 253; and labour and delivery, 140, 147; mastectomy and, 343-4; obesity and, 245, 248, 249, 250; osteoporosis and, 275, 283, postnatal, 153; pregnancy and, 122, 132; sexual problems and, 381; sleeplessness and, 233-4; wrinkles and, 239-40

External version, childbirth and, 159

Eyebrows, avoiding dyes and tints for, 229

Eyelid repair (blepharoplasty), 241

Eye problems; gonorrhea and pregnancy and, 183; infections, mascara use and, 230-1; marijuana use and glaucoma, 257-8; the pill and, 46, 50; in pregnancy, 135, 183; routine exams, 391, 392

Facial care, 238-41; cosmetic surgery, 238-41; discolouration, 240; eyelid repair, 240; hair removal, 226-8; make-up, 228; (see also Cosmetics); wrinkles, 239-40

Fallopian tubes, 18-19, 20, 21, 38, 94, 209; abnormalities and infertility, 92, 94, 107-8; clips or rings, laparoscopy and, 85-6; conception and, 113; effect of oestrogen and progesterone on, 21; infection, gonorrhea and, 299; insufflation, 100, 103; IUD and 60; pregnancy (see Tubal pregnancy); sterilization and (see Tubal sterilization); surgery to correct ligation or scarring, 107-8; surgery to remove, 165

False pregnancy, 161

Family groups, and birth defects, 210-13

Family health history, record-keeping and, 390

Family Planning Association, 380

Fantasies, sexual, 376; rape and, 383

Fat (weight gain). See Obesity; Weight gain and loss

Fatigue, 259; after abortion, 197; Lack of exercise and, 259; poor nutrition and, 259; in pregnancy, 118, 134

Fats, blood. See Blood fats

Fats dietary, 245, 252 (see also Blood fats; Lipoproteins); cholesterol, 251-2; recommended daily allowances, 260

Feet and ankles, pregnancy and oedema of, 134

Ferning test, 22

Ferrous gluconate, 120

Ferrous sulfate, 120

Fertility, 91-111; drugs, 105-6, 160; infertility and 91-111; IUD use and, 60; miscarriage and, 161-2; multiple births, 160; tests, 99-104

Fertilization: cell division immediately after, 209; infertility problem, 98, 113-14; in vitro, 110-11; role of chromosomes in, 207-9, 212-13

Fetal monitoring, 145-6, 171, 172, 179, 183-5; high-risk pregnancies and, 179, 183-5; tests used in late pregnancy, 183-5

Fetoscopy, 218

Fetus, 114-16; abortions, 186-205; alcoholism and, 256; amniocentesis and (see Amniocentesis); birth defects and (see Birth defects); conception and pregnancy and, 114-16, 157-85; drug use and fetal damage, 221, 222 (see also under Pregnancy); effect of the pill on, 52; genetics and antenatal diagnosis, 206-22; infections and fetal damage, 219-22; labour and delivery and, 138-41 (see also Delivery; Labour);

medically high-risk pregnancies and, 179-85; miscarriage and, 161-2 (see also Miscarriage); monitoring (see Fetal monitoring); nourishment in uterus, 115-16; organic differentiation in, 114-15 (see also Differentiation, cellular and organic)
Fibroadenomas, 341
Fibrocystic disease of the breast, 340
Fibroid tumours, uterine, 326-7; hysterectomy for, 326; infertility and, 95, 102, 108; myomectomy for, 327; the pill and, 46, 50-51; symptoms of, 326
Fimbria, 20; fimbriectomy sterilization, 86
Fingernails, infections and, 231
Fish eating, 246
Fistula, bladder, hysterectomy and, 324
Flagyl, for trichomoniasis, 293
Fluoridation, 242
Foams, creams and jellies, spermicidal, 65, 66-8; use of diaphragm with, 65
Folic acid; and deficiency anaemia, 174, 359; need in pregnancy, 120, 174; recommended daily allowance, 262
Follicles, 18 (see also FSH; FSH-RF); ovarian, 18-20
Folliculitis, 295
Food. See Nutrition
Food additives and preservatives, 246; and genetic mutations, 208
Food substances—recommended daily allowances (table), 260-2
Forceps, use in childbirth of, 147, 148
Foreign objects in vagina, 266-7, 268
Formaldehyde, toothpastes with, 243
Franklin, Rosalind, 332
Freckles, 240
Frigidity, sexual, 377
Frozen shoulder, mastectomy and, 344
FSH (Follicle Stimulating Hormone) 18, 19, 96, 105, 106, 271
FSH-RF (Follicle Stimulating Hormone-Releasing Factor), 18, 19, 38, 106
Fundus, in puberty, 16

Galactorrhea, 51
Gallstones, the pill and, 49
General anaesthesia. See Anaesthetics
Genes, 207-12 (see also Genetic and antenatal diagnosis; Heredity); recessive and dominant, and inherited characteristics, 211-13
Genetics and antenatal diagnosis, 206-22 (see also Heredity); amniocentesis and genetic testing, 214-18; birth defects congenital or inherited, 210-14 (see also specific conditions); chromosomal disorders, 212-13; chromosomes and genes and, 207-9, 211-14; drug use and pregnancy dangers and, 182; immature delivery and, 164; infections and birth defects, 219, 220-2; infertility problems and, 95, 110; inherited characteristics and, 210-14; mutations and, 208, 210
Genitals (genital region), 92 (see also specific areas, organs, problems); abnormalities and infertility; 92, genital herpes, 183, 295, 349; herpes simplex, 295; swelling and discharge in newborn girls, 264; venereal disease, 298-303
German measles. See Rubella
Germ cells, 212
Gestational diabetes, 179
Gingivitis, 126, 244
Ginseng extract, hot flashes, and, 280
Glandular fever, the pill and, 49

Glaucoma, 46, 258; marijuana use and, 258
Gold-salts injection, arthritis, and, 363-4
Gonadotropins, 105, 160
Gonorrhea, 72, 293, 298-300, 386; and arthritis, 369; and pregnancy risks, 183; preventing 300, symptoms in men, 299; symptoms in women, 299
Granuloma inguinale, 302
Green leafy vegetables, folic-acid deficiency anaemia and, 174, 359
Group medical practice, 4-5
Group sex, 376
G-6-P-D deficiency anaemia, 357
Gum problems: gingivitis, 244; pregnancy and 126; pyorrhea, 244, smoking and, 244
Gynaecologists (see also Obstetricians-gynaecologists): and examinations in adolescence, 27-28

Habitual abortion, infertility and, 95-6, 107
Haematocrit, 356
Haematoma, 88
Haemoglobin, 116, 356, 358
Haemophilia, 210, 212, 216, 217
Haemophilia vaginitis, 293
Haemorrhage (see also Bleeding): abortions and, 198; postnatal, 160-1
Haemorrhoids, 371; in pregnancy, 128
Hair (hair care) 226-8, 228-9; changes in menopause, 275; changes in pregnancy, 129-30 depilatories, 227; dye use and cautions, 129-30, 229; electrolysis, 227; facial, 227; hair loss, the pill and, 44; oily, 228, 229 ; protein conditioners, 228; removal, 226-8; shampoos and rinses, 229; shaving, 227; tweezing, 227; waxing, 227
Hardening of the arteries. See Arteriosclerosis
Having children, 112-85
HCG (human chorionic gonadotropin), 106, 107, as infertility vaccine, 80; and pregnancy, 117; tests for detecting, 117; for weight loss, 249
Headaches: the pill and, 44, 45, 50; and pregnancy, 134
Health (health care). See Wellness and well-woman care; specific aspects
Health farms, 250
Health foods, 246
Heart attacks (see also Heart disease): fear of sex, 382; oestrogen (the pill) and, 45, 48, 50, 281-2; strenuous now-and-then exercise and, 253
Heartbeat (heart rate), 127; Caesarean section and, 171; fetal monitoring and, 146, 171, 183-4; increase during pregnancy of, 126
Heartburn, in pregnancy, 126
Heart disease (heart problems), 180, 236; (see also Cardiovascular disease; Heart attacks); alcohol use and, 256; and fetal death, 163; oestrogen, (the pill) and, 45, 48, 50, 281-2; pregnancy risks and, 180; rheumatic fever, 368; stress and, 259
Heat, decrease in sperm count and, 75
Height/weight chart for women, 250
Henna, use of, 229
Hepatitis, 302; and arthritis, 369; the pill and, 45, 49
Heredity (see also Genetics and antenatal diagnosis): and anaemia, 358 (see also Sickle-cell anaemia); and first menstruation, 14; inherited characteristics, 210-13; osteoporosis and, 282-3; and premature menopause, 277; Tay-Sachs disease (see Tay-Sachs disease); and tooth decay, 243; and varicose veins, 373-4; and wrinkles, 239

Rh disease, 176-8, 185, 197; detection and treatment of, 119, 177, 185, 197; prevention of, 178

Rheumatoid arthritis, 360-5; aspirin for, 362; surgery for, 365; treatment for, 361-6

Rhinoplasty ("nose job"), 239

Rhythm method of birth control, 75-80; calendar and temperature forms of, 77-8; cervical mucus method, 78-9; effectiveness of 76-7

Rhytidectomy ("face lift"), 240

Riboflavin, recommended daily allowance of, 262

Ritodrine, 168

"Rooming in," childbirth and breast-feeding and, 151, 156

Rosacea, the pill and, 45

Round ligament pains, 131

Rubella (German measles), 210, 219-20; and arthritis, 369; pregnancy risks and, 182, 220; when to be vaccinated, 220

Rupture of the membranes. See membranes

Saccharin, use of, 247

Saddle block, 143-4

Saf-T-Coil, 56

Salicylimide, 248

Salivation, increase in pregnancy of, 126

Salt: care in use of, 246; pregnancy and, 134

Sanitary napkins, 237

Scabies, 303

Scars; Caesarean section and, 170-1 laparotomy, 82-3

Scrotal problems, infertility and, 96

Second medical opinions, 6, 320, 390

Sedatives, 233-4

Self-help groups, patients and, 10

Semen, infertility and, 103-4, 110-11 (see also Sperm); analysis, 103-4

Sequential birth-control pills, 40-1

Sex determination (gender identity) 209, confusion as to sex of a baby, 265; sex chromosomes and, 209, 216, 265; Shettles theory of 221

Sex-linked genetic disorders, 212-13 (see also specific kinds); amniocentesis and, 124, 216

Sexual activity, 373-88 (see also specific aspects, kinds, problems); and abortions, 186-205; adolescence and puberty and, 11-12, 26-7; after childbirth, 152; and birth control, 35-90; and cervical cancer, 348; and cystitis, 304, 305; female arousal and orgasm and, 373-5, 376, 378, 382-3; herpes virus and, 295-6; infertility and, 98-9, 100, 102; libido and (see Libido); pregnancy and, 28-30, 122-3; sexual dysfunction and, 377-9; sexual health and, 373-88; and venereal disease, 298-303; (see also Venereal disease)

Sexual dysfunction (sexual problems), 377-9 (see also specific aspects, kinds); causes, 377; female problems and, 377-9; male problems and, 379; physical illness and, 382-3; rapists and, 383; sex therapy and, 380, 381, 383; treatment of, 379-83

Shampoos, 228-9; "baby," 229

Shaving, 227

Sheath. See Birth control

Shettles theory of sex determination, 221

Shortness of breath in pregnancy, 128

"Siamese twins," 159

Sickle-cell anaemia, 45, 110, 119, 210, 214, 217-18, 358; pregnancy risks and, 180; test for and prevention of, 217-18, 358

Silastic implants, 80

Silicon plugs, 80

Silicone, breast surgery and use of, 241, 345

Skin (skin care and changes): cosmetics and (see Cosmetics); cosmetic surgery, 238-42; face lift, 240; facial discolourations, 240-1; menopause and, 274; the pill and, 45; pregnancy and, 129; wrinkles, 239-40

Sleeping positions , pregnancy and, 116

Sleeplessness (disturbed sleep, insomnia), 233-4; exercise and therapy for, 233-4; major causes, 234; pregnancy and, 134-5; sedatives, 233

Smear test, 101, 119, 349; abnormal results, steps after, 349; and cancer detection, 340, 349 (see also specific kinds); routine check, 390, 391; and vaginitis, 288, 291

Smoking, 253-5; and breast-feeding, 155; chest X rays, 391; dangers, 253-5; and dental care, 244; marijuana, 257-8; and miscarriage, 162; the pill and, 45, 48; pregnancy and, 116, 162, 181, 254; quitting, 254-5; and wrinkles, 239

Soap and water, hygiene and, 224, 226; vaginitis and, 287, 288

Speculum, 189

Sperm (see also Semen; Sperm problems; specific problems); acid phosphotase, rape evidence and, 386; birth control and, 35-90; capacitation, 38, 92, 98, 113; and conception, 113; heat and ultrasound to decrease, 75; and sex chromosomes, 209; vasectomy and, 88-9

Spermicidal creams, foams and jellies, 66-8; use with diaphragm, 65

Sperm problems (sperm production): antisperm antibodies and, 92, 97, 98-9, 102, 103-4; artificial insemination and, 109-10; chromosomal disorders, 212-13; infertility and, 92, 97, 98-9, 103-4; semen analysis and, 103-4; sperm banks and donors, 89, 110; test-tube babies, 110-11

Spherocytosis, 357

Sphingomyelin, 185

Spina bifida, 217-18

Spinal block, 143

Spontaneous abortion, 131, 161-2

Squamous cell cancer, vaginal, 354

Stein-Leventhal Syndrome. See Polycystic ovarian syndrome

Steptoe, Dr. Patrick, 80, 110-11

Sterility. See Infertility; Sterilization, voluntary

Sterilization, voluntary, 80-9; recommendations, 80

Steroids (see also Corticosteroids); candidiasis and, 289; oral contraceptives and, 36

Stomach cancer, 180; pregnancy and, 180

Stool softeners, bulk, 235

Strep throat, rheumatic fever and, 367-8

Stress (see also Emotional changes: Tension): and fatigue and disease, 259; menopause and, 273, 284-5

Stress incontinence, 309, 310

Stress testing, use in late pregnancy of, 184

Stretch marks, pregnancy and, 129

Stroke: the pill (oestrogen) and, 48, 253, 281-2; smoking and the pill, and 253

Subdermal birth-control pellets, 55

Subtotal hysterectomy (supracervical), 320, 328

Sugar (carbohydrates), 243, 247 (see also Carbohydrates); diabetes test, 119; lactose intolerance, 252; substitutes, 247; and tooth decay, 243

422